Physiology of Sport and Exercise Study Guide

Christine M. Drews

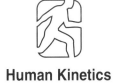

Human Kinetics

Library of Congress Cataloging-in-Publication Data

Drews, Christine M., 1965-
    Physiology of sport and exercise study guide / Christine M. Drews.
      p. cm
    Includes bibliographical references and index.
    ISBN 0-7360-0090-9
    1. Exercise--Physiological aspects.   2. Sports--Physiological
aspects. I. Wilmore, Jack H., 1938-   Physiology of sport and
exercise. II. Title.
QP301.W6749   1999 Suppl.   99-22719
612'.044--dc21   CIP

ISBN: 0-7360-0090-9

Content Consultants: Cheryl J. Cohen and Jack H. Wilmore; **Developmental Editor:** Julie Rhoda; **Assistant Editors:** Sandra Merz Bott, John Wentworth, and Susan Hagan; **Copyeditor:** Arlene Miller; **Proofreader:** Myla Smith; **Graphic Designer and Cover Designer:** Stuart Cartwright; **Graphic Artists:** Angela Snyder and Yvonne Griffith; **Photographer (cover):** © Sherri Meyer; **Mac Illustrator:** Sharon Smith; **Printer:** United Graphics

Special thanks to Brenda Jean Salogga, who created activities 7.6, 7.7, 8.3, and 11.1 (hyperbaric).

Printed in the United States of America   10 9 8 7 6 5 4 3 2

Human Kinetics
Web site: www.humankinetics.com

United States: Human Kinetics, P.O. Box 5076, Champaign, IL 61825-5076
800-747-4457
e-mail: humank@hkusa.com

Canada: Human Kinetics, 475 Devonshire Road Unit 100, Windsor, ON N8Y 2L5
800-465-7301 (in Canada only)
e-mail: hkcan@mnsi.net

Europe: Human Kinetics, P.O. Box IW14, Leeds LS16 6TR, United Kingdom
+44 (0)113 278 1708
e-mail: humank@hkeurope.com

Australia: Human Kinetics, 57A Price Avenue, Lower Mitcham, South Australia 5062
08 8277 1555
e-mail: humank@hkaustralia.com

New Zealand: Human Kinetics, P.O. Box 105-231, Auckland Central
09-309-1890
e-mail: hkp@ihug.co.nz

CONTENTS

Chapter 20 Cardiovascular Disease and Physical Activity 329

Chapter 21 Obesity, Diabetes, and Physical Activity 341

TO THE STUDENT

Physiology of Sport and Exercise introduces you to the wonders of the human body and how your body responds to the demands of physical activity. At times, the many details and scientific processes presented might be overwhelming and confusing. This Student Study Guide is designed to assist you in learning, understanding, and applying the main concepts of each chapter.

We have included a variety of activities to help *Physiology of Sport and Exercise* come to life. We hope that through analyzing case studies, conducting experiments, jogging around campus, and exploring physiology-related sites on the Internet, you will see how important the physiology of sport and exercise is to our daily lives. Who knows? In addition to helping you learn the material in order to do well in this class, perhaps this guide will help you grow to truly enjoy the fascinating science of exercise and sport physiology. If so, be sure to let your professor or teaching assistant know so he or she can help you plan for further education in this area.

The physiology of sport and exercise is complex and amazing. We hope this study guide makes the complex clear and the amazing useful to your life. Now, let's get that heart pumping and your muscles working as we tackle the first activity.

TO THE INSTRUCTOR

This study guide is designed to do more than help your students pass your tests. It is designed to assist them in learning, understanding, and applying the main concepts presented in *Physiology of Sport and Exercise*. As such, it contains a wide variety of activities—from those that require only rote memorization to those that challenge students to assimilate complex concepts and apply them to exercise and sport situations.

This guide has been written with a variety of institutions and curricula in mind. Whether you are at a small college with classes of 25 students and no laboratory equipment or at a large university teaching mass lectures of 150 students, this study guide will complement your teaching.

Because this study guide contains activities for all levels of students and for a variety of class sizes, it is imperative that you assist your students in knowing which activities they should do. You may reserve more difficult activities for upperclassmen or honors students, and you may want to modify assignments to fit your class size, for instance, not asking 150 students to turn in a report.

In addition to supporting your teaching of *Physiology of Sport and Exercise*, we hope this guide will help students grow to truly appreciate the fascinating science of exercise and sport physiology.

INTRODUCTORY ACTIVITY

A Good Workout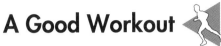

Do this activity before reading *Physiology of Sport and Exercise*.

In its most basic sense, exercise and sport physiology is the study of how the body responds, adjusts, and adapts to physical activity. Whether you've exercised on your own or played on a sports team, you have probably recognized some of these changes without realizing you were thinking about physiology. Do this activity to see what physiological adaptations you can identify. After you have completed this course, we will come back to this activity to see what you have learned.

Choose your favorite physical activity, whether it be running, cycling, doing areobics, playing basketball, or whatever you find most enjoyable. Spend a few minutes warming up, and then do this activity at a relatively high intensity for about 15 minutes. End your workout by cooling down for a couple of minutes. Pay close attention to how different parts of your body react and adapt to the physical activity.

In the spaces below, record your observations of what you think the following systems did while you exercised and how they adapted to the warm-up, more intense exercise, and cool-down:

Muscles

Nervous system

Heart

Lungs

Now take a moment to think about what the exercise environment was like. Was it hot or cold? At high altitude or low altitude? What do you think your body did to adjust to this environment?

How did the fact that you are male or female; young or old; physically trained or untrained; and of your particular body composition affect your body's reaction to this bout of physical activity? (Body composition refers to the amount of fat mass versus fat-free mass, which includes bone, muscle, organs, and connective tissue.)

Although we asked you to exercise at a high intensity, you might have walked at a fairly low intensity; run at a high intensity; or played basketball, which might have been intermittently high and low in intensity. How did the intensity of your physical activity seem to affect your body's reaction?

What, if anything, had you eaten in the four hours prior to this bout of physical activity? How did what you had eaten or not eaten seem to affect your body's response to this physical activity?

Based on your body's reaction to this bout of physical activity, do you think you are in shape or out of shape?

Are you currently participating in some type of regular fitness program? If so, describe it.

How does what you know about cardiovascular disease, obesity, and diabetes affect how frequently you exercise and what types of physical activities you do?

Through this course, you will learn the detailed answers to these questions. *Physiology of Sport and Exercise* will take you on a fascinating journey of how your body adapts to exercise and what factors affect those adaptations.

Throughout this study guide you will see the following icons used to denote the types of activities:

 Application

 Calculation

 Case study

 Computer

 Design/creativity

 Experiment

 Flowchart/process

 Memory

 Movement

 Observation

 Pencil/paper

 Putting it all together

 Research

 Self-reflection

 Textbook

An Introduction to Exercise and Sport Physiology

concepts

- Exercise physiology has evolved from its parent discipline, physiology. It is concerned with the study of how the body adapts physiologically to the acute stress of exercise, or physical activity, and the chronic stress of physical training. Sport physiology grew out of exercise physiology. It applies exercise physiology to problems unique to sports.

- The current state of knowledge in exercise and sport physiology builds on the past and is merely a bridge to the future—many questions remain unanswered.

- The Harvard Fatigue Laboratory (HFL) became the mecca of exercise physiology in the late 1920s until its closure in 1947. Founded by L.J. Henderson and directed by D.B. Dill, this laboratory trained most of those who became world leaders in exercise physiology through the 1950s and 1960s. Most contemporary exercise physiologists can trace their roots back to the HFL.

- *Acute responses* to physical activity are the body's immediate responses to an individual bout of physical activity. *Chronic adaptations* to physical activity are the responses the body makes over time to the stress of repeated exercise bouts.

- The basic training principles of individuality, specificity, disuse, progressive overload, hard/easy, and periodization can be used to impact the body's chronic adaptations to physical activity.

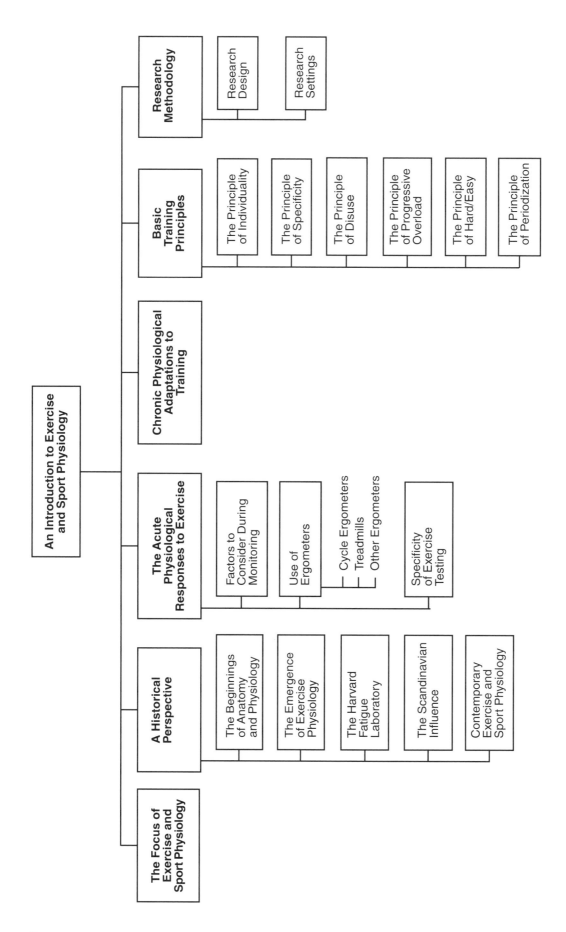

An Introduction to Exercise and Sport Physiology

- The Focus of Exercise and Sport Physiology

- A Historical Perspective
  - The Beginnings of Anatomy and Physiology
  - The Emergence of Exercise Physiology
  - The Harvard Fatigue Laboratory
  - The Scandinavian Influence
  - Contemporary Exercise and Sport Physiology

- The Acute Physiological Responses to Exercise
  - Factors to Consider During Monitoring
  - Use of Ergometers
    - Cycle Ergometers
    - Treadmills
    - Other Ergometers
  - Specificity of Exercise Testing

- Chronic Physiological Adaptations to Training

- Basic Training Principles
  - The Principle of Individuality
  - The Principle of Specificity
  - The Principle of Disuse
  - The Principle of Progressive Overload
  - The Principle of Hard/Easy
  - The Principle of Periodization

- Research Methodology
  - Research Design
  - Research Settings

Activity 0.1

Browsing the Web

Do this activity before reading the intro- duction to *Physiology of Sport and Exercise*.

Exercise and sport physiology is one of the largest and most popular subdisciplines of the field of physical activity. Conduct a web search to discover answers to the questions below. Be sure to record the URLs of the Web sites you found most helpful.

- What kind of education do you need to become an exercise or sport physiologist?

- What do exercise and sport physiologists seem to study?

- What types of career opportunities are available for exercise and sport physiologists?

- What are the major professional organizations to which exercise and sport physi- ologists belong?

Key Individuals in the History of Exercise and Sport Physiology

Activity 0.2

Do this activity after reading pages 3-10 of *Physiology of Sport and Exercise.*

The information in *Physiology of Sport and Exercise* represents the lifelong efforts of many outstanding scientists who have helped piece together the puzzle of human move- ment. What we consider as original or new is most often an assimilation of previous findings. Read pages 3-10 in the textbook, noting the scientists mentioned, the work they did, and other important events in the history of exercise and sport physiology.

On the next page is a time line recognizing key individuals in the development of exercise and sport physiology. In the right-hand column, write the major contributions these individuals made to the field.

Key Individuals in the History of Exercise and Sport Physiology

Date	Individual	Contribution to field
1543	Andreas Vesalius	
1889	Fernand LaGrange	
1921	Archibald V. Hill	
1927	Lawrence J. Henderson	
1927	D.B. Dill	
Late 1930s	Hohwü-Christensen and Ole Hansen	
1947	HFL was closed	
1927-1968	Peter Karpovich	
1941-1971	Thomas K. Cureton	
1950s and 1960s	Per-Olof Åstrand	
1960s		Until the late 1960s, most exercise physiology studies focused on the whole body's response to exercise. Due to technological advances exercise physiology research took on a more biochemical approach. Electronic analyzers to measure respiratory gases were developed; radio-telemetry was developed and used tomonitor heart rate and body temperature during exercise.
Mid-1960s	John Holloszy and Charles "Tip" Tipton	
Around 1966	Jonas Bergstrom	
Late 1960s	Bengt Saltin and Jonas Bergstrom	
Late 1960s	Reggie Edgerton and Phil Gollnick	

Activity 0.3

Acute Responses and Chronic Adaptations

Do this activity after reading pages 11-19 of *Physiology of Sport and Exercise.*

Acute responses to physical activity are the body's immediate responses to an individual bout of physical activity. *Chronic adaptations* to physical activity are the responses the body makes over time to the stress of repeated exercise bouts.

Choose one of the following options and, on separate paper, answer the questions that follow.

Option 1: Ergometer Workout. At the fitness facility of your choice, run on a treadmill, cycle on a cycle ergometer, or row on a rowing machine. Do this activity at a high intensity for as long as is comfortable for you. If you are an avid runner, cyclist, or rower, there's no need to push to your ultimate limit (we don't want you spending more than an hour at this); instead, run, cycle, or row until you feel your body responding to this intensive exercise.

- What acute responses did your body seem to make to this single bout of physical activity?

- If you were to run, cycle, or row on an ergometer at a high intensity for as long as you could three times a week for six weeks, what chronic adaptations do you think your body would make to this activity?

Option 2: Taking a Run. Find time in your schedule to go for a run. Run for as long as is comfortable for you. If you are an avid runner, there's no need to push to your ultimate limit (we don't want you taking the time to run 10 or more miles); instead, run until you feel your body responding to this intensive exercise.

- What acute responses did your body seem to make to this single bout of physical activity?

- If you were to run as far as you could three times a week for six weeks, what chronic adaptations do you think your body would make to this activity?

Option 3: For Those With Disabilities or Injuries. If a disability or injury prevents you from doing one of the above activities, choose an activity of your liking that will physically challenge you in a similar way. Do this activity for as long as is comfortable. Then answer these questions:

- What activity did you do?

- What acute responses did your body seem to make to this single bout of physical activity?

- If you were to do this activity three times a week for six weeks, what chronic adaptations do you think your body would make to this activity?

Activity 0.4

Factors That Alter Acute Responses

Do this activity after reading pages 11-12 of *Physiology of Sport and Exercise.*

If you were to participate in an exercise physiology research study at this very point in time, in the very place where you are currently sitting, how would the following factors affect the outcome of the study? Write your answers on a separate piece of paper.

Environmental conditions

- Temperature

- Humidity

- Altitude

- Noise

Diurnal variation (see page 12 of the textbook for more information)

Gender

Sleep patterns

Activity 0.5

Case Study of Basic Training Principles

Do this activity after reading pages 17-19 of *Physiology of Sport and Exercise.*

Review pages 17-19 in the textbook. Notice that chronic physiological adaptations to physical activity can be affected by several training principles. Read the case study that follows, keeping in mind the training principles mentioned in the text.

Sharon was a starter on her high school volleyball team. She was a strong server, regularly serving aces, so her coach usually put her into the rotation right before they needed to score a few points off some good serves. Sharon had always loved sports; she picked them up quickly, and it was easy for her to gain strength and aerobic capacity after working out in the right ways for just a few practices.

Even though she was a starter, Sharon had trouble with digs—she just didn't react quickly enough to spikes from the other team. Her coach noticed this and told her to practice by bumping the ball up high on the gym wall and then returning it quickly to the wall again. Sharon did this for 20 min every practice, but she couldn't figure out how this was going to help her respond to spikes that came in at different angles and faster speeds. While Sharon worked on returning spiked balls, the rest of the team did short sprints across the gym with periodic rests in order to improve their speed and endurance. About midway through the season, Sharon noticed that she felt winded after even short runs and dives toward the ball, and she felt like she had less power in her legs.

On her own, Sharon began doing interval training after practice. She would sprint a few times across the gym, recover for a few seconds, and then sprint again. Soon, she was able to run faster and take fewer rests, and she didn't get nearly as winded during her games.

After a few weeks of doing her self-directed interval training every day, Sharon felt like she wasn't improving anymore. She seemed to have plateaued. Was she working too hard? Not hard enough? Sharon wasn't sure what she should do now.

By the end of the season, Sharon was just plain worn out. Her team's practices and rigorous game schedule combined with her own everyday workout had been grueling. Sharon wondered why that hadn't been enough. Why, when they were now entering the most important part of the season and had a chance to make it past regionals, was Sharon not at her best physical condition of the entire season?

On a separate piece of paper, describe what evidence of each of the training principles you see in the case study about Sharon. For each principle, comment on what Sharon or her coach should have done differently and what they did well.

- The principle of individuality
- The principle of specificity
- The principle of disuse
- The principle of progressive overload
- The principle of hard/easy
- The principle of periodization

Do this activity after reading pages 20-21 of *Physiology of Sport and Exercise*.

Activity 0.6

Research Methodology

Throughout *Physiology of Sport and Exercise*, you will see references to research studies that have led to our understanding of how the body functions during physical activity and how this functioning is altered by training. To more easily interpret these studies, you should be able to discern what type of research design was used and in what setting the research took place. Look at the figures on the next page and then answer the questions that follow.

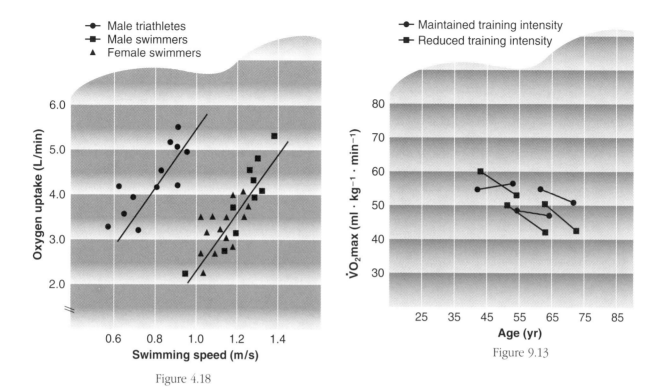

Figure 4.18

Figure 9.13

Which of the figures above shows a

cross-sectional research design? _____

longitudinal research design? _____

study that was likely done in a controlled laboratory setting? _____

study that was likely done in the field? _____

Sample Test Questions for the Introduction

Test yourself on your knowledge of this chapter by taking this self-test. Write the correct answers on a separate sheet of paper.

Multiple Choice

1. One day last week, Jenna went hiking in the woods and noticed that her heart beat faster and her respiration rate increased as she climbed some steep hills. Jenna was noticing

   a. chronic adaptations to physical activity;   b. diurnal variation;   c. the principle of periodization;   d. acute adaptations to physical activity.

2. If a discus thrower emphasizes distance running in his training program, he is not correctly incorporating the principle of

   a. disuse;   b. progressive overload;   c. specificity;   d. individuality.

3. Dr. Jones is studying the effects of distance cycling on aerobic capacity. She recruits 60 subjects for her study: Group A has had no distance training, group B cycles 48 km (30 mi) per week, and group C cycles 96 km (60 mi) per week. She then compares the results of all three groups, basing her conclusions on how much cycling was done. Dr. Jones has used a _____ design for her research study.

   a. longitudinal; b. symmetrical; c. cross-sectional; d. diurnal

True-False

4. Acute adaptations are the ways in which the body responds over time to the stress of repeated exercise bouts.

5. A treadmill would be the most appropriate ergometer to use to test swimmers.

6. For most exercise physiology research studies, laboratory tests are more accurate than field tests.

Fill in the Blank

7. If a person stops training, his or her state of fitness will drop to a level that meets only the demands of daily use. This is called the principle of _____.

8. In 1921, _____ was awarded the Nobel Prize for his findings on energy metabolism.

Short Answer

9. What are several environmental conditions that could affect your response to an acute bout of exercise?

10. What steps should a researcher take to control a study for diurnal variation? Why is this important to do?

11. What are ergometers, and why are they useful in physiology research?

Essay

12. Describe the history of the Harvard Fatigue Laboratory and the impact it has had on exercise and sport physiology. What were some of the areas of research emphasized by HFL personnel?

13. Name some of the equipment that was developed in the 1960s due to technological advances. How did this equipment help to change and advance the study of exercise and sport physiology?

14. How is the philosophy of the principle of hard/easy similar to the philosophy underlying the principle of periodization?

Answers to Selected Introduction Activities

0.2   Key Individuals in the History of Exercise and Sport Physiology

Date	Individual	Contribution to field
1543	Andreas Vesalius	Published *Fabrica Humani Corporis [Structure of the Human Body]*, an anatomy text that occasionally attempted to explain the function of organs
1889	Fernand LaGrange	Published *Physiology of Bodily Exercise*
1921	Archibald V. Hill	Received Nobel Prize for findings on energy metabolism
1927	Lawrence J. Henderson	Founded Harvard Fatigue Laboratory (HFL)
1927	D.B. Dill	Named director of HFL
Late 1930s	Hohwü-Christensen and Ole Hansen	Conducted studies of carbohydrate and fat metabolism during exercise
1947	HFL was closed	
1927-1968	Peter Karpovich	Introduced the field of exercise physiology to physical education during his tenure at Springfield College
1941-1971	Thomas K. Cureton	Directed the exercise physiology laboratory at the University of Illinois at Urbana-Champaign and taught many of today's leaders in physical fitness and exercise physiology
1950s and 1960s	Per-Olof Åstrand	Conducted numerous studies of physical fitness and endurance capacity
1960s	Until the late 1960s, most exercise physiology studies focused on the whole body's response to exercise. Due to technological advances exercise physiology research took on a more biochemical approach. Electronic analyzers to measure respiratory gases were developed; radio-telemetry was developed and used tomonitor heart rate and body temperature during exercise.	
Mid-1960s	John Holloszy and Charles "Tip" Tipton	Used rats and mice to study muscle metabolism and to examine factors related to fatigue
Around 1966	Jonas Bergstrom	Reintroduced the biopsy needle to sample muscle tissue
Late 1960s	Bengt Saltin and Jonas Bergstrom	Used the needle biopsy procedure to study the effects of diet on muscle endurance and nutrition
Late 1960s	Reggie Edgerton and Phil Gollnick	Used rats to study the characteristics of individual muscle fibers and their responses to training

0.5   Case Study of Basic Training Principles

Individuality: Sharon's body adapts quickly to training. She shows great improvement after participating in a given program; she is a "responder."

Specificity: Sharon's coach did not understand the principle of specificity well enough to construct a good practice drill for reacting to spikes. Because a spiked ball will come in faster and at different angles than the ball Sharon is bumping to the wall, the drill Sharon was told to do will not improve her ability to respond to spikes.

Disuse: While Sharon is practicing bumping the ball against the wall, she is missing out on interval training. Her cardiorespiratory system succumbs to disuse, and she begins to feel more winded during the games; she feels less power in her legs because her leg muscles have not gotten the workout they need.

Progressive overload: When Sharon begins her own interval training to improve her speed and endurance, she actually implements the principle of progressive overload without knowing it. Each day she sprints faster (increasing intensity) and with fewer rests (increasing duration) than on the previous day.

Hard/easy: Unfortunately, Sharon and her coach are not aware of this principle. Sharon goes all-out every practice and never gives her body a break. By the end of the season, she is fatigued and not in her best physical condition.

Periodization: Sharon's coach does not seem to be aware of this principle. There is no mention of the gradual cycling of specificity, intensity, and volume of training in this case study. Therefore, Sharon does not achieve her peak level of fitness by the end of the season, when every game counts.

0.6 Research Methodology

cross-sectional: 4.18 * *longitudinal:* 9.13 * *controlled laboratory setting:* both * *field setting:* neither

Answers to Selected Introduction Test Questions

Multiple Choice

1. d; 2. c; 3. c

True-False

4. False; 5. False; 6. True

Fill in the Blank

7. disuse; 8. Archibald V. Hill

Short Answer and Essay

For questions 9 to 14, check your answers against the explanations given in the textbook.

Muscular Control of Movement

concepts

- A single muscle cell is known as a muscle fiber. The sarcomere is the smallest functional unit of a muscle and is composed of two protein filaments, myosin and actin, which are responsible for muscle contraction.

- A motor unit consists of a single motor neuron and all the muscle fibers it supplies.

- The sequence of events leading to muscle action is complex, ending when the Ca^{2+} binds to troponin on the actin filament, and the troponin pulls tropomyosin off the active sites, allowing myosin heads to attach to the actin filament.

- Most skeletal muscles contain both slow-twitch (ST) fibers and fast-twitch (FT) fibers. FT fibers are better than ST fibers for anaerobic activity, with FT_a fibers being most useful for explosive bouts of exercise. ST fibers have high aerobic endurance and are well suited to endurance activities.

- The three main types of muscle action are concentric, in which the muscle shortens; static, in which the muscle acts but the joint angle is unchanged; and eccentric, in which the muscle lengthens.

- The amount of force produced depends on the number of motor units activated, the type of motor units activated, the size of the muscle, the muscle's initial length when activated, the angle of the joint, and the muscle's speed of action.

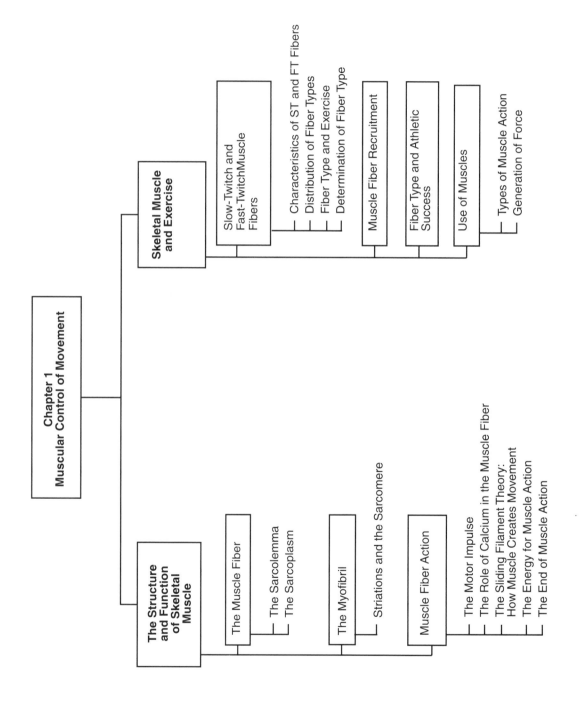

**Chapter 1
Muscular Control of Movement**

**The Structure
and Function
of Skeletal
Muscle**

The Muscle Fiber
- The Sarcolemma
- The Sarcoplasm

The Myofibril
- Striations and the Sarcomere

Muscle Fiber Action
- The Motor Impulse
- The Role of Calcium in the Muscle Fiber
- The Sliding Filament Theory: How Muscle Creates Movement
- The Energy for Muscle Action
- The End of Muscle Action

**Skeletal Muscle
and Exercise**

Slow-Twitch and Fast-TwitchMuscle Fibers
- Characteristics of ST and FT Fibers
- Distribution of Fiber Types
- Fiber Type and Exercise
- Determination of Fiber Type

Muscle Fiber Recruitment

Fiber Type and Athletic Success

Use of Muscles
- Types of Muscle Action
- Generation of Force

Activity 1.1

How Do Muscles Work?

Do this activity before reading chapter 1 of *Physiology of Sport and Exercise.*

Exercise requires movement of the body, which is accomplished through the action of skeletal muscles. This chapter looks at the structure and function of skeletal muscles. To get you thinking about these muscles and how they work, answer the questions below (on separate paper). After you have finished studying this chapter, we will return to this activity to see what understanding you have gained about skeletal muscle.

1. To observe the importance of your muscles to your everyday life, list all of the movements you can think of that your muscles have contributed to in the last hour. Be sure to include both large-muscle movements and small-muscle movements.

2. From what you know from past experience, do your muscles seem better at (a) sustaining low-intensity endurance activities like walking or running long distances, (b) performing shorter, high-intensity endurance activities like running the mile or swimming the 400 m, or (c) doing highly explosive events like the 100-m dash and the 50-m sprint swim? Give examples to prove your point.

3. When performing movements, our muscles either shorten, lengthen, or remain the same in length. Pick up a heavy object—a standard dumbbell, a paperweight, a small heavy book—in one hand. Describe what your biceps muscle seems to do as you bend your elbow, bringing the object closer to your chest. Do you think your biceps shortened, lengthened, or stayed the same? Now lower the object in a controlled manner. What type of muscle action took place—did your biceps shorten, lengthen, or remain the same? Now bend your elbow at a 90-degree angle and hold the object away from your body with sustained effort. What does your biceps seem to be doing now—shortening, lengthening, or remaining the same?

4. Holding the same object as in number 3, move your arm and the object in different ways, trying to discern what factors help you to generate more force. At what elbow angle does your arm seem the strongest? How far from your body is the object when your arm seems the strongest? Does your arm seem to exert more force when you move the object faster or slower? How does the weight of the object seem to impact this?

Activity 1.2

Structure of Skeletal Muscle

Do this activity after reading pages 29-34 of *Physiology of Sport and Exercise.*

The following exercises test your knowledge of the structure of skeletal muscle. For your studying benefit, do these exercises without looking in your textbook. Once you have completed this activity, check your labels against the textbook to see how you did and what you need to study.

1. The drawing at the top of the next page shows the basic structure of muscle. Fill in the blanks with the correct names of the parts of the muscle.

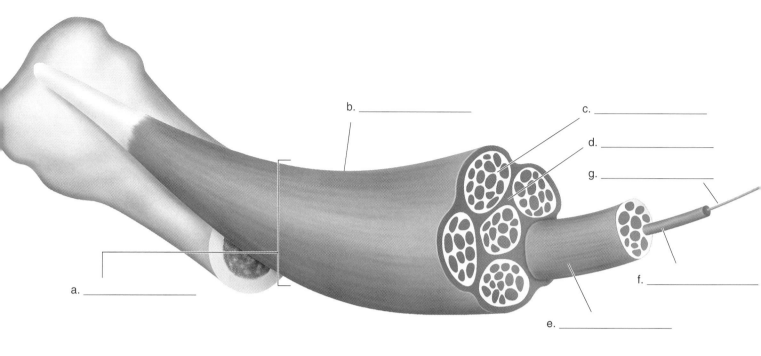

b. _____

c. _____

d. _____

g. _____

a. _____

e. _____

f. _____

2. The drawing below shows a single muscle fiber. Fill in the blanks with the correct names of the parts of the muscle fiber.

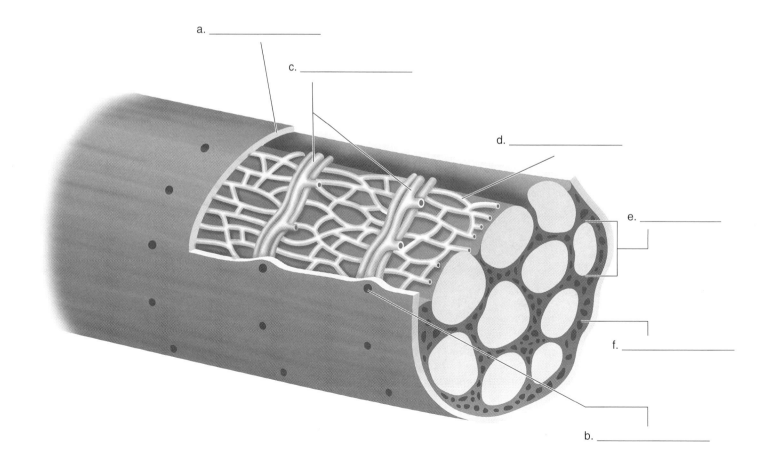

a. _____

c. _____

d. _____

e. _____

f. _____

b. _____

3. The drawing below shows the sarcomeres, the basic functional unit of a myofibril. Label this drawing to show the sarcomeres, Z disks, H zones, I bands, A bands, actin, and myosin.

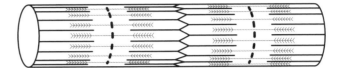

4. The drawing below shows portions of actin and myosin filaments. Circle and label the myosin molecule, the myosin filament, and the actin filament. Then fill in the blanks with the correct names of the parts of these molecules and filaments.

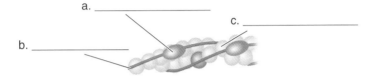

a. _____

c. _____

b. _____

Activity 1.3

What Makes Muscles Move?

Do this activity after reading pages 34-37 of *Physiology of Sport and Exercise.*

Muscle action begins with a motor nerve impulse from the brain or spinal cord, which initiates a complex process, and ends when the removal of calcium causes the myosin and actin filaments to return to their original relaxed state. Review pages 34-37 of *Physiology of Sport and Exercise*. Draw a flowchart that illustrates the step-by-step process of muscle fiber action. Briefly describe each step and draw an arrow connecting it to the next step.

A key theory in muscle action is the sliding filament theory, which attempts to explain how muscle fibers shorten. In the space below, describe in your own words what is happening in this illustration:

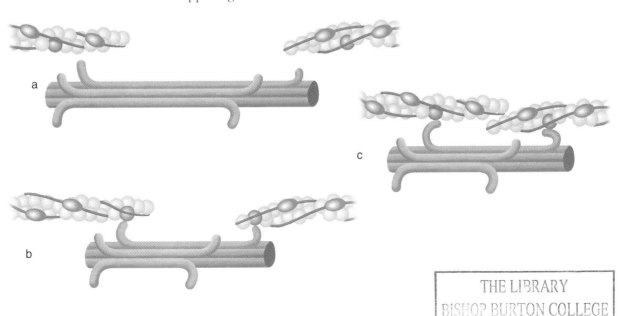

Activity 1.4

Fast-Twitch and Slow-Twitch Muscle Fibers

Do this activity after reading pages 37-43 of *Physiology of Sport and Exercise*.

In the blank preceding each of the following statements, write "FT," "ST," or "Both," to indicate which fiber type the statement describes (FT = Fast-twitch muscle fibers; ST = Slow-twitch muscle fibers).

_____ Are contained in most skeletal muscles.

_____ Take longer than other muscle fibers to reach peak tension.

_____ Predominantly have a slow form of myosin ATPase.

_____ Predominantly have a fast form of myosin ATPase.

_____ Have a more highly developed sarcoplasmic reticulum, which helps deliver calcium into the muscle cell when stimulated.

_____ Have a motor neuron with a small cell body and innervate a cluster of 10 to 180 muscle fibers.

_____ Reach peak tension faster and collectively generate more force than other fiber types.

_____ Has three subtypes.

When challenged with a question in exercise and sport physiology, you can usually figure out the answer using basic information and logic. To check your understanding of the fiber types, complete the table that follows, writing the appropriate information in each column. Do this without looking in your textbook. Once you have completed the exercise, check your answers against the textbook.

Characteristic	Fiber type		
	ST	FTa	FTb
Fibers per motor neuron [provide approximate range of numbers of fibers]			
Motor neuron size [small, medium, or large?]			
Nerve conduction velocity [slow, medium, or fast?]			
Contraction speed (ms) [provide approximate speed]			
Type of myosin ATPase [slow, medium, or fast?]			
Sarcoplasmic reticulum development [low, moderate, or high?]			
Motor unit force [low, moderate, or high?]			

Characteristic	Fiber type		
	ST	FTa	FTb
Aerobic (oxidative) capacity [low, moderate, or high?]			
Anaerobic (glycolytic) capacity [low, moderate, or high?]			

Activity 1.5

Muscle Fiber Types and Physical Activity

Do this activity after reading pages 42-45 of *Physiology of Sport and Exercise*.

Find at least five photos showing physical activities: Go online to Web sites containing site URL, newspaper, or name of magazine). Then, based on what you have learned about slow-twitch and fast-twitch muscle fibers, identify the probable primary fiber type in the key body part of the particular movement shown. We've listed some possible Web sites to explore as well as one example to get you started.

Possible Web sites to visit:

http://www.cnnsi.com—CNN's and *Sports Illustrated*'s joint site

http://www.adventuretime.com—the Web site of *AdventureTime Magazine*, including stories and photos of adventure and extreme sports, such as whitewater rafting and rock climbing

http://www.justwomen.com—news and information on women's sports

http://www.runnersweb.com—links to running and triathlon online magazines

http://www.insidetr.com—news and information on triathlons

http://www.greatoutdoors.com—from the Outdoor Life Network and Cox Interactive Media, including photos and information on such outdoor sports as snowboarding, kayaking, and windsurfing

http://www.espn.com—the Web site of the ESPN broadcasting network

http://www.usatoday.com—the Web site of the nationally distributed newspaper (check out the sports section online)

http://www.humankinetics.com—includes the latest releases from this publisher of physical activity resources as well as links to the best physical activity Web sites.

Photo description	Where found	Analysis of fiber type
Mark McGwire, hitting 62nd home run	Cover of 9/8/98 *Sports Illustrated*	Primarily FT fibers in arms in order to hit ball forcefully enough to produce home runs.
1.		
2.		
3.		
4.		
5.		

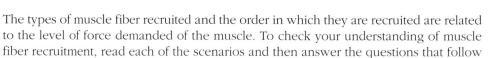

Activity 1.6

Muscle Fiber Recruitment

Do this activity after reading pages 43-44 of *Physiology of Sport and Exercise.*

The types of muscle fiber recruited and the order in which they are recruited are related to the level of force demanded of the muscle. To check your understanding of muscle fiber recruitment, read each of the scenarios and then answer the questions that follow (on separate paper).

Scott is a swimmer on his university's swim team. Before each competition, he spends some time walking around the pool area, getting psyched for the event. He swings his arms a little, shakes his legs, and just generally tries to loosen up. Soon he's in position on the starting blocks, waiting for the sound of the starting gun. The gun fires, and Scott dives off the block into the water, swimming his best event—the 50-m freestyle.

1. As Scott was loosening up and walking around the pool area, which muscle fibers were creating the force needed?

2. During Scott's warm-up phase, were all the muscle fibers that had been stimulated acting maximally?

3. When Scott dove into the pool and swam the 50-m freestyle, which muscle fibers were added to the workforce?

4. How did Scott's body produce the force to spring off the blocks and swim a fast freestyle? What did the number of activated muscle fibers and the size of the motor neuron have to do with this?

Tera is running her first marathon. She has trained well for the event, and she finds that the first 15 or so miles are not so bad. She has been running at a comfortable pace for her, trying to set a pace that she can maintain for the entire race. Around the 15-mi mark, Tera feels a sense of fatigue. She drinks more, keeps running at the same pace, and over time the fatigue passes. Around the 22-mi mark, Tera is surprised to find herself overwhelmingly fatigued. She feels as if she has "hit the wall" and must actually "will" herself to keep up her pace and finish the marathon. The last 4 miles are grueling, but Tera does it. She collapses at the finish line, exhausted but exhilarated.

5. During the first few miles of Tera's marathon, which muscle fiber types were primarily doing the work?

6. Describe what likely happened around the 15-mi mark? Which muscle fibers were depleted? What were they depleted of? What muscle fiber type was likely recruited?

7. In the final miles of the marathon, Tera felt extreme exhaustion. What was likely happening in terms of muscle fiber recruitment during these last few miles?

Activity 1.7

Identifying Types of Muscle Action

Do this activity after reading pages 46-48 of *Physiology of Sport and Exercise.*

The three main types of muscle action are concentric, in which the muscle shortens; isometric, or static, in which the muscle acts but the joint angle is unchanged; and eccentric, in which the muscle lengthens. In many activities, all three types of actions occur in the execution of a smooth, coordinated movement. For the sake of learning about these actions, though, see if you can spot the individual types of muscle action in everyday activities.

Find a place to observe people—perhaps sit on a bench near a walkway on campus, go to a restaurant or shopping mall, or attend a sporting event. Look for examples of concentric, eccentric, and static (isometric) muscle actions and write about them on a separate piece of paper. Try to find at least 10 examples of the various muscle actions. We've listed one example to get you started.

Type of muscle action	Example from your observations
Static (isometric)	Waitress holding heavy tray steady, filled with plates, with elbows bent

Roles of Muscles and Factors That Affect Force Generation

Activity 1.8

Do this activity after reading pages 45-49 of *Physiology of Sport and Exercise.*

Muscles involved in a movement can be classed as agonists (prime movers), antagonists (opponents), or synergists (assistants). The amount of force produced depends on the number of motor units activated, the type of motor units activated, the size of the muscle, the muscle's initial length when activated, the angle of the joint, and the muscle's speed of action.

Find a place to ride a bicycle—either go to a fitness facility and cycle on a cycle ergometer or exercise cycle, or ride a touring bicycle or mountain bike around campus or on trails somewhere. Take a look at the questions in this activity before you begin to cycle so you know what to observe as you do this activity.

If an injury or disability prevents you from cycling, choose another physical activity that you think will help you learn the same concepts and answer the questions as best you can. Be sure to write down the name of the activity you chose to do.

Using the diagram of leg muscles below, identify which muscles served as the agonists, the antagonists, and the synergists during the downstroke of your biking.

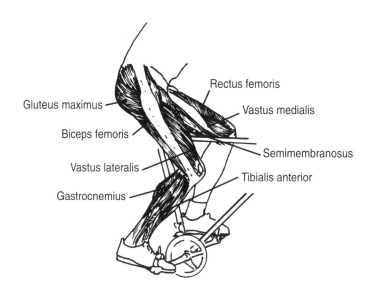

Gluteus maximus

Rectus femoris

Biceps femoris

Vastus medialis

Vastus lateralis

Semimembranosus

Gastrocnemius

Tibialis anterior

Adapted, with permission, from "Effects of Saddle Height and Pedaling Cadence on Power Output and Efficiency" by R.J. Gregor and S.G. Rugg. In *Science of Cycling* (p. 74) by E.R. Burke (Ed.), 1986, Champaign, IL: Human Kinetics. Copyright 1986 by Edmund Burke.

Downstroke

Agonists: _____

Antagonists: _____

Synergists: _____

1. Based on the speed with which you cycled and the settings on the cycle ergometer or the type of terrain (hilly or flat) you cycled on, describe in general how the likely number of motor units and the type of motor units recruited for this activity affect the amount of force you are able to produce while cycling.

2. Describe how the size of your leg muscles affects the amount of force produced. How does this compare with the size and force capabilities of other muscles in your body?

3. While you are cycling, is there any evidence of increased force generation by stretching a muscle prior to contracting it? If so, describe this. If not, describe an activity that would illustrate this phenomenon.

4. What seems to be the optimal angle of the knee joint for maximizing the amount of force generated?

5. How does the speed of your muscle actions affect the amount of force they are generating while cycling?

Putting It All Together: Muscular Control of Movement

Activity 1.9

Do this activity after completing chapter 1 of *Physiology of Sport and Exercise*.

Now that you have studied this chapter, it is time to see how much you have learned about the muscular control of movement. Look back at activity 1.1 and record your answers to the following questions on a separate sheet of paper.

1. The first thing you did in activity 1.1 was to list all of the muscle movements you had made in the last hour. Without their complex structure, muscles would not be able to accomplish all of these movements. Describe in detail the structure of skeletal muscle and how a muscle fiber is triggered to act.

2. Secondly, we asked if your muscles seem better at (a) sustaining low-intensity endurance activities like walking or running long distances, (b) performing shorter,

high-intensity endurance activities like running the mile or swimming the 400 m, or (c) doing highly explosive events like the 100-m dash and the 50-m sprint swim. What do your responses tell you about the fiber type that seems predominant in your muscles? What are the characteristics of this fiber type? How does this help to explain the physical activities at which you are most successful?

3. Thirdly, we asked you to do a biceps curl with a heavy object and to hold it in a sustained manner. (a) What type of action did your biceps perform when you bent your elbow and brought the object close to your chest? (b) What type of action did your biceps muscle perform when you lowered the object? (c) When you held the object with sustained effort, what type of muscle action was your biceps performing? Explain the underlying mechanisms of each of these muscle actions.

4. Finally, in activity 1.1, you experimented with force generation. Now that you have studied this chapter, you have a much better idea about what helps to increase a muscle's force generation. How perceptive were your responses in activity 1.1? Explain in detail the factors that impact force generation.

Sample Test Questions for Chapter 1

Test yourself on your knowledge of this chapter by taking this self-test. Write the correct answers on a separate sheet of paper.

Multiple Choice

1. Smooth muscle is called

   a. voluntary muscle and composes most of the heart's structure.
   b. involuntary muscle and is found in the walls of most blood vessels and the walls of most internal organs.
   c. voluntary muscle and is found in the walls of most blood vessels.
   d. involuntary muscle and composes most of the heart's structure.

2. Cardiac muscle is called

   a. involuntary muscle and is found in the heart, the blood vessels, and in the walls of many internal organs.
   b. voluntary muscle and is found in the heart and in the blood vessels.
   c. involuntary muscle and is found only in the heart.
   d. voluntary muscle and is found only in the heart.

3. Skeletal muscle is called

   a. voluntary muscle and is attached to and moves the skeleton;
   b. voluntary muscle and is attached to both the skeleton and to internal organs;
   c. involuntary muscle and is attached to and moves the skeleton;
   d. involuntary muscle and is attached to both the skeleton and to internal organs.

4. When movement takes place, the muscles involved play these three roles.

    a. agonists, antagonists, and concentrics
    b. agonists, eccentrics, and synergists
    c. synergists, eccentrics, and concentrics
    d. agonists, antagonists, and synergists

5. Which of the following items best describes the three main types of muscle action?

    a. concentric, in which the muscle decelerates; static (isometric), in which the muscle speed stays the same; and eccentric, in which the muscle accelerates;
    b. concentric, in which the muscle shortens; static (isometric), in which the muscle acts but the joint angle is unchanged; and eccentric, in which the muscle lengthens;
    c. concentric, in which the muscle acts in a circular fashion; dynamic, in which joint movement is produced; and eccentric, in which the muscle lengthens;
    d. concentric, in which the muscle weakens; static (isometric), in which the muscle strength stays the same; and eccentric, in which the muscle strengthens.

6. Which of the following items does *not* help increase force production?

    a. using an optimal joint angle when performing the movement
    b. recruiting more motor units
    c. stretching the muscle to a length approximately 20% greater than its resting length
    d. executing the movement more slowly, even in eccentric actions

True-False

7. FT_a fibers are the most frequently recruited muscle fibers.

8. Myosin ATPase is the enzyme that splits ATP to release energy for driving contraction; it does not help facilitate relaxation.

9. FT fibers have a fast form of ATPase, which means ATP is split more rapidly in FT fibers than in ST fibers.

10. FT fibers have a more highly developed sarcoplasmic reticulum than do ST fibers.

11. People who have a predominance of FT fibers in their leg muscles tend to be better at aerobic endurance activities than people who have a high percentage of ST fibers.

12. ST fibers have a high oxidative capacity.

13. FT motor units have less force generation potential than ST motor units.

14. Recent research has shown that muscle fiber composition is genetically determined and cannot be modified at all through training or inactivity.

Fill in the Blank

15. Agonists are also called _____.

16. _____ are muscles that assist the antagonists.

17. Antagonists are muscles that _____ the prime movers.

Short Answer

18. Explain the all-or-none response.

19. Explain the relationship between force development and the recruitment of ST, FT_a, and FT_b fibers.

20. Explain how fatigue affects muscle fiber recruitment in aerobic endurance events.

Essay

21. Describe in detail the structure of skeletal muscle. Include these terms in your description: epimysium, fasciculus, perimysium, muscle fibers, endomysium, sarcolemma, sarcoplasm, transverse tubules, sarcoplasmic reticulum, myofibril, sarcomere, actin filaments, myosin filaments, titin, tropomyosin, and troponin.

22. Describe the sequence of events involved in muscle fiber action, from the events that lead to muscle action to those that end muscle action.

Answers to Selected Chapter 1 Activities

1.2   Structure of Skeletal Muscle

1. a. muscle;   b. epimysium;   c. endomysium;   d. perimysium;   e. fasciculus   f. muscle fiber;   g. my/ofibril

2. a. sarcolemma;   b. opening into T tubule;   c. transverse tubules;   d. sarcoplasmic reticulum;   e. myofibril;   f. sarcoplasm

3. See figure 1.5 in the textbook for correct labeling.

4. Top left = myosin filament

   Bottom left = myosin filament

   Right = actin filament

   a. tail;   b. myosin head;   c. myosin heads;   d. troponin;   e. tropomyosin;   f. actin

1.3   What Makes Muscles Move?

See page 35 of the textbook for a good summary of the steps the flowchart should include and page 36 for an explanation of the sliding filament theory.

1.4   Fast-Twitch and Slow-Twitch Muscle Fibers

Fill in the blanks: Both, ST, ST, FT, FT, ST, FT, FT

Table:

Fibers per motor neuron: 10-180, 300-800, 300-800

Motor neuron size: Small, Large, Large

Nerve conduction velocity: Slow, Fast, Fast

Contraction speed (ms): 110, 50, 50

Type of myosin ATPase: Slow, Fast, Fast

Sarcoplasmic reticulum development: Low, High, High

Motor unit force: Low, High, High

Aerobic (oxidative) capacity: High, Moderate, Low

Anaerobic (glycolytic) capacity: Low, High, High

1.6 Muscle Fiber Recruitment

1. As Scott was warming up, primarily ST fibers were recruited to create the force needed.

2. Yes, all of Scott's muscle fibers that had been stimulated were acting maximally. This is an example of the all-or-none response.

3. Scott's FT_a and FT_b fibers were activated to produce the force he needed to spring from the blocks and swim all out.

4. Scott's nervous system activated more muscle fibers in order to produce more force. In addition, motor units with larger neurons (FT_a and FT_b motor units) were now recruited.

5. The ST and some FT_a muscle fibers were the primary muscle fibers used during the first few miles of the marathon.

6. Around the 15-mi mark, Tera's ST muscle fibers and the FT_a muscle fibers that had been recruited were depleted of glycogen, their primary fuel supply, and more FT_a fibers were recruited to maintain muscle tension.

7. By the last few miles of the marathon, both the ST and the FT_a fibers had become exhausted, and FT_b fibers were probably recruited to help Tera finish the race.

1.8 Roles of Muscles and Factors That Affect Force Generation

Agonists: Rectus femoris, vastus medialis, vastus lateralis, and gastrocnemius

Antagonists: Biceps femoris and tibialis anterior

Synergists: Semimembraneous and other muscles that assist the prime movers

1. If you pedaled fast or had to deal with hilly terrain—meaning your muscles needed to generate a great deal of force—your nervous system probably recruited a high number of motor units, and both ST and FT_a motor units were likely activated. FT_b motor units might have been recruited if you gave an all-out effort, such as climbing a steep hill, or if you cycled to exhaustion.

If you pedaled at a leisurely rate or on flat terrain, and not for a very long period of time—so your need for force generation was minimal—your nervous system probably recruited fewer motor units, and it is likely that only ST units and perhaps some FT_a motor units were activated.

2. The thigh muscles are quite large compared to other muscles in the body and therefore can produce a great amount of force.

3. There is no real evidence of this stretch-shortening phenomenon in bicycling. However, plyometrics training, which takes advantage of the eccentric action to stretch muscles in order to produce a more forceful concentric action, can help cyclists improve their muscular strength in explosive-type actions, such as sprinting up a short hill or accelerating at the start of a sprint.

4. While this might vary individually, most cyclists attain peak force when the force applied is close to a 90-degree angle with the crank arm, which corresponds to the knee being bent at about 90 degrees.

5. Because the downstroke is an eccentric action of the leg muscles, the faster the pedaling, the greater the force generation.

Answers to Selected Chapter 1 Test Questions

Multiple Choice

1. b;   2. c;   3. a;   4. d;   5. b;   6. d

True-False

7. False;   8. False;   9. True;   10. True;   11. False;   12. True;   13. False;   14. False

Fill in the Blank

15. prime movers;   16. synergists;   17. oppose

Short Answer and Essay

For questions 18 to 22, check your answers against the explanations given in the textbook.

Neurological Control of Movement

concepts

- The basic unit of the nervous system is the neuron, which is an individual nerve fiber (nerve cell) composed of three regions: the cell body, the dendrites, and the axon.

- Neurons communicate with one another across sites of impulse transmission called synapses; motor neurons communicate with muscle fibers at neuromuscular junctions.

- The central nervous system is made up of the brain and the spinal cord.

- The peripheral nervous system can be subdivided into the sensory and motor divisions. The sensory division carries information from the sensory receptors toward the central nervous system; the motor division carries motor impulses out from the central nervous system to the muscles.

- Sensory-motor integration is the process by which the peripheral nervous system relays sensory input to the central nervous system, and the central nervous system interprets this information and then sends out the appropriate motor signal to elicit the desired motor response.

- The level of nervous system control varies in response to sensory input according to the complexity of movement necessary. Simple reflexes are handled by the spinal cord, whereas complex reactions require involvement of the brain.

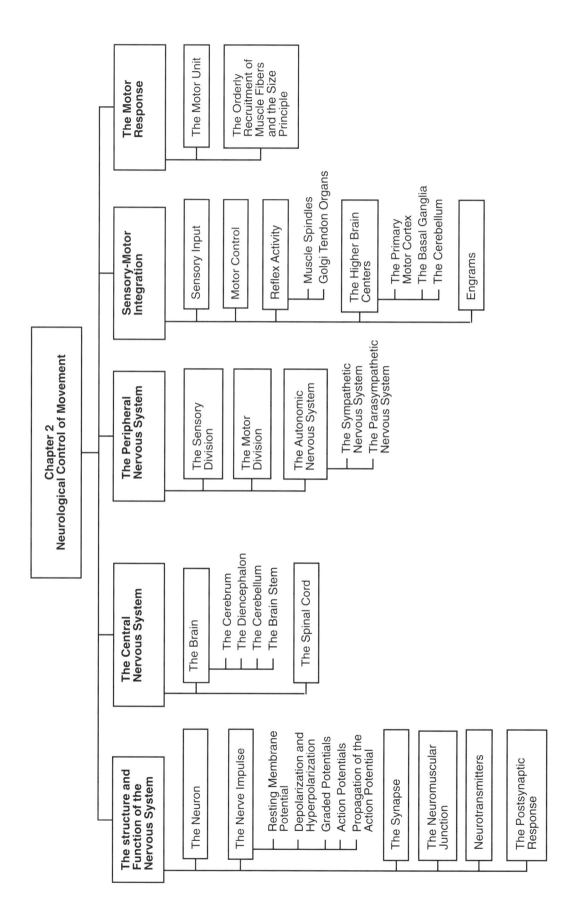

Chapter 2
Neurological Control of Movement

The structure and Function of the Nervous System

The Neuron

The Nerve Impulse
— Resting Membrane Potential
— Depolarization and Hyperpolarization
— Graded Potentials
— Action Potentials
— Propagation of the Action Potential

The Synapse

The Neuromuscular Junction

Neurotransmitters

The Postsynaptic Response

The Central Nervous System

The Brain
— The Cerebrum
— The Diencephalon
— The Cerebellum
— The Brain Stem

The Spinal Cord

The Peripheral Nervous System

The Sensory Division

The Motor Division

The Autonomic Nervous System
— The Sympathetic Nervous System
— The Parasympathetic Nervous System

Sensory-Motor Integration

Sensory Input

Motor Control

Reflex Activity
— Muscle Spindles
— Golgi Tendon Organs

The Higher Brain Centers
— The Primary Motor Cortex
— The Basal Ganglia
— The Cerebellum

Engrams

The Motor Response

The Motor Unit

The Orderly Recruitment of Muscle Fibers and the Size Principle

What Does the Nervous System Do?

Activity 2.1

Do this activity before reading chapter 2 of *Physiology of Sport and Exercise.*

Your nervous system is made up of two divisions: the central nervous system, which includes the brain and the spinal cord, and the peripheral nervous system, which includes all nerve cells outside the central nervous system. Together, the central and peripheral nervous systems control and regulate the internal environment and voluntary movement. In this activity, you will begin to explore some of the functions of the nervous system. When you finish the chapter, we will revisit this activity to see how much more you understand about this subject.

Make a list of the major movements you have done over the last hour. These might include climbing a flight of stairs, walking to or from class, opening a door, sitting down or standing, throwing a football, and so forth.

Now choose one of these movements to analyze, and answer the questions that follow on a separate sheet of paper.

Movement chosen: _____

1. What sounds did your nervous system need to interpret in order for you to perform the movement well?

2. What visual cues did your nervous system need to interpret in order for you to perform the movement well?

3. What cues from the sense of touch did your nervous system need to interpret in order for you to perform the movement well?

4. What adjustments in heart rate and respiratory rate did your body make in response to this movement?

5. Did performing this movement affect your thirst level? How?

6. Would you describe this movement as a simple movement or as a complicated one, requiring thought processes? Explain.

7. How much conscious thought did you have to give to this movement? Explain.

8. Given the knowledge you have right now, explain as best you can how your nervous system senses information, interprets it, and then communicates to your muscles exactly when and how much to act.

Activity 2.2

The Neuron

Do this activity after reading pages 54-56 (top) of *Physiology of Sport and Exercise.*

The fundamental functional unit of the nervous system is the neuron. The drawing below shows the basic structure of a neuron. Fill in the blanks with the correct names of the parts of the neuron. Then in the space provided on the next page, explain the function of select parts of the neuron.

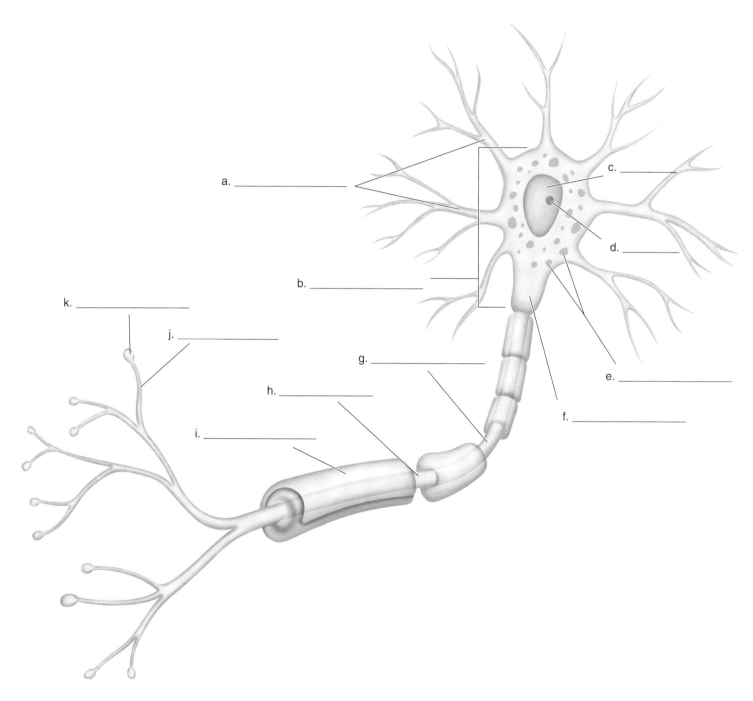

a. _____

c. _____

d. _____

b. _____

k. _____

j. _____

g. _____

e. _____

h. _____

f. _____

i. _____

Part	Function
Dendrite	_____
	_____
Axon	_____
	_____
Synaptic knobs	_____
	_____

Activity 2.3

The Nerve Impulse

Do this activity after reading pages 56-60 of *Physiology of Sport and Exercise.*

A nerve impulse—an electrical charge—is the signal that passes from one neuron to the next and finally to an end organ (such as a group of muscle fibers) or back to the central nervous system. Review pages 56-60 of *Physiology of Sport and Exercise.* Draw a flowchart that illustrates the step-by-step process of a nerve impulse. Briefly describe each step and draw an arrow connecting it to the next step. Be sure to include information about the myelin sheath and its role in conduction. Note that at some point you will have separate branches in your flowchart for graded potentials and action potentials.

Communication Among Neurons and Muscle Fibers

Activity 2.4

Do this activity after reading pages 60-64 of *Physiology of Sport and Exercise.*

Review pages 60-64 in *Physiology of Sport and Exercise* to be sure you have a complete understanding of the synapse, the neuromuscular junction, neurotransmitters, and the postsynaptic response.

With a small group of your classmates, construct a model that depicts neurons communicating via synapses and neuromuscular junctions. You might use clay, wood, cardboard, marbles, liquids for neurotransmitters, and so forth. An extra challenge is to depict the concept of summation through your model. Be ready to demonstrate your model to the class by the date your instructor specifies.

The Central Nervous System

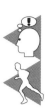

Do this activity after reading pages 64-67 of *Physiology of Sport and Exercise.*

The central nervous system is made up of the brain and the spinal cord and houses more than 100 billion neurons. The drawings below show the major parts of the central nervous system. Fill in the blanks with the correct labels, and then answer the questions that follow.

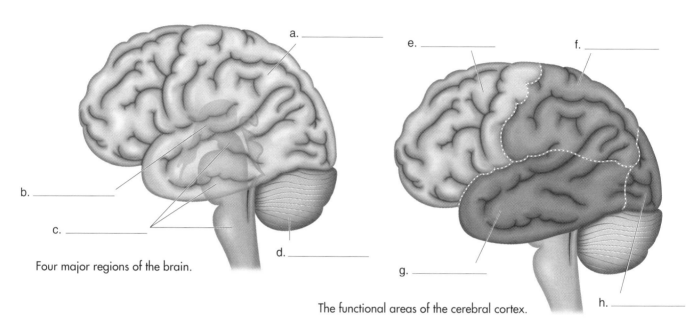

a. _____

b. _____

c. _____

d. _____

Four major regions of the brain.

e. _____

f. _____

g. _____

h. _____

The functional areas of the cerebral cortex.

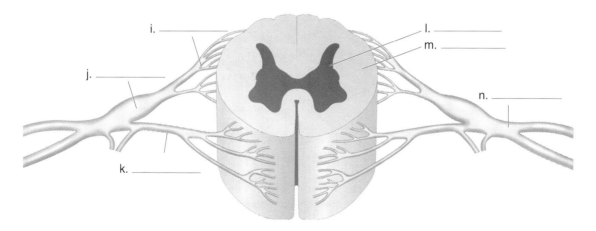

i. _____

j. _____

k. _____

l. _____

m. _____

n. _____

A cross section of the spinal cord illustrating spinal nerves.

Choose a physical activity of your choice to perform for a few minutes. Any activity will work: playing on a sports team, walking or running, playing catch, bowling, dancing, and so on. Prior to doing the activity, look over the questions that follow so you know what to notice as you perform the activity.

1. What were the primary sounds that you heard and needed to interpret (perhaps the calls of a teammate, the sounds of traffic, the noises in a fitness facility)?

   Which portion of the central nervous system (CNS) dealt with this auditory input and its interpretation?

2. What did you see and need to interpret as you performed this physical activity (e.g., the speed and angle of the ball, the car coming down the street)?

   Which portion of the CNS dealt with this visual input and its interpretation?

3. How did your body need to adjust to its surroundings (e.g., shifting to deal with changes in the terrain, avoiding bumping into other people, adjusting your response in order to aim the ball in the right direction)?

   Which portion of the CNS dealt with this general sensory input from receptors in the skin and from proprioceptors in the muscles, tendons, and joints, and allowed you to be constantly aware of your surroundings and your relationship to them?

4. What adjustments did your body make in heart rate, respiration, body temperature, and thirst?

   Which portion of the CNS regulated these changes in your body's internal environment?

5. Which individual muscle movements needed to be coordinated together and smoothed out in order to produce coordinated movement during this activity?

   Which portion of the CNS maintained coordination and caused your muscles to respond appropriately?

6. What decisions did your CNS need to make about your movement (e.g., whether to speed up, stand, run, reach)?

   Which portion of the CNS decided what movements to make and when to make them?

7. What movements of a repetitive and sustained nature did you perform (e.g., arm-swinging while walking)?

   Which portion of the CNS initiated such repetitive and sustained movements and thus controlled complex semivoluntary movements?

> **Activity 2.6**

The Peripheral Nervous System

Do this activity after reading pages 67-70 of *Physiology of Sport and Exercise*.

The peripheral nervous system contains 43 pairs of nerves: 12 pairs of cranial nerves that connect with the brain and 31 pairs of spinal nerves that connect with the spinal cord. Spinal nerves directly supply the skeletal muscles. The peripheral nervous system has two major divisions: the sensory division and the motor division.

Think back to the physical activity you did in activity 2.5, and answer the questions below (on separate paper).

1. While performing this activity, what kind of sensory information did the sensory neurons communicate to the central nervous system? Think through what might have been changing in your blood and lymph vessels, your internal organs, your special sense organs, your skin, and your muscles and tendons.

2. What do you suppose each of the following receptors sensed as you performed this physical activity? Give examples specific to the activity you performed.

   Mechanoreceptors

   Thermoreceptors

   Nociceptors

   Photoreceptors

   Chemoreceptors

3. Imagine that your joint kinesthetic receptors, muscle spindles, and Golgi tendon organs had not sufficiently sensed joint angles and rates of change in these angles, the amount your muscles stretched, and the amount of tension your muscles applied to your tendons. Give specific examples of how this would have affected your ability to perform this physical activity.

4. Review the roles of the sympathetic and parasympathetic nervous systems (pp. 69-70). Describe the effects you think each had on your physical activity. How did each system respond to your physical activity? Which of these nervous systems seemed more dominant during your physical activity? If you experienced the fight-or-flight response during your activity, explain what situation caused this and how your body responded.

Activity 2.7

Sensory-Motor Integration

Do this activity after reading pages 70-78 of *Physiology of Sport and Exercise.*

For your body to respond to sensory stimuli, the sensory and motor divisions of your nervous system must function together in a specific sequence of events.

Draw two flowcharts, one that illustrates the step-by-step process of a motor reflex, and one that depicts the control and coordination of movement through the higher brain centers. Briefly describe each step and draw an arrow connecting it to the next step.

For the motor reflex, be sure to start at the point of sensory input, to include the role of muscle spindles and Golgi tendon organs, and to end with the point of motor response. For the complex activity (with control through higher brain centers), be sure to include the role of the primary motor cortex, the basal ganglia, and the cerebellum.

For each flowchart (the reflex and the more complex activity), consider choosing a specific example (e.g., hitting finger with hammer, returning a tennis serve) and using that example throughout the flowchart.

Researching Neuromuscular Diseases and Disorders

Activity 2.8

Do this activity after reading chapter 2 of *Physiology of Sport and Exercise.*

When your nervous system works well, you may take for granted how miraculous it is. But when something in your nervous system goes awry, the consequences can be dire, and you realize how important this physiological system is to your everyday life.

Research a central nervous system disease, a nervous system abnormality, a neuromuscular disease, or a peripheral nervous system disease. You might research one of the diseases listed here or another one that you find interesting:

- Multiple sclerosis or other demyelinating diseases
- Guillain-Barré syndrome
- Amyotrophic lateral sclerosis (ALS), also called Lou Gehrig's disease
- Cerebral palsy
- Polio
- Reflex sympathetic disorder (RSD)
- Meningitis

    Write a report that summarizes the following:

- The definition of the disease
- The causes of the disease
- Diagnosis and treatment of the disease
- The effects the disease has on the neurological system; focus especially on how this disease relates to information you have learned in this chapter
- The symptoms of the disease; focus especially on how the disease affects a person's motor control and muscle movement
- The progression of the disease

Be sure to document your sources. If you know someone who has the disease you are researching, interview this person to find out what he or she knows about the disease, how it affects his or her everyday functioning, and how he or she adapts activities to cope with the disease. Include your findings from this personal interview in your report.

Turn in your report to your instructor or, if your instructor prefers, present your report orally to the class.

Putting It All Together: Neurological Control of Movement

Activity 2.9

Do this activity after reading chapter 2 of *Physiology of Sport and Exercise*.

In activity 2.1, before you studied this chapter, you hypothesized about how your nervous system senses information, interprets it, and then communicates to your muscles exactly when and how much to act. Look back at your responses to that activity. Now we'll see how much better you understand this complex process.

Choose either the same physical activity you chose for activity 2.1 or another major movement you have done over the last hour. On a separate piece of paper, explain in great detail the process your nervous system went through during that movement. Be sure to include the following information in your discussion:

- The role the central nervous system played, including discussion of the cerebrum, the diencephalon, the cerebellum, the brain stem, and the spinal cord
- The role the peripheral nervous system played, including the sensory division, the motor division, and the autonomic nervous system
- How the sensory and motor systems communicated with each other
- How nerve impulses travel within neurons and to other neurons or muscle fibers (include concepts of resting membrane potential, depolarization and hyperpolarization, graded potentials, action potentials, synapses, neuromuscular junctions, neurotransmitters, and summation)
- How your muscles responded to motor impulses once they reached the muscle fibers, including discussion of the motor unit and the recruitment of muscle fibers

Sample Test Questions for Chapter 2

Test yourself on your knowledge of this chapter by taking this self-test. Write the correct answers on a separate sheet of paper.

Multiple Choice

1. Which of the following items best describes dendrites?
   a. They are the neuron's receivers, they carry the impulses away from the cell body, and most neurons contain many of them.
   b. They are the neuron's receivers, they carry the impulses toward the cell body, and most neurons contain many of them.

c. They are the neuron's transmitters, they carry the impulses away from the cell body, and most neurons contain only one of them.

d. They are the neuron's transmitters, they carry the impulses toward the cell body, and most neurons contain only one of them.

2. Which of the following sentences is *not* true of an action potential?

a. Any time depolarization reaches or exceeds the threshold, an action potential will result.

b. An action potential is a rapid and substantial depolarization of the neuron's membrane.

c. An action potential always begins as a graded potential.

d. An action potential is usually just a local event, so that the depolarization does not spread very far along the neuron.

3. The velocity of a nerve impulse transmission is primarily determined by

a. myelination and diameter of the neurons.

b. absolute refractory and relative refractory.

c. number of muscle fibers per motor neuron.

d. sodium concentration.

4. Which of the following sentences is *not* true of the brain stem?

a. All sensory and motor nerves pass through it as they relay information between the brain and the spinal cord.

b. It contains the major autonomic regulatory centers that exert control over the respiratory and cardiovascular systems.

c. It is the site of origin of both the cranial nerves and the spinal nerves.

d. The reticular formation runs the entire length of the brain stem and influences nearly all areas of the central nervous system.

5. This nervous system prepares your body to face a crisis, regulating the fight-or-flight response.

a. the parasympathetic nervous system

b. the central nervous system

c. the sympathetic nervous system

d. Tthe sensory-motor nervous system

6. The autonomic nervous system regulates all of the following functions *except*

a. heart rate.

b. respiration.

c. blood distribution.

d. motor control.

7. Which of the following statements is true of muscle spindles?

a. They sense tension in muscles; they inhibit the contracting muscles, and they excite the antagonist muscles.

b. They supply information on the length and contractile state of the muscle, as well as the rate at which those states are changing.

c. They initiate movements of a sustained and repetitive nature.

d. They are the center of conscious motor control.

True-False

8. Depolarization occurs any time the charge difference in a neuron increases, moving from the resting membrane potential to an even more negative number.

9. Neurons communicate with one another across sites of impulse transmission called neuromuscular junctions.

10. A nerve impulse can be transmitted across a synapse in only one direction.

11. An incoming impulse—that is, an impulse being received by a neuron or a muscle fiber—can be only excitatory.

12. The sum of all changes in the membrane potential must equal or exceed the threshold in order to cause sufficient depolarization to generate an action potential.

13. The central nervous system transmits information to various parts of the body through the motor, or efferent, division of the peripheral nervous system.

14. Sensory impulses that terminate in the spinal cord typically result in a conscious movement.

Fill in the Blank

15. Muscles controlling fine movements have _____ [a small number of, many] muscle fibers per motor neuron. Muscles with more general functions have _____ [a small number of, many] fibers per motor neuron.

16. The neurotransmitters most important to regulation of exercise are _____ _____ and _____.

17. The _____ keeps a running total of the neuron's responses to all incoming impulses.

18. The _____ regulates what sensory input reaches your conscious brain.

19. Neurons in the _____ let us consciously control movement of our skeletal muscles.

Short Answer

20. Describe the sequence of events in an action potential.

21. Define and explain the role of the myelin sheath.

22. Explain the role of neurotransmitters, sodium, and potassium at a neuromuscular junction.

23. Explain in detail the role of the cerebellum in coordinating movement.

24. Define engrams.

Essay

25. What is the resting membrane potential? What is it caused by? How is a constant resting membrane potential maintained?

26. Explain in detail the process of sensory-motor integration.

Answers to Selected Chapter 2 Activities

2.2   The Neuron

a. Dendrites;   b. Cell body;   c. Nucleus;   d. Nucleolus;   e. Nissl bodies;   f. Axon hillock;   g. Axon;   h. Node of Ranvier;   i. Myelin sheath;   j. Axon terminal;   k. Synaptic knob

Part	Function
Dendrite	The neuron's receivers. Most impulses coming into the nerve enter the neuron via the dendrites. The dendrites then carry the impulses toward the cell body.
Axon:	The neuron's transmitter. It conducts impulses away from the cell body.
Synaptic knobs	These knobs are on the tips of the axon terminals and house vesicles (sacs) filled with chemicals known as neurotransmitters. The neurotransmitters are used for communication between a neuron and another cell.

2.5   The Central Nervous System

a. Cerebrum;   b. Diencephalon;   c. Brain stem;   d. Cerebellum;   e. Frontal lobe;   f. Parietal lobe;   g. Temporal lobe;   h. Occipital lobe;   i. Dorsal (sensory) root;   j. Dorsal root ganglion;   k. Ventral (motor) root;   l. Gray matter;   m. White matter;   n. Spinal nerve

1. Temporal lobe;
2. Occipital lobe;
3. Primary sensory cortex in the parietal lobe;
4. Diencephalon;
5. Cerebellum;
6. Primary motor cortex in the frontal lobe;
7. Basal ganglia in the cerebral white matter

Answers to Selected Chapter 2 Test Questions

Multiple Choice

1. b;   2. d   3. a   4. c;   5. c;   6. d;   7. b

True-False

8. False;   9. False;   10. True;   11. False;   12. True;   13. True;   14. False

Fill in the Blank

15. a small number of, many;   16. acetylcholine and norepinephrine;   17. axon hillock;   18. thalamus;   19. primary motor cortex

Short Answer and Essay

For questions 20 to 26, check your answers against the explanations given in the textbook.

Neuromuscular Adaptations to Resistance Training

concepts

- Muscular power is the product of the strength and the speed of a movement. It is the key component for most athletic performances.

- Although most muscle hypertrophy probably results from an increase in the size of individual muscle fibers (fiber hypertrophy), some evidence suggests that an increase in the number of muscle fibers (fiber hyperplasia) might also be involved.

- Early gains in strength appear to be more influenced by neural factors, but later long-term gains are largely the result of hypertrophy (increases in muscle size).

- The factors that cause muscle soreness may be necessary to maximize the resistance training response. Acute muscle soreness occurs late in an exercise bout and during the immediate recovery period. Delayed-onset muscle soreness (DOMS) occurs a day or two after the exercise bout, results primarily from eccentric actions, and might be caused by structural damage to muscle cells and inflammatory reactions within the muscles.

- The ability of a muscle or muscle group to generate force varies throughout the full range of movement.

- Resistance training should be as sport specific as possible. At least part of the training should involve movements that closely mimic, in both pattern and speed, those needed for the athlete's sport or activity.

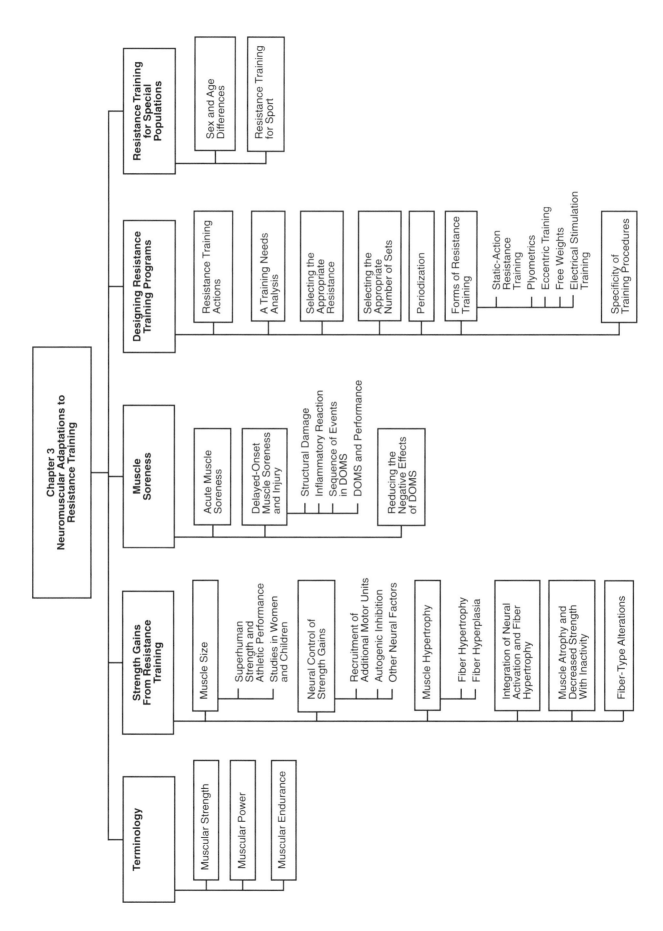

Chapter 3
Neuromuscular Adaptations to Resistance Training

Terminology
- Muscular Strength
- Muscular Power
- Muscular Endurance

Strength Gains From Resistance Training
- Muscle Size
  - Superhuman Strength and Athletic Performance
  - Studies in Women and Children
- Neural Control of Strength Gains
  - Recruitment of Additional Motor Units
  - Autogenic Inhibition
  - Other Neural Factors
- Muscle Hypertrophy
  - Fiber Hypertrophy
  - Fiber Hyperplasia
- Integration of Neural Activation and Fiber Hypertrophy
- Muscle Atrophy and Decreased Strength With Inactivity
- Fiber-Type Alterations

Muscle Soreness
- Acute Muscle Soreness
- Delayed-Onset Muscle Soreness and Injury
  - Structural Damage
  - Inflammatory Reaction
  - Sequence of Events in DOMS
  - DOMS and Performance
- Reducing the Negative Effects of DOMS

Designing Resistance Training Programs
- Resistance Training Actions
- A Training Needs Analysis
- Selecting the Appropriate Resistance
- Selecting the Appropriate Number of Sets
- Periodization
- Forms of Resistance Training
  - Static-Action Resistance Training
  - Plyometrics
  - Eccentric Training
  - Free Weights
  - Electrical Stimulation Training
- Specificity of Training Procedures

Resistance Training for Special Populations
- Sex and Age Differences
- Resistance Training for Sport

How Does the Neuromuscular System Adapt to Resistance Training?

Activity 3.1

Do this activity before reading chapter 3 of *Physiology of Sport and Exercise.*

Nearly everyone can improve his or her strength through resistance training. Interestingly, with long-term training, many adaptations occur in the neuromuscular system. This chapter will examine those changes and apply them specifically to sport situations. Before you read the chapter, take a look at the case study below and answer the questions that follow it. After you have studied the chapter, we will revisit this case study to see what you have learned.

John, a freshman at a small regional college, is an offensive lineman on the football team. He knows he barely made the cut for the team and needs to make some improvements, but he is not quite sure what to do. Though he is the same size or even bigger than some of his opponents, John often loses the battle with the defensive lineman he is blocking. He seems to be able to react quickly and exert his force with a lot of speed, but he just can't keep his opponents from breaking through the line. In high school, John relied on his natural body size and weight to win these battles, but now that he is facing stronger opponents, he wonders if he should be doing something to train specifically for this.

1. Which area does John need to focus most on improving—his strength, his power, or his endurance?

2. What is the best way for John to improve in this area?

3. If you were to design a resistance training program for John, which muscle groups would you concentrate on?

4. Which resistance training exercises would you build into John's program?

5. How much of an improvement would you expect John to see from strength training?

6. With what you know now, what is your best explanation for the physiological causes of the strength gains John would make? (What would be changing within his muscles and his nervous system to cause strength gains?)

Assessing Your Muscular Strength, Power, and Endurance

Activity 3.2

Do this activity after reading pages 84-86 of *Physiology of Sport and Exercise.*

Muscular strength is the maximum amount of force that a muscle or muscle group can generate. Muscular power is the product of strength and speed of movement. Muscular endurance is the ability to sustain repeated muscle actions or a single static action.

In this activity you will assess your own muscular strength, power, and endurance in doing the single-arm biceps curl. It is preferable that you do this in a weight-training or fitness facility with standard weights. However, if this is impossible, you may use other items (cans or jars filled with rocks or sand) as substitutes for weights, but you must be able to measure the exact weight of these items. If a disability or injury prevents you from doing the single-arm biceps curl, choose another movement to use in assessing your muscular strength, power, and endurance.

Proper Form for Single-Arm Biceps Curl

Grasp a dumbbell in one hand. Your palm should be facing away from the front of your body. Stand erect with feet shoulder-width apart, knees slightly flexed. Allow the dumbbell to hang near your thigh, with your elbow fully extended. Raise the dumbbell in an arc by flexing your arm at the elbow. Keep your upper arm and elbow stationary. Maintain your body position. Do not swing the dumbbell upward; rather move it in a controlled manner, with only your arm doing the work. Using a full range of motion, raise the dumbbell toward your anterior deltoid. Lower the dumbbell slowly and under control until the elbow is fully extended. Do not jerk or bounce the dumbbell at the bottom of the movement.

Muscular Strength

Assess your biceps strength by determining your one-repetition maximum (1-RM). Select a weight that you know you can lift at least one time. After warming up, try to execute several repetitions. If you can perform more than one repetition, add weight and try again to execute several repetitions. If you can tell that your muscles are tiring out, take a break long enough for them to regain full strength. Continue adding weight until you are unable to lift the weight more than a single repetition. This last weight, which you are able to lift only once, is your 1-RM.

Fill in your 1-RM here: _____

Muscular Power

Muscular power is very difficult to measure. This activity is included to give you an idea of the differences among strength, power, and endurance; however, the results of this muscular power activity should not be viewed as entirely accurate.

After having determined your muscular strength, find a friend or classmate who has the same or a very similar 1-RM. Find a weight that is 50% of your 1-RM. Compare your power levels by seeing who can perform the biceps curl (from the starting position with your elbow fully extended, through the upward and downward phases, and to the ending position with your elbow fully extended again) more quickly with 50% of your 1-RM. Have a third person observe the two of you as you perform your biceps curl as quickly as possible. Be sure to keep correct form during this attempt in order to prevent injury. The third person should not only evaluate who performs the biceps curl faster, but also about how much faster that person does it. (For instance, was it twice as fast? Just barely faster?)

The person who could lift the same weight yet do it more quickly has a biceps with more muscular power.

Whose biceps has more muscular power? _____

What aspects of you as individuals might account for your differences or similarities in muscular power?

Muscular Endurance

Find a weight that is 75% of your 1-RM. See how many repetitions of the single-arm biceps curl you can perform with this weight.

Weight used: _____

Number of repetitions you are able to perform: _____

Compare this to others' endurance levels. What might cause some of the differences in your levels of endurance?

| Activity 3.3 | # What Causes Strength Gains? |

Do this activity after reading pages 86-96 of *Physiology of Sport and Exercise.*

Resistance training programs can produce substantial strength gains. Within 3 to 6 months, you can see from 15% to 100% improvement, and sometimes even more. How do you become stronger? Read the following case study and then answer the questions that follow on separate paper.

Samantha, a high school sophomore, has played softball for several years. A highly successful player, she was on a string of winning teams her first few years, occasionally made it to the all-star game in her community, and has been selected to be on a traveling team the last three years. Despite these high honors, upon entering her sophomore year in high school, Samantha could tell she would have to improve her hitting power and her running speed if she was to remain at the top of her game.

So Samantha set out to gain strength and power through a well-planned resistance training program. Her coach helped her design the plan, and then Samantha, self-motivated as she was, stuck to the plan for eight weeks, working out three times a week. Samantha didn't think the program was nearly as difficult as she had thought it would be, and she was surprised that by the end of only eight weeks, she had increased her arm strength 25% and her leg strength 50%. What surprised her most was that even though she had obviously gained strength, her muscles weren't bulging as she had feared they might. Samantha was thrilled when she started seeing some slight improvement in her game. Her batting felt stronger, and she thought she was running the bases slightly faster. She determined that she would stick with this resistance training plan—it seemed to be paying off!

1. Review pages 86-96 in your textbook. As Samantha followed through on her resistance training program, what physiological adaptations might have occurred to allow Samantha to gain greater levels of strength?

2. How is it that Samantha could gain strength without significant hypertrophy?

| Activity 3.4 | **Observing Muscle Atrophy** |

Do this activity after reading pages 94-95 of *Physiology of Sport and Exercise.*

Muscles atrophy—decrease in size and strength—when they become inactive, as with injury or disuse. For this activity, find a place to observe people who might be experiencing atrophy—a hospital, a nursing home, a park or restaurant frequented by older people, or a rehabilitation facility where athletes or others are working to regain strength. Write your answers to the following questions on a separate piece of paper.

1. Note evidence you see of muscle atrophy. Give specific examples from your observation. Be sure to cite evidence of atrophy only, not of unrelated symptoms of old age, illness, or injury.

2. Review pages 94 to 95 of your textbook. What causes atrophy?

3. When a trained muscle suddenly becomes inactive through immobilization—let's say you break your ankle and wear a cast for several weeks—when during this period are strength decreases most dramatic?

4. Which fiber type does atrophy most affect? Why? Describe the physiological changes that occur in the muscle fiber with atrophy.

5. Describe the results of a recovery from atrophy. Can muscles recover completely from atrophy? How long does this recovery take?

Activity 3.5

Muscle Soreness

Do this activity after reading pages 96-100 of *Physiology of Sport and Exercise*.

Muscle soreness can be present during the later stages of an exercise bout and the immediate recovery period, between 12 and 48 h after a strenuous bout of exercise, or both. Review pages 96-100 in *Physiology of Sport and Exercise*. Think back to activity 3.2. If you did not complete that activity, do the biceps curl exercises now.

1. Which type of muscle soreness did you experience after assessing your muscle strength, power, and endurance in activity 3.2?

2. If someone felt immediate soreness during and immediately after activity 3.2, what were the likely causes of this acute muscle soreness?

3. If someone felt sore a day or two after this exercise, what were the possible causes of this delayed-onset muscle soreness (DOMS)?

4. If you experienced muscle soreness after completing activity 3.2, which action of that activity caused this soreness?

Activity 3.6	# Pros and Cons of Forms of Resistance Training

Do this activity after reading pages 100-102 and 103 (bottom)-105 of *Physiology of Sport and Exercise*.

Each form of resistance training has advantages and disadvantages. Reread pages 100-102 and 103-105 and then fill out the table below with what you have learned.

Form of resistance training	Advantages	Disadvantages
Static-action resistance training (isometric training)		
Plyometrics		
Eccentric training		
Electrical stimulation training		
Variable resistance devices		
Isokinetic devices		
Free weights		

Designing Your Own Resistance Training Program

Activity 3.7

Do this activity after reading pages 100-107 of *Physiology of Sport and Exercise.*

Designing an appropriate resistance training program is quite complex and takes much skill. Even after years of experience, seasoned strength-training professionals find new ways to modify programs to meet an athlete's goals. However, in order to help you learn the basic concepts of designing a resistance training program, you are going to design a basic program for yourself based on your personal goals. Because this chapter concentrates on resistance training for sport, we will focus on training for sport here, too.

As you do this activity, if you desire more information on a certain area, you may want to consult other resources, such as these:

Fleck, S.J., and Kraemer, W.J. 1997. *Designing resistance training programs.* 2nd ed. Champaign, IL: Human Kinetics.

Baechle, T.R., and Earle, R.W. (Eds.). 2000. *Essentials of strength training and conditioning.* 2nd ed. Champaign, IL: Human Kinetics.

1. Decide what sport or physical activity you are going to train for. Write that activity here: _____

2. Conduct a training needs analysis.

   a. What muscle groups do you need to train?

   b. What energy system should be stressed (aerobic, anaerobic)?

   c. What type of muscle action (e.g., concentric, static or isometric, eccentric) should be used?

   d. What are the primary sites of concern for injury prevention?

3. Select the appropriate exercises based on your needs analysis and the sport or activity you are training for. Write those exercises here:

4. Select the order in which you will perform these exercises. Number the exercises listed above in the order in which you will perform them. Then briefly explain your reasoning for this order.

5. Select the appropriate resistance (the percentage RM) for each exercise, based on whether you desire to improve your muscular strength, endurance, or power. For each exercise in question 4, write the percentage RM you are going to use. Then briefly explain your reasoning for your selections.

6. Select the appropriate number of sets and rest periods for each exercise. Decide whether you will rest between sets or between exercises, and how long your rest periods will be. Record your decisions for each exercise below.

7. Now fill in the table on the next page to see how all of your decisions fit into a whole resistance training program.

8. How does your gender, age, and athletic involvement impact your program?

9. If you were training year-round for this particular sport or physical activity, how would you adjust this program over time (see the section on periodization in the text)?

Resistance Training Program

Exercises in preferred order	Muscle groups involved	Energy system stressed	Type of muscle action	Percentage RM to be used	Number of sets	Rest periods *Between sets?* *Between exercises?* *For how long?*

Activity 3.8

Do this activity after
reading chapter 3 of
*Physiology of Sport
and Exercise*.

Putting It All Together: Neuromuscular Adaptations to Resistance Training

In this chapter, you have learned about the role of resistance training in increasing muscular strength and improving performance. We have examined how muscle strength is gained through both muscular and neural adaptations, what factors can lead to muscle soreness, and how to design an appropriate resistance training program that will meet the specific needs of the individual athlete.

Now let's revisit the case study we started this chapter with—remember our offensive lineman named John?—and see how all of this information works together to plan a successful resistance-training program.

> John, a freshman at a small regional college, is an offensive lineman on the football team. He knows he barely made the cut for the team and needs to make some improvements, but he is not quite sure what to do. Though he is the same size or even bigger than some of his opponents, John often loses the battle with the defensive lineman he is blocking. He seems to be able to react quickly and exert his force with a lot of speed, but he just can't keep his opponents from breaking through the line. In high school, John relied on his natural body size and weight to win these battles, but now that he is facing stronger opponents, he wonders if he should be doing something to train specifically for this.

Answer the following questions on a separate piece of paper.

1. Does John need to gain muscular strength, power, or endurance in order to keep his spot on the football team? Explain your answer.

2. With this goal and John's playing position in mind, design a resistance training program for John.

   First, perform a needs analysis for John:

   a. Which major muscle groups does John need to concentrate on?

   b. What type of muscle action (e.g., concentric, static or isometric, eccentric) should be used? Why?

   c. What energy system would you stress? Why?

   d. What are the primary sites of concern for injury prevention?

   Based on your needs analysis, design the specifics of the program:

   e. Which exercises would you include in John's resistance training program?

   f. What order would you put them in?

   g. How would you structure the number of sets and the number and length of rest periods?

   h. How much resistance—what percentage RM—would you have John use?

3. Discuss the physiological changes that could lead to John's strength gains as he continues with this resistance-training program. You should include discussion of muscle size, neural control, and muscle hypertrophy.

4. Once John has met his training goals, how should he adjust his training program?

5. When John first starts to train, he will likely experience some delayed-onset muscle soreness (DOMS). Explain the physiological mechanisms underlying this phenomenon. How should John adjust his training program when he experiences DOMS?

6. Is it possible that John's fiber types might be altered through this training program? Why or why not? What would be the possible reasons for fiber-type alteration?

Sample Test Questions for Chapter 3

Test yourself on your knowledge of this chapter by taking this self-test. Write the correct answers on a separate sheet of paper.

Multiple Choice

1. The maximal force a muscle or muscle group can generate is termed
   a. muscular power.
   b. muscular endurance.
   c. muscular strength.
   d. muscular weight.

2. Which of the following items is *not* a neural adaptation that may cause gains in strength?
   a. changes in the firing frequency or discharge rates of motor units
   b. additional motor unit recruitment, perhaps with synchronization
   c. Reduction in coactivation of antagonist muscles
   d. Gradually increased neurological inhibition of such mechanisms as the Golgi tendon organs.

3. This type of muscle action is most likely to increase a muscle fiber's cross-sectional area.
   a. eccentric
   b. concentric
   c. static or isometric
   d. asymmetric

4. Which of the following sentences is *not* true regarding fiber-type alterations?
   a. Fast-twitch muscle fibers can become more oxidative with aerobic training.
   b. Short-term fiber-type alterations are the result of transient muscle hypertrophy.
   c. One fiber type might actually be converted to the other type as a result of cross-innervation or chronic, low-frequency nerve stimulation.
   d. Generally, the fiber types transition from FT_b to FT_a and from FT_a to ST.

5. Which of the following is *not* true of delayed-onset muscle soreness (DOMS)?
   a. In the short term, DOMS reduces the force-generating capacity of the affected muscles.
   b. DOMS is most likely necessary to maximize the training response.
   c. Intense concentric exercise is the most likely cause of DOMS.
   d. DOMS may actually result from structural damage in the muscle.

True-False

6. Muscle strength is related only to muscle size.

7. Muscles can completely recover from atrophy once activity resumes.

8. Delayed-onset muscle soreness is caused in part by actual damage to the muscle.

9. Early gains in strength appear to be more influenced by hypertrophy, but later long-term gains are largely the result of neural factors.

10. Strength development is optimized by many repetitions and low resistance, whereas muscular endurance is optimized by few repetitions and high resistance.

11. To prevent injury, women should not use the same resistance training techniques that men use.

12. Your strength varies throughout the full range of motion.

13. Children and the elderly can gain muscular strength and muscle mass through resistance training.

Fill in the Blank

14. The equation for *power* is _____.

15. The more technical name for jump training is _____.

16. Strength gains from resistance training are highly specific to the _____ and the _____ of the training.

Short Answer

17. Define *transient hypertrophy*.

18. How can a person prevent losses in strength gained through resistance training once the goals for strength development have been achieved?

19. Define periodization and list the five phases and their characteristics.

Essay

20. Compare and contrast fiber hypertrophy and fiber hyperplasia. Explain the possible physiological mechanisms underlying each.

21. Define atrophy and explain the physiological changes that take place when atrophy occurs.

22. Explain the possible causes of delayed-onset muscle soreness and the possible sequence of events leading to this type of soreness.

23. Compare and contrast the advantages and disadvantages of free weights, variable-resistance devices, and isokinetic devices.

Answers to Selected Chapter 3 Activities

3.3   What Causes Strength Gains?

1. **Possible neural factors:** Recruitment of additional motor units to act synchronously, facilitating contraction and increasing the muscle's ability to generate force; recruitment of additional motor units, though not necessarily synchronously; a gradual reduction or counteraction of the inhibitory impulses of the Golgi tendon organs; a reduction in the coactivation of antagonist muscles; increased firing frequency or discharge rates of motor units; changes in the morphology of neuromuscular junctions that might relate to a muscle's force-producing capacity.

   Possible hypertrophy factors: Though the hypertrophy might not have been significant enough for Samantha to observe, she might have undergone slight hypertrophy because either fiber hyperplasia or fiber hypertrophy. Fiber hyperplasia is an increase in the number of muscle fibers. It is postulated that individual muscle fibers do have the capacity to divide and split into daughter cells, each of which can then develop into a functional muscle fiber. Satellite cells, which are the myogenic stem cells involved in skeletal muscle regeneration, are likely involved in the generation of new muscle fibers. These cells are typically activated by muscle injury, which might, in fact, occur in intense resistance training.

Fiber hypertrophy is an increase in the size of existing individual muscle fibers and could be caused by more myofibrils, more actin and myosin filaments, more sarcoplasm, more connective tissue, or any combination of these. Individual fiber hypertrophy appears to result from a net increase in muscle protein synthesis and might be related to levels of the hormone testosterone.

2. The neural control of Samantha's muscle must have been altered, allowing greater force production without noticeable hypertrophy. In addition, early gains in strength appear to be more influenced by neural factors; it could be that Samantha has not trained long enough to experience strength gains from hypertrophy.

3.4   Observing Muscle Atrophy

1. Responses will vary.

2. Atrophy results from lack of muscle use and the consequent loss of muscle protein that accompanies the inactivity.

3. Strength decreases are most dramatic during the first week of immobilization, averaging 3% to 4% per day.

4. Atrophy affects primarily the slow-twitch fibers. Researchers have observed disintegrated myofibrils, streaming Z disks, and mitochondrial damage in ST fibers. When the muscle atrophies, both the cross-sectional fiber area and the percentage of ST fibers decrease.

5. Muscles can recover from atrophy when activity is resumed. The recovery period is substantially longer than the period of immobilization, but shorter than the original training period.

3.5   Muscle Soreness

1. Answers will vary.

2. The pain probably resulted from accumulation of the end products of exercise, such as H^+, and from tissue edema, which is caused by fluid shifting from the blood plasma into the tissues.

3. DOMS is not fully understood. However, possible causes include structural damage to muscle cells and inflammatory reactions within the muscles. A proposed model of the sequence of events leading to DOMS includes (1) structural damage, (2) impaired calcium availability leading to necrosis, (3) accumulation of irritants, and (4) increased macrophage activity.

4. The soreness was probably a result of the eccentric action, when the muscles were lengthening as the weight was lowered.

Answers to Selected Chapter 3 Test Questions

Multiple Choice

1. c;   2. d;   3. a;   4. b;   5. c

True-False

6. False;   7. True;   8. True;   9. False;   10. False;   11. False;   12. True;   13. True

Fill in the Blank

14. power = (force × distance)/time;   15. plyometrics;   16. speed, movement patterns

Short Answer and Essay

For questions 17 to 23, check your answers against the explanations given in the textbook.

Metabolism and Basic Energy Systems

concepts

- The formation of ATP provides the cells with a high-energy compound for storing and conserving energy.

- ATP is generated through three energy systems: (1) the ATP-PCr system, (2) the glycolytic system, and (3) the oxidative system. The ATP-PCr and glycolytic systems are major contributors of energy during the early minutes of high-intensity exercise, while the oxidative system yields more energy and is the primary method of energy production during endurance events.

- Our muscles' oxidative capacity depends on their oxidative enzyme levels, their fiber-type composition, and oxygen availability.

- The most common methods for estimating anaerobic effort involve the examination of either the excess postexercise oxygen consumption or the lactate threshold. Lactate threshold, when expressed as a percentage of $\dot{V}O_2max$, is one of the best determinants of an athlete's pace in endurance events.

- Your metabolism increases with increased exercise intensity, but your oxygen consumption is limited. Its peak value is $\dot{V}O_2max$.

- Fatigue may be caused by (1) depletion of PCr or glycogen, which impairs ATP production; (2) the accumulation of hydrogen generated by lactic acid, which impairs the cellular processes that produce energy and muscle contraction; (3) failure of neural transmission; or (4) the central nervous system's responses to the psychological trauma of exhaustive exercise.

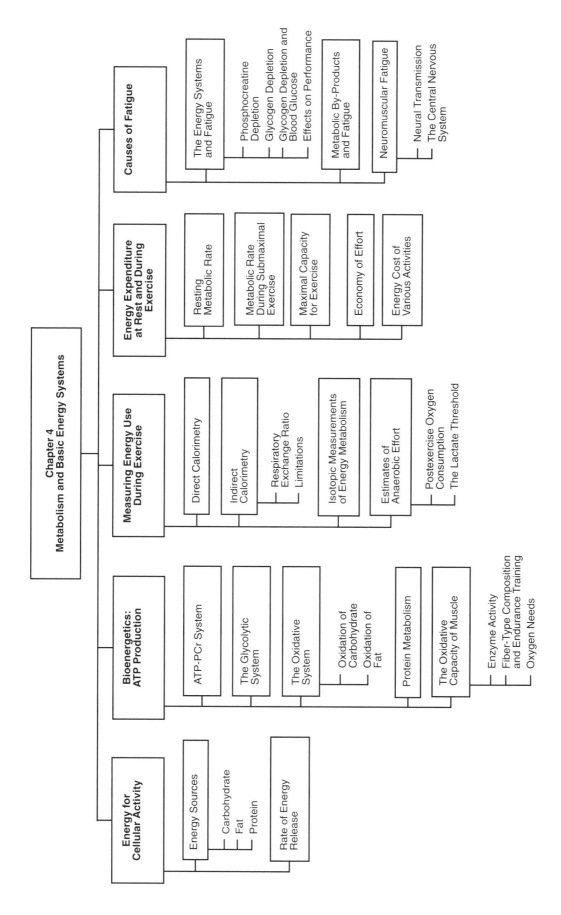

Chapter 4
Metabolism and Basic Energy Systems

Energy for Cellular Activity

- Energy Sources
  - Carbohydrate
  - Fat
  - Protein
- Rate of Energy Release

Bioenergetics: ATP Production

- ATP-PCr System
- The Glycolytic System
- The Oxidative System
  - Oxidation of Carbohydrate
  - Oxidation of Fat
- Protein Metabolism
- The Oxidative Capacity of Muscle
  - Enzyme Activity
  - Fiber-Type Composition and Endurance Training
  - Oxygen Needs

Measuring Energy Use During Exercise

- Direct Calorimetry
- Indirect Calorimetry
  - Respiratory Exchange Ratio
  - Limitations
- Isotopic Measurements of Energy Metabolism
- Estimates of Anaerobic Effort
  - Postexercise Oxygen Consumption
  - The Lactate Threshold

Energy Expenditure at Rest and During Exercise

- Resting Metabolic Rate
- Metabolic Rate During Submaximal Exercise
- Maximal Capacity for Exercise
- Economy of Effort
- Energy Cost of Various Activities

Causes of Fatigue

- The Energy Systems and Fatigue
  - Phosphocreatine Depletion
  - Glycogen Depletion
  - Glycogen Depletion and Blood Glucose
  - Effects on Performance
- Metabolic By-Products and Fatigue
- Neuromuscular Fatigue
  - Neural Transmission
  - The Central Nervous System

Activity 4.1

Energy Sources and Their Uses

Do this activity after reading pages 116-119 of *Physiology of Sport and Exercise.*

Typically 60% to 70% of the total energy expended by the human body is degraded to heat, while the remaining energy is used for muscular activity and cellular operations. Read pages 116 to 119 in your textbook, and then do the activities that follow.

What Is Energy Used For?

List the uses of energy mentioned in this chapter (see page 116):

1.

2.

3.

How Is the Energy Supplied?

Complete the table below about energy sources.

Energy source	Amount of energy provided	Accessibility as an energy source	Conversion process to form ATP
	9 kcal/g		
Carbohydrate			Carbohydrate to glycogen stored in muscles and liver, converted to glucose as needed, and metabolized.
		Least accessible	

Activity 4.2

Pathways of ATP Production

Do this activity after reading pages 120-129 of *Physiology of Sport and Exercise.*

The formation of ATP provides the cells with a high-energy compound for storing and conserving energy. ATP is generated through three energy systems: (1) the ATP-PCr system, (2) the glycolytic system, and (3) the oxidative system. The ATP-PCr and glycolytic systems are major contributors of energy during the early minutes of high-intensity exercise, while the oxidative system yields more energy and is the primary method of energy production during endurance events. Draw the following flowcharts on separate pieces of paper.

1. Draw a flowchart to illustrate how the ATP-PCr system maintains ATP levels. Begin with the PCr molecule, include the release of energy, and end with the creation of ATP.

2. Draw a flowchart to illustrate how the glycolytic system produces ATP. You do not need to include all of the chemical reactions, but do list all of the general steps. At the very least, include the roles of glycogen, glucose, ATP, glucose-6-phosphate, glycolytic enzymes, pyruvic acid, and lactic acid.

3. Draw a flowchart that shows both the oxidation of carbohydrate and the oxidation of fat. Remember that at some points, these processes share the same pathways and will combine in your flowchart. Again, the complex chemical processes are not required, but the general steps of the oxidative system should be shown.

Activity 4.3

ATP Production and Exercise

Do this activity after reading pages 120-129 of *Physiology of Sport and Exercise.*

The method by which your body generates ATP is determined by the type of exercise you perform and depends on the length and intensity of the activity and, in turn, the availability of oxygen. To broaden your understanding of ATP production and exercise, read the case studies and answer the questions that follow them (on separate paper).

Stephen is a long jumper on his high school's track team. His strength seems to be his sprint speed, but he has struggled occasionally with getting a powerful enough take-off from the board leading into the jump. Last season, his coach started incorporating plyometrics into his training program, and Stephen seems to have really improved his ability to attack the board in order to achieve height and length in the jump. The combination of his sprinting speed and powerful jumping abilities have made Stephen a solid long jumper.

1. Which energy system does Stephen's body primarily use during the long jump?

2. Does this system produce ATP with or without the aid of oxygen? Therefore, what do we call this type of metabolism?

3. What type of energy-storing molecule does this energy system use, and what is its role in creating ATP?

4. For how long can this system maintain an adequate ATP level? Describe the progression of ATP and PCr stores as this system's capacity is taxed.

5. Suppose that next season, Stephen switches to the 800-m dash, an event that average high schoolers run in a little over two min. In terms of his prior training and his energy systems, what part of the 800 m would Stephen be well trained for? What would he likely find difficult? Why?

Sarah has been training for the 5,000 m for several years. Now a college sophomore, it seems that her hard work might pay off; she has qualified for the Junior Nationals and even has a chance to medal. When she first started training in high school, she found that she was exhausted even 2 laps into the 12.5-lap race. But after adding some variation into her training program—interspersing her usual easy two-mi run with some longer runs and harder days—she found her endurance really improved and she no longer faded in the final minutes of the event. Her time improved from 21:07 to 19:50 in one season.

6. During the early minute or two of the 5,000 m, what energy systems are likely providing most of Sarah's energy? Which energy system is the primary source of Sarah's energy during the majority of her running of the 5,000 m? Describe what causes this transition to take place.

7. Does the primary system Sarah's body uses during the 5,000-m run produce ATP with or without the aid of oxygen? Therefore, what do we call this type of metabolism?

8. What are the sources of energy in this ATP-producing system? Which of these sources is the preferred fuel during high-intensity exercise? Why?

9. What physiological changes may have caused an increase in oxidative capacity and therefore an improvement in Sarah's time over one season?

Evaluating Different Measures of Energy Use

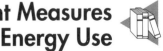

Activity 4.4

Do this activity after reading pages 130-137 of *Physiology of Sport and Exercise.*

Energy use cannot be directly measured, but numerous indirect laboratory methods have been developed to calculate the rate and quantity of energy expenditure when the body is at rest and while it is exercising. Review pages 130 to 137 in your textbook, and then fill in the table on the next page with the correct information.

Activity 4.4 **Evaluating Different Measures of Energy Use**

Name of method	Basic approach of method	Advantages	Disadvantages
Direct calorimetry			
Indirect calorimetry			
Carbon 13			
Doubly labeled water			
Excess postexercise oxygen consumption			
Lactate threshold			

Activity 4.5

Determining Endurance Performance Success

Do this activity after reading pages 138-144 of *Physiology of Sport and Exercise*.

Although we can never fully predict a person's athletic success and must be careful not to limit someone's performance or training based only on objective tests, several variables do seem to impact performance outcomes. Read the following case study about two endurance swimmers and evaluate who you think might be the better performer.

> Shanese and Erika are both endurance swimmers. They have been training side by side under the same coach's tutelage for five years, and though their technique differs slightly, it is very similar.
>
> Shanese weighs 58 kg (128 lb). Her $\dot{V}O_2$max is 2.2 L/min. Shanese can perform at about 80% of her $\dot{V}O_2$max. Shanese's lactate threshold is slightly higher than Erika's is. About 67% of Shanese's muscle fibers appear to be ST fibers.
>
> Erika weighs 55.5 kg (122 lb). Her $\dot{V}O_2$max is 2.5 L/min. Erika can perform at 70% of her $\dot{V}O_2$max. About 63% of Erika's muscle fibers appear to be ST fibers.

Based on the information provided, do you expect Shanese or Erika to swim the 5-km open water event faster? (This event is completed in about one hour by the best in the world.) Explain your reasoning in detail, discussing all of the variables presented in the case study.

Activity 4.6

Causes of Fatigue

Do this activity after reading pages 145-151 of *Physiology of Sport and Exercise*.

Sensations of fatigue are markedly different when exercising to exhaustion in events lasting for less than a minute than during prolonged exhaustive muscular effort, such as running a marathon. We typically use the term *fatigue* to describe general sensations of tiredness accompanying decrements in muscular performance. But what causes this fatigue? Many questions about fatigue remain unanswered, but we will explore some possible causes in this activity.

Push-Up Test. The purpose of this activity is to assess your upper body endurance and then to examine the possible causes of fatigue. Perform push-ups to exhaustion. Keep track of both the number of push-ups done and the overall time it takes for you to reach exhaustion. If an injury or disability prevents you from doing push-ups, choose another activity that will help you to evaluate the same issues.

If possible, perform the push-ups on a mat; a thick towel will work, too. Females may perform the test with the knees bent and touching the ground. Be sure that your shoulders through your buttocks to your knees form a straight line (the tendency is to incorrectly bend at the buttocks). Males should perform the push-ups with the toes touching the ground. Do as many push-ups as you can until you can do no more. Just as you think you can do no more, tell yourself "You can do it" or "Keep going" and see how many more push-ups you can complete. Once you can do no more, stop the activity and answer the following questions (on separate paper).

1. a. How many push-ups did you do?
   b. How long (in overall time) did it take for you to reach exhaustion?
   c. What sensations caused you to cease doing push-ups?

2. Describe your pace throughout this activity. For example, did you start out fast and then slow down because of early fatigue? Did you maintain a steady, slow pace throughout the activity?

3. Based on the length of this activity and the pace you used, what was the likely role of phosphocreatine depletion and glycogen depletion during your push-up test?

4. Which of your muscle groups felt the most fatigue?

5. How might metabolic by-products have influenced your rate of fatigue? Discuss the possible role of lactic acid and hydrogen ion buildup.

6. Although studies in this area are speculative, describe the possible neural mechanisms that could contribute to fatigue.

7. a. How many push-ups did you complete after you gave yourself verbal encouragement?

   b. Were these push-ups done just as fast as the previous ones or at a slower pace?

   c. How does your answer help to prove or disprove the theory that the central nervous system might be related to neuromuscular fatigue?

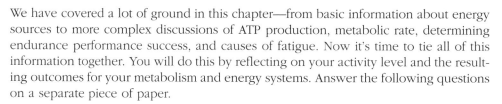

Putting It All Together: Metabolism and Basic Energy Systems

Activity 4.7

Do this activity after reading chapter 4 of *Physiology of Sport and Exercise.*

We have covered a lot of ground in this chapter—from basic information about energy sources to more complex discussions of ATP production, metabolic rate, determining endurance performance success, and causes of fatigue. Now it's time to tie all of this information together. You will do this by reflecting on your activity level and the resulting outcomes for your metabolism and energy systems. Answer the following questions on a separate piece of paper.

1. a. List all the foods you have eaten in the last 24 h—be sure to list the exact foods and how much of each food you have eaten.

   b. What percentage of these foods are carbohydrates? fats? proteins?

2. a. List all the foods you have eaten in the last 24 h—be sure to list the exact foods and how much of each food you have eaten.

   b. What about during short but intense bursts of muscle action?

   c. How about during prolonged, less intense exercise?

3. Explain the role of ATP in energy production. Describe the ATP-PCr system, the glycolytic system, and the oxidative system, including the chemical pathways through which ATP is produced in each system.

4. Think through the activity level of your lifestyle and jot a few notes in response to the following questions:

How often do you exercise?

How long are your exercise sessions?

What is your preferred exercise or sport?

Is this preferred exercise or sport anaerobic/aerobic? high-intensity/low-intensity? sprintlike/endurance-like?

Based on your activity level and the types of activities you do, which of your energy systems do you think is best developed? Back up your assertion with thoughtful reasonings based on what you have learned in this chapter.

5. Which types of activities—aerobic or anaerobic—are you least successful at? How might this relate to the energy system that you stress the most in your lifestyle?

6. Based on your activity level and whether you are aerobically or anaerobically trained, what generalizations can you make about your muscles' oxidative capacity? Be sure to comment on enzyme levels, fiber-type composition, and oxygen availability.

7. Imagine that you are participating in a major competition in your sport tomorrow, or that you are participating in a hard workout of your favorite type of exercise tomorrow. What would be the consequences of inadequate carbohydrate intake?

8. Think about your preferred form of exercise or sport.

   a. What would be the most *accurate* method of measuring energy usage during this physical activity? Why?

   b. What would be the most *practical* method of measuring energy usage during this physical activity? Why?

   c. If you were a coach of this exercise or sport and you had no laboratory equipment, how would you judge the energy usage of your athletes?

9. Imagine that we are using indirect calorimetry to measure your respiratory exchange ratio (RER). We find that you are releasing 6 CO_2 molecules and consuming 7 O_2 molecules.

   a. Given these figures, calculate your RER.

   b. What food mixture is being oxidized?

   c. What type of activity does this mean you are likely performing?

10. a. Based on your activity level and whether you are aerobically or anaerobically trained, at what percentage of your $\dot{V}O_2$max do you think your lactate threshold is?

   b. Imagine that we measured your lactate threshold and found it to be at 75% of your $\dot{V}O_2$max. What type of training would this suggest you had done? What types of events would you be capable of performing well in?

11. Would you expect your basal metabolic rate (BMR) to be average, below average, or above average? Explain your answer. Remember to take into account your amount of fat-free mass, your body's surface area, your age, your body temperature, your stress level, and activities that may affect the amount of thyroxine and epinephrine produced.

12. a. When you participate in your preferred form of exercise or sport, at what point do you begin to experience fatigue?

   b. Based on what you have learned in this chapter, and taking into account the energy systems taxed during your preferred form of physical activity, what are the possible causes of this fatigue?

Sample Test Questions for Chapter 4

Test yourself on your knowledge of this chapter by taking this self-test. Write the correct answers on a separate sheet of paper.

Multiple Choice

1. Energy for muscular activity and cellular operations is primarily derived from

   a. carbohydrate, fat, and sodium.
   b. carbohydrate, fat, and protein.
   c. carbohydrate, iron, and water.
   d. carbohydrate, protein, and water.

2. Which training strategy would most improve oxidative capacity of muscle?

   a. adding plyometrics to the training program
   b. eating more carbohydrates
   c. adding endurance training to the training program
   d. drinking fluids before training

3. A high lactate threshold indicates

   a. very good endurance capabilities.
   b. a high consumption of fat.
   c. a high rate of protein metabolism.
   d. greater muscular strength.

4. Which of the following items does *not* affect a person's basal metabolic rate?

   a. age
   b. body temperature
   c. calcium consumption
   d. fat-free mass

5. If maximal adaptation to $\dot{V}O_2$max is achieved within 8 to 12 wk of training, yet endurance performance continues to improve, which is most likely the cause for continued improvement?

   a. improved economy of effort
   b. adaptations of slow-twitch muscle fibers
   c. adaptations of fast-twitch muscle fibers
   d. increases in the lactate threshold

True-False

6. Because its rate of energy production is so fast, fat is the preferred source of energy to meet the energy demands of intense muscular contraction.

7. When phosphorylation occurs without the aid of oxygen, it is called aerobic metabolism.

8. A 100-m sprinter uses primarily the ATP-PCr system.

9. The glycolytic system has a tremendous energy-yielding capacity, so it is the primary method of energy production during endurance events.

10. The healthy body uses little protein during rest and exercise.

Fill in the Blank

11. By definition, one kilocalorie equals the amount of heat energy needed to raise _____ kg of water _____ °C at _____ °C.

12. Glycogen is stored in _____ or in _____ until needed.

13. Muscle's oxidative capacity depends on _____, _____, and _____.

14. The temporary elevation of oxygen consumption upon stopping exercise is termed _____.

15. The rate at which your body uses energy is your _____.

Short Answer

16. Explain the role of ATP.

17. Define the respiratory exchange ratio and explain what it helps to measure.

18. Explain the possible reasons for excess postexercise oxygen consumption (EPOC).

Essay

19. Explain how energy (ATP) is produced via glycolysis, and describe the role of the glycolytic system during exercise.

20. Compare and contrast the oxidation of carbohydrate and fat.

21. Describe protein metabolism.

22. Discuss the possible reasons for fatigue mentioned in the textbook.

Answers to Selected Chapter 4 Activities

4.1 Energy Sources and Their Uses

What Is Energy Used For?

1. Growth and repair, such as building muscle mass during training and repairing muscle damage after exercise or injury.

2. Active transport of many substances, such as glucose and calcium across cell membranes.

3. Myofibrils use some of the energy released in our bodies to cause the sliding of the actin and myosin filaments, resulting in muscle action and force generation.

How Is the Energy Supplied?

Energy source	Amount of energy provided		Accessibility as an energy source	Conversion process to form ATP
Fat	**9 kcal/g**	Very accessible		Triglyceride to glycerol and free fatty acids. Only FFAs are used to form ATP.
Carbohydrate	4.1 kcal/g	Most accessible		**Carbohydrate to glycogen stored in muscles and liver, converted to glucose as needed, and metabolized.**
Protein	4.1 kcal/g	**Least accessible**		Protein to glucose or free fatty acids through glucogenesis and lipogenesis, respectively.

4.3   ATP Production and Exercise

1. Stephen's body likely maintains his ATP levels via the ATP-PCr system.

2. This system produces ATP without the aid of oxygen, though oxygen can be present. Metabolism without the aid of oxygen is called anaerobic metabolism.

3. The ATP-PCr system uses the molecule phosphocreatine to rebuild ATP for maintaining a relatively constant supply of ATP. The creatine kinase enzyme acts on PCr to separate P_i from creatine. The energy released can then be used to couple P_i to an ADP molecule, forming ATP.

4. On its own, the ATP-PCr system can sustain your muscles' energy needs for only 3 to 15 s during an all-out sprint. During the first few s of all-out, intense muscular activity, ATP is maintained at a relatively constant level. But the PCr level declines steadily as it is used to replenish depleted ATP, and soon it is at too low a level to create more ATP. At exhaustion, both ATP and PCr levels are very low and unable to provide the energy for further muscle movement.

5. If Stephen switches to the 800 m, he will find that his training is initially inadequate for the event. Although the first few seconds of the race will feel good to him, Stephen will likely find that the length of the event taxes energy systems that he has not fully trained, that is, the glycolytic and oxidative systems. Before he has fully trained for the event, he will probably find that he is a strong starter and a weak finisher—that is, his untrained energy systems will fail him, and he will not produce enough ATP to complete the race with a strong finish.

6. During the early minute or two of the 5,000 m, the ATP-PCr and glycolytic systems are providing most of Sarah's energy. Early into the race, the PCr stores are depleted and cannot produce more ATP. Her glycolytic system becomes the primary energy producer for the next few min, but as her lactic acid levels rise, the resulting acidification of muscle fibers inhibits further glycogen breakdown and decreases the fibers' calcium-binding capacity, impeding muscle contraction. It is likely that at this point, Sarah's oxidative system becomes the primary ATP-producing system. This aerobic metabolism is the primary method of energy production during Sarah's event.

7. The oxidative system produces ATP with the aid of oxygen; therefore, this form of metabolism is called aerobic metabolism.

8. Fat, carbohydrate, and protein can all be metabolized aerobically, but it is likely carbohydrate and fat that contribute the most to Sarah's efforts. Although fat provides more kilocalories of energy per gram than carbohydrate, fat oxidation requires more oxygen than carbohydrate oxidation does. Therefore, carbohydrate is the preferred fuel during high-intensity exercise.

9. It is possible that Sarah's addition of longer runs into her training program enhanced the oxidative capacity of all of her muscle fibers, especially her FT fibers; improved the gas exchange in her lungs; and increased her oxidative enzyme activity. All of these physiological changes may have contributed to an improved oxidative capacity and therefore an improvement in Sarah's times.

4.4 Evaluating Different Measures of Energy Use

Name of method	Basic approach of method	Advantages	Disadvantages
Direct calorimetry	Place the athlete inside an airtight chamber with copper tubing in walls through which water is passed. Heat produced by body warms the water. Metabolism is calculated from resulting values.	Measures heat directly.	Expensive to construct and use. Slow to generate results. Cannot follow rapid changes in energy release.
Indirect calorimetry	Heat production is calculated from the respiratory exchange of CO_2 and O_2.	Less expensive and more practical than direct calorimetry.	Equipment is cumbersome and limits movement. Not accurate for nonsteady-state exercise; RER artificially elevated by hyperventilation; ignores protein metabolism.
Carbon 13	Isotopes are infused into an individual and their movements and distribution are traced. The rates at which they are cleared can be used to calculate CO_2 production and then caloric expenditure.	Less easily traced than radioactive isotopes would be.	Isotope turnover is relatively slow. Therefore, this method is not suited for measurement of acute exercise metabolism.
Doubly labeled water	Subject ingests water labeled with two isotopes. The ^2H diffuses throughout the body's water. The ^{18}O diffuses throughout both the water and the bicarbonate stores. The rates at which the two isotopes leave the body are used to calculate CO_2 production and then energy expenditure.	98% accuracy rate. Low risk. Well-suited for determining day-to-day energy expenditure.	Isotope turnover is slow. Measurement must be conducted over several weeks. Not well suited for measurements of acute exercise metabolism.
Excess postexercise oxygen consumption	Upon ending exercise, the amount of oxygen consumption in excess of what is needed at rest is measured.	Helps to explain anaerobic processes, which many other methods ignore.	Traditionally, it has been thought that the amount of anaerobic activity that had occurred could be estimated from the

(continued)

(continued)

Name of method	Basic approach of method	Advantages	Disadvantages
			EPOC. Recent studies indicate that the EPOC reflects much more than the physiological processes involved in anaerobic metabolism, so the true basis for the EPOC is unclear.
Lactate threshold	Blood samples are taken to measure arterialized blood lactate. The point at which blood lactate appears to increase above resting levels is termed the lactate threshold.	May represent a significant shift toward anaerobic glycolysis, which forms lactate.	Anaerobic metabolism in muscle might be occurring well before the lactate threshold. A clear breakpoint is not always apparent and arbitrary value might need to be used.

4.5   Determining Endurance Performance Success

Not all reasonings are given here, but in summary, Shanese will likely swim the 5-km open water event faster. Because swimming is a nonweight-bearing sport, their slight differences in body weight will not affect their performance as much as their $\dot{V}O_2$max will. Even though Erika has a higher $\dot{V}O_2$max, she can perform at only 1.70 L/min over a long distance, while Shanese can perform at 1.76 L/min. This, along with her higher lactate threshold and higher percentage of ST fibers, gives Shanese a slight edge over Erika.

4.6   Causes of Fatigue

1. Answers will vary.

2. Answers will vary.

3. If the beginning pace was too rapid, the available ATP and PCr quickly decreased, leading to fatigue within the first 30 s. Even if the pace was not too rapid, the intensity of this activity was likely very high for untrained participants, and it was likely completed in less than two min, meaning that PCr levels had been depleted early in this activity and were unable to produce more ATP. The glycolytic system had probably become the primary energy producer after the first few s of exercise. And though muscle glycogen probably declined rapidly during the last s of this activity, it is likely that the muscle glycogen stores were not totally depleted.

4. Although answers may vary, the fatigue most likely was felt in the triceps, chest, or shoulders.

5. Low muscle pH is the major limiter of performance and the primary cause of fatigue during maximal, all-out exercise lasting more than 20 to 30 s. Lactic acid is a by-product of anaerobic glycolysis. When not cleared, the lactic acid dissociates,

converting to lactate and causing an accumulation of hydrogen ions. This H^+ accumulation causes muscle acidification. Buffers minimize the disrupting influence of the H^+, but the H^+ still causes a change in pH, which adversely affects energy production and muscle contraction. Depending on the pH level, this lowering of the pH can inhibit the action of PFK, an important glycolytic enzyme; stop any further glycogen breakdown; or interfere with the coupling of the actin-myosin cross-bridges, decreasing the muscle's contractile force.

6. See the list on page 151 of your textbook for possible neural transmission mechanisms leading to fatigue.

7. Answers will vary, but if the verbal reinforcement did seem to help you to do more push-ups, and if these were slower than the push-ups completed earlier on, this is at least anecdotal evidence that the central nervous system is a possible site of fatigue.

Answers to Selected Chapter 4 Test Questions

Multiple Choice

1. b;   2. c;   3. a;   4. c;   5. d

True-False

6. False;   7. False;   8. True;   9. False;   10. True

Fill in the Blank

11. one, one, fifteen;   12. the liver, muscle;   13. oxidative enzyme levels, fiber-type composition, and oxygen availability;   14. excess postexercise oxygen consumption (EPOC);   15. metabolic rate

Short Answer and Essay

For questions 16 to 22, check your answers against the explanations given in the textbook.

Hormonal Regulation of Exercise

concepts

- The endocrine system includes all tissues or glands that secrete hormones. The endocrine system is responsible for fine-tuning the body's physiological responses to any disturbance of its equilibrium and has longer lasting and more general effects than does the nervous system.

- Hormones are generally secreted into the blood and then circulated through the body to exert an effect only on their target cells. They act by binding in a lock-and-key manner with specific receptors found only in the target tissues.

- Plasma glucose is increased by the combined actions of several hormones that promote glycogenolysis and gluconeogenesis, thus increasing the amount of glucose available for use as a fuel source.

- When carbohydrate reserves are low, fat metabolism is increased by the combined actions of several hormones that promote fat oxidation.

- The endocrine system plays a major role in monitoring fluid levels and correcting imbalances, and in regulating electrolyte imbalance. The two primary hormones involved in this regulation are aldosterone and antidiuretic hormone (ADH).

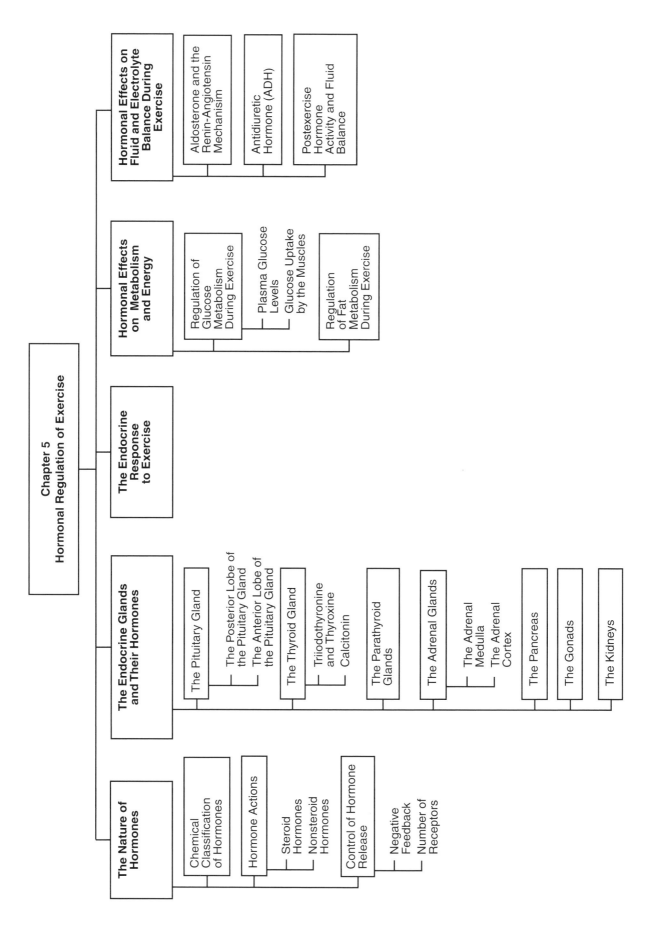

Chapter 5
Hormonal Regulation of Exercise

The Nature of Hormones
- Chemical Classification of Hormones
- Hormone Actions
  - Steroid Hormones
  - Nonsteroid Hormones
- Control of Hormone Release
  - Negative Feedback
  - Number of Receptors

The Endocrine Glands and Their Hormones
- The Pituitary Gland
  - The Posterior Lobe of the Pituitary Gland
  - The Anterior Lobe of the Pituitary Gland
- The Thyroid Gland
  - Triiodothyronine and Thyroxine
  - Calcitonin
- The Parathyroid Glands
- The Adrenal Glands
  - The Adrenal Medulla
  - The Adrenal Cortex
- The Pancreas
- The Gonads
- The Kidneys

The Endocrine Response to Exercise

Hormonal Effects on Metabolism and Energy
- Regulation of Glucose Metabolism During Exercise
  - Plasma Glucose Levels
  - Glucose Uptake by the Muscles
- Regulation of Fat Metabolism During Exercise

Hormonal Effects on Fluid and Electrolyte Balance During Exercise
- Aldosterone and the Renin-Angiotensin Mechanism
- Antidiuretic Hormone (ADH)
- Postexercise Hormone Activity and Fluid Balance

Activity 5.1

Endocrine Glands

Do this activity after reading pages 157-158 of *Physiology of Sport and Exercise*.

The endocrine system includes all tissues or glands that secrete hormones. Endocrine glands secrete their hormones directly into the blood, where the hormones are transported to specific target cells—cells that possess specific hormone receptors. Below is an illustration of the major endocrine organs. Fill in the blanks with the correct names of the endocrine organs.

For your studying benefit, do this activity without looking in your textbook. Once you have completed this activity, check your labels against the textbook to see how you did and what you need to study.

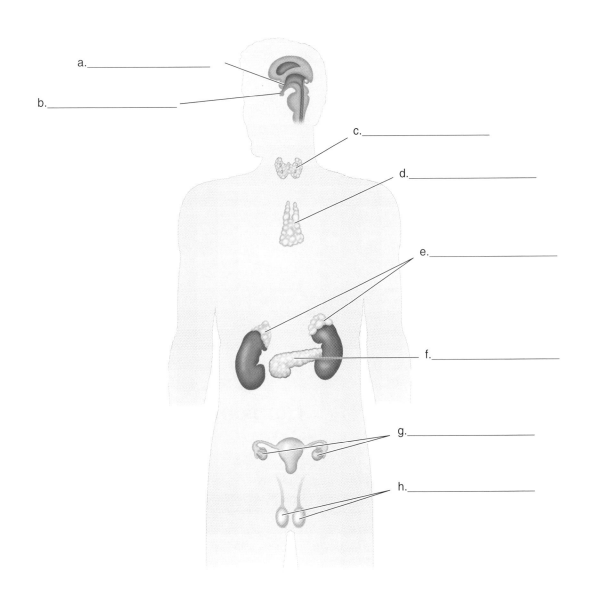

a._____

b._____

c._____

d._____

e._____

f._____

g._____

h._____

Activity 5.2

Steroid and Nonsteroid Hormones

Do this activity after reading pages 159-161 of *Physiology of Sport and Exercise*.

Hormones can be categorized as two basic types: steroid hormones and nonsteroid hormones. Each type of hormone has a distinct chemical makeup, is secreted from different endocrine glands, and controls the actions of cells in a particular way. To ensure that you know the characteristics of the two types of hormones, review pages 159-161 in *Physiology of Sport and Exercise* and complete the table below.

	Characteristics (Lipid soluble? Diffuse through cell membranes?)	Where secreted from	Mechanism of action
Steroid hormones			
Nonsteroid hormones			

Activity 5.3

Hormones and Their Functions

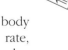

Do this activity after reading pages 163-171 of *Physiology of Sport and Exercise*.

The endocrine system is extremely complex. From promoting development of body tissues and sex characteristics to mobilizing glycogen and increasing the heart rate, hormones work to control the most basic of body functions as well as the complex interactions that occur during physical activity.

Without looking in your textbook, (1) try to match the hormones listed with the endocrine glands that release them. You may use the letters for the endocrine glands more than once. (2) Then match the hormone with its major functions. You will use the letters for each function only once. (3) Finally, even though you have not studied this yet, look over the list you have created and asterisk the hormones you think are most related to responses to exercise. This will get you thinking about the next topic in the textbook.

Note that the hormones and functions continue on to page 80.

Hormone

1. Calcitonin

   Gland: _____

   Function: _____

2. Epinephrine

   Gland: _____

   Function: _____

3. Estrogen

   Gland: _____

   Function: _____

4. Renin

   Gland: _____

   Function: _____

5. Growth hormone (GH)

   Gland: _____

   Function: _____

6. Oxytocin

   Gland: _____

   Function: _____

7. Thyroxine and triiodothyronine

   Gland: _____

   Function: _____

8. Adrenocorticotropin (ACTH)

   Gland: _____

   Function: _____

9. Glucocorticoids (cortisol)

   Gland: _____

   Function: _____

10. Insulin

    Gland: _____

    Function: _____

11. Testosterone

    Gland: _____

    Function: _____

12. Prolactin

    Gland: _____

    Function: _____

13. Parathyroid hormone (PTH, or parathormone)

    Gland: _____

    Function: _____

Endocrine gland

a. Anterior lobe of pituitary

b. Posterior lobe of pituitary

c. Thyroid

d. Parathyroid

e. Adrenal medulla

f. Adrenal cortex

g. Pancreas

h. Testes (gonads)

i. Ovaries (gonads)

j. Kidneys

Function

a. Assists in blood pressure control

b. Controls blood glucose levels by lowering glucose levels; increases use of glucose and synthesis of fat

c. Increases the rate of cellular metabolism; increases rate and contractility of the heart

d. Assists in controlling water excretion by the kidneys; elevates blood pressure by constricting blood vessels

e. Controls the amount of thyroxin and triiodothyronine produced and released by the thyroid gland

f. Promotes development and enlargement of all body tissues up through maturation; increases rate of protein synthesis; increases mobilization of fats and use of fat as an energy source; decreases rate of carbohydrate use

g. Assists in the development of female and male sex characteristics

h. Mobilizes glycogen; increases skeletal muscle blood flow; increases heart rate and contractility; increases oxygen consumption

i. Stimulates breast development and milk secretion

j. Depresses the secretion of both insulin and glucagon

k. Promotes secretion of estrogen and progesterone and causes the follicle to rupture, releasing the ovum; causes testes to secrete testosterone

l. Controls the secretion of hormones from the adrenal cortex

m. Controls calcium-ion concentration in the blood

n. Promotes development of male sex characteristics, including growth of testes, scrotum, and penis, growth of facial hair, and change in voice; promotes muscle growth

o. Constricts arterioles and venules, thereby elevating blood pressure

p. Stimulates contraction of uterine muscles; promotes milk secretion

q. Produces erythrocytes

r. Increases sodium retention and potassium excretion through the kidneys

(continued)

Hormone

14. Thyrotropin (thyroid-stimulating hormone, TSH)

    Gland: _____

    Function: _____

15. Norepinephrine

    Gland: _____

    Function: _____

16. Glucagon

    Gland: _____

    Function: _____

17. Follicle-stimulating hormone (FSH)

    Gland: _____

    Function: _____

18. Erythropoietin

    Gland: _____

    Function: _____

19. Antidiuretic hormone (ADH, or vasopressin)

    Gland: _____

    Function: _____

20. Somatostatin

    Gland: _____

    Function: _____

21. Mineralocorticoids (aldosterone)

    Gland: _____

    Function: _____

22. Androgens and estrogens

    Gland: _____

    Function: _____

23. Luteinizing hormone (LH)

    Gland: _____

    Function: _____

Function

s. Promotes development of female sex organs and characteristics; provides increased storage of fat; assists in regulating the menstrual cycle

t. Increases blood glucose; stimulates the breakdown of protein and fat

u. Controls metabolism of carbohydrates, fats, and proteins; promotes anti-inflammatory action

v. Initiates growth of follicles in the ovaries and promotes secretion of estrogen from the ovaries; promotes development of sperm in testes

w. Controls calcium-ion concentration in extracellular fluid through its influence on bone, intestine, and kidneys

---

Activity 5.4

Hormones and Exercise

Do this activity after reading pages 172-181 of *Physiology of Sport and Exercise.*

The endocrine system plays a key role in maintaining homeostasis amidst the internal chaos created during physical activity. After reading each scenario in this activity, write down the names of the hormones most significant to that situation. And although we don't ask you to do so here, be sure you know the mechanisms through which these hormones work.

1. Sue is a long-distance cyclist. Today she is cycling in °C (90 °F) heat and is sweating a lot. She is worried about dehydrating.

    _____

2. Marquez lifts weights three days a week. He has noticed an increase in the size of his muscles.

    _____

3. Dave is an endurance swimmer. He is particularly concerned with knowing that once his glucose stores run low, his body will successfully switch to fat oxidation.

    _____

    _____

4. John, an avid skier from the Midwest, is thrilled to be going to college in Colorado. Every weekend he can, he goes skiing. The first few weeks in Colorado, he noticed a marked difference in his aerobic capacity. Although he was surprised to notice this in simple activities like walking to class, he found an even greater difference when skiing. He figures this has something to do with the altitude shift from skiing the hills of Wisconsin to skiing the mountains of Colorado.

    _____

    _____

5. As a person who has type II diabetes, Tim is well aware that his body easily frees glucose from storage (glycogenolysis) but has difficulty transporting the glucose into the muscle fibers (gluconeogenesis). This causes elevated blood sugars. Tim has read that exercise enhances the binding of this hormone to receptors on the muscle fibers, improving the action of this hormone and lowering elevated blood sugars, so he has made physical activity a key part of his lifestyle.

    _____

    _____

6. Aleshia runs the 400 m. As with almost any athlete, it is crucial to Aleshia's performance that glucose be freed from its storage as glycogen in the liver and muscles so it can be used to produce energy.

    _____

    _____

7. Brenda runs the 800 m for her junior college track team. She notices that in the last few m of a race, when she's giving all she has to beat her competitors, her heart rate increases greatly. She has also read that her cellular metabolism increases in those last few s when her body needs extra energy.

    _____

Activity 5.5

Hormonal Dysfunction

Do this activity after reading chapter 5 of *Physiology of Sport and Exercise.*

When our endocrine system maintains homeostasis, we hardly even notice that it is working. But when an imbalance occurs in our endocrine system, the symptoms are difficult to miss, and we realize how important this physiological system is to our everyday life.

For extra understanding on this subject, research an endocrine disorder—either one listed here or another one that you find interesting.

- Diabetes
- Hypoglycemia
- Hyperthyroidism
- Hyperparathyroidism
- Cushings syndrome

Write a report that summarizes the definition, causes, diagnosis, symptoms, and treatment of the disorder as well as any implications this disorder has for exercise.

Be sure to document your sources. You might want to check out these Web sites for some preliminary information:

http://www.endocrineweb.com   http://www.endo-society.org

Activity 5.6

Putting It All Together: Hormonal Regulation of Exercise

Do this activity before reading chapter 5 of *Physiology of Sport and Exercise.*

In this chapter, you have learned how the endocrine system, through its release of hormones, constantly monitors your body's internal milieu, noting the changes that occur and responding quickly to ensure that homeostasis is not drastically disrupted. In this activity, you will actually put your endocrine system to the test and then reflect on all of the actions it took to maintain this internal balance.

Choose a physical activity of your choice—whether it be a sport like basketball or soccer or an exercise like aerobics, walking, or bicycling. Do this activity at as high an intensity as you can for 30 min. Then answer the following questions on a separate piece of paper.

If you have an injury or disability that prevents you from exercising strenuously, simply answer the questions based on an imagined exercise bout.

1. Describe which hormones were likely released during your exercise session. For each hormone, explain which endocrine gland released it, what the likely cause of release was, and what the likely effects of the hormone release were.

2. How did the hormones activate changes in the cells? (Comment on target cells, direct gene activation, and the second messenger mechanism.)

3. How did your endocrine system regulate your metabolism and energy systems during this exercise bout? Be sure to comment on plasma glucose levels, glucose uptake by your muscles, and regulation of fat metabolism; and be sure to consider that your exercise session was only 30 min in length.

4. How did your endocrine system regulate your fluid and electrolyte balance during this exercise bout? Be sure to comment on aldosterone and the renin-angiotensin mechanism as well as ADH.

5. a. Now that you have finished your exercise bout, what hormonal adaptations caused by the exercise are still in place?

   b. If you were involved in heavy training—say two hours of high-intensity exercise five days a week for a year—what adaptations in plasma volume could you expect to experience?

Sample Test Questions for Chapter 5

Test yourself on your knowledge of this chapter by taking this self-test. Write the correct answers on a separate sheet of paper.

Multiple Choice

1. Which of the following sentences is an example of the negative feedback system?

   a. A cell responds to the prolonged presence of large amounts of insulin by increasing its number of available insulin receptors.
   b. The pituitary gland acts as the relay between the central nervous system and the peripheral endocrine glands.
   c. When plasma glucose concentration returns to normal, insulin release is inhibited until the plasma glucose level rises again.
   d. Muscular activity promotes sweating.

2. When an increased amount of a specific hormone causes a decrease in the number of cell receptors available to it, the cell

   a. overresponds to that hormone.
   b. cannot respond to that hormone.
   c. becomes more sensitive to that hormone.
   d. becomes less sensitive to that hormone.

3. The pituitary gland is largely controlled by

   a. the thyroid.   c. the posterior lobe.
   b. the hypothalamus.   d. the pancreas.

4. Which two hormones work together to increase the rate and force of heart contraction, increase glycogenolysis, redistribute blood to the skeletal muscles, increase blood pressure, and increase respiration?

   a. mineralcorticoids and glucocorticoids   c. estrogen and progesterone
   b. ADH and PTH   d. epinephrine and norepinephrine

5. During exercise,

   a. glucagon, epinephrine, norepinephrine, and cortisol secretion increase.
   b. glucagon secretion decreases but epinephrine, norepinephrine, and cortisol secretion increase.
   c. glucagon secretion increases but epinephrine, norepinephrine, and cortisol secretion decrease.
   d. epinephrine and norepinephrine secretion increase, but glucagon and cortisol secretion decrease.

True-False

6. Steroid hormones are lipid soluble and have difficulty crossing cell membranes.

7. Each hormone is highly specific for a single type of receptor and binds only with its specific receptors, thus affecting only tissues that contain those specific receptors.

8. Up-regulation refers to a cell responding to the prolonged presence of large amounts of a hormone by increasing its number of available receptors.

9. An increased concentration of electrolytes in blood plasma caused by sweating is an example of hemodilution.

Fill in the Blank

10. _____ is a powerful anabolic agent that promotes muscle growth and hypertrophy by facilitating amino acid transport into the cells.

11. _____ is a hormone released from the kidneys and is very important in our adaptation to training and altitude.

12. _____ accelerates lypolysis, releasing free fatty acids into the blood so they can be taken up by the cells and used for energy production.

Short Answer

13. List the major endocrine organs.

14. Explain what a target cell is.

15. In type II diabetes, high blood sugars represent insulin resistance—that is, the pancreas produces enough insulin, but the target cells are not sensitive enough to the hormone. From what you know from reading this chapter, how could exercise benefit a person with type II diabetes?

Essay

16. Compare and contrast direct gene activation versus the formation of a second messenger.

17. What are prostaglandins? Where do they exert their effects? What are some of their functions?

18. Describe how the renin-angiotensin mechanism affects blood pressure during exercise.

19. Explain why most athletes involved in heavy training have an expanded plasma volume, which dilutes various blood constituents.

20. Describe how ADH promotes water conservation during exercise.

Answers to Selected Chapter 5 Activities

5.1   Endocrine Glands

a. Hypothalamus;   b. Pituitary gland;   c. Thyroid and parathyroid glands;   d. Thymus gland;   e. Adrenal glands;   f. Pancreas;   g. Ovaries;   h. Testes

5.2 Steroid and Nonsteroid Hormones

	Characteristics (Lipid soluble? Diffuse through cell membranes?)	Where secreted from	Mechanism of action
Steroid hormones	Chemical structure similar to cholesterol. Lipid soluble. Diffuse easily through cell membranes.	Adrenal cortex, ovaries, testes, placenta	**Direct gene activavation:** The hormone passes into the cell membrane and binds to its specific receptors inside the cell. The hormone-receptor complex then enters the nucleus and activates the cell's DNA, which forms mRNA. The mRNA then enters the cytoplasm where it promotes protein synthesis.
Nonsteroid hormones	Not lipid soluble. Cannot easily cross cell membranes. Subdivided into two groups: protein or peptide hormones and amino acid-derivative hormones	Amino acid hormones are secreted by the thyroid and the adrenal medulla.	**Second messenger:** The nonsteroid hormone binds to its receptor outside the cell, on the cell membrane, and triggers a series of enzymatic reactions that lead to the formation of an intracellular second messenger. The second messenger can then produce specific physiological responses.

5.3 Hormones and Their Functions

The asterisked items are the hormones researchers think are most related to exercise.

1. Calcitonin; *Gland:* c, Thyroid; *Function:* m, Controls calcium-ion concentration in the blood

*2. Epinephrine; *Gland:* e, Adrenal medulla; *Function:* h, Mobilizes glycogen; increases skeletal muscle blood flow; increases heart rate and contractility; increases oxygen consumption

3. Estrogen; *Gland:* i, Ovaries; *Function:* s, Promotes development of female sex organs and characteristics; provides increased storage of fat; assists in regulating the menstrual cycle

4. Renin; *Gland:* j, Kidneys; *Function:* a, Assists in blood pressure control

*5. Growth hormone (GH); *Gland:* a, Anterior lobe of pituitary; *Function:* f, Promotes development and enlargement of all body tissues up through maturation; increases rate of protein synthesis; increases mobilization of fats and use of fat as an energy source; decreases rate of carbohydrate use

6. Oxytocin; *Gland:* b, Posterior lobe of pituitary; *Function:* p, Stimulates contraction of uterine muscles; promotes milk secretion

*7. Thyroxine and triiodothyronine; *Gland:* c, Thyroid; *Function:* c, Increases the rate of cellular metabolism; increases rate and contractility of the heart

8. Adrenocorticotropin (ACTH); *Gland:* a, Anterior lobe of pituitary; *Function:* l, Controls the secretion of hormones from the adrenal cortex

*9. Glucocorticoids (cortisol); *Gland:* f, Adrenal cortex; *Function:* u, Controls metabolism of carbohydrates, fats, and proteins; promotes anti-inflammatory action

*10. Insulin; *Gland:* g, Pancreas; *Function:* b, Controls blood glucose levels by lowering glucose levels; increases use of glucose and synthesis of fat

*11. Testosterone; *Gland:* h, Testes; *Function:* n, Promotes development of male sex characteristics, including growth of testes, scrotum, and penis, growth of facial hair, and change in voice; promotes muscle growth

12. Prolactin; *Gland:* a, Anterior lobe of pituitary; *Function:* i, Stimulates breast development and milk secretion

*13. Parathyroid hormone (PTH or parathormone); *Gland:* d, Parathyroid; *Function:* w, Controls calcium-ion concentration in extracellular fluid through its influence on bone, intestine, and kidneys

14. Thyrotropin (thyroid-stimulating hormone, TSH); *Gland:* a, Anterior lobe of pituitary; *Function:* e, Controls the amount of thyroxin and triiodothyronine produced and released by the thyroid gland

*15. Norepinephrine; *Gland:* e, Adrenal medulla; *Function:* o, Constricts arterioles and venules, thereby elevating blood pressure

*16. Glucagon; *Gland:* g, Pancreas; *Function:* t, Increases blood glucose; stimulates the breakdown of protein and fat

17. Follicle-stimulating hormone (FSH); *Gland:* a, Anterior lobe of pituitary; *Function:* v, Initiates growth of follicles in the ovaries and promotes secretion of estrogen from the ovaries; promotes development of sperm in testes

*18. Erythropoietin; *Gland:* j, Kidneys; *Function:* q, Produces erythrocytes

*19. Antidiuretic hormone (ADH, or vasopressin); *Gland:* b, Posterior lobe of pituitary; *Function:* d, Assists in controlling water excretion by the kidneys; elevates blood pressure by constricting blood vessels

20. Somatostatin; *Gland:* g, Pancreas; *Function:* j, Depresses the secretion of both insulin and glucagon

*21. Mineralocorticoids (aldosterone); *Gland:* f, Adrenal cortex; *Function:* r, Increases sodium retention and potassium excretion through the kidneys

22. Androgens and estrogens; *Gland:* f, Adrenal cortex; *Function:* g, Assists in the development of female and male sex characteristics

23. Luteinizing hormone (LH); *Gland:* a, Anterior lobe of pituitary; *Function:* k, Promotes secretion of estrogen and progesterone and causes the follicle to rupture, releasing the ovum; causes testes to secrete testosterone

5.4   Hormones and Exercise

1. ADH, aldosterone;   2. GH, testosterone;   3. cortisol, epinephrine, norepinephrine, growth hormone;   4. erythropoietin;   5. insulin;   6. glucagon, epinephrine, norepinephrine, cortisol;   7. triiodothyronine, thyroxine

Answers to Selected Chapter 5 Test Questions

Multiple Choice

1. c;   2. d;   3. b;   4. d;   5. a

True-False

6. False;   7. True;   8. True;   9. False

Fill in the Blank

10. Growth hormone;   11. Erythropoietin;   12. Cortisol

Short Answer and Essay

For questions 13 to 20, check your answers against the explanations given in the textbook.

Metabolic Adaptations to Training

concepts

- Aerobic training results in enlargement of ST fibers, an increase in the number of capillaries supplying each muscle fiber, increased myoglobin content, an increase in the number and size of mitochondria, and increased activity of enzymes, all of which lead to enhanced functioning of the oxidative system and improved endurance.

- With aerobic training, the body becomes much more efficient at using fat as an energy source for exercise. This allows muscle and liver glycogen to be used at a slower rate.

- The aerobic system is best trained by expending about 5,000 to 6,000 kcal/wk (high volume) and by including high-intensity bouts in the training, whether the intensity is gained through interval or continuous training.

- Anaerobic training results in strength gains, improved efficiency of movement through optimized fiber recruitment, increased muscle aerobic capacity, and improved muscle buffering capacity.

- The easiest method for monitoring training adaptations is comparing blood lactate values taken after a fixed-pace activity at various times during a training period.

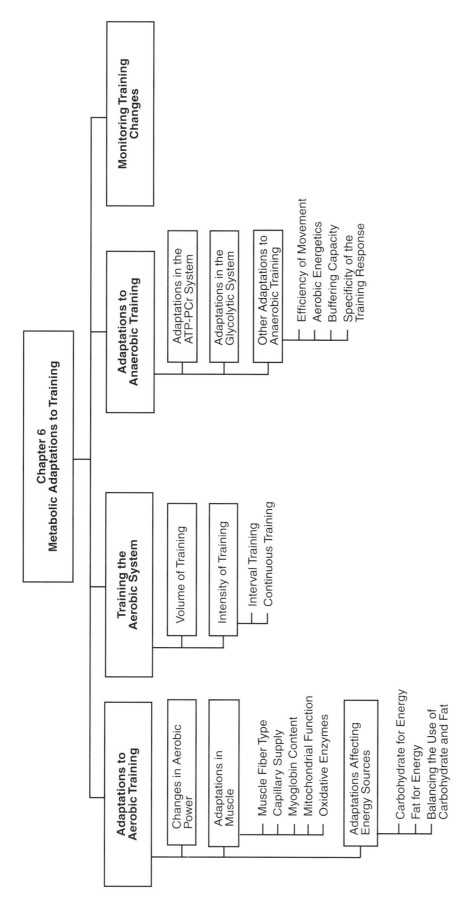

Chapter 6
Metabolic Adaptations to Training

Adaptations to Aerobic Training

Changes in Aerobic Power

Adaptations in Muscle
- Muscle Fiber Type
- Capillary Supply
- Myoglobin Content
- Mitochondrial Function
- Oxidative Enzymes

Adaptations Affecting Energy Sources
- Carbohydrate for Energy
- Fat for Energy
- Balancing the Use of Carbohydrate and Fat

Training the Aerobic System

Volume of Training

Intensity of Training
- Interval Training
- Continuous Training

Adaptations to Anaerobic Training

Adaptations in the ATP-PCr System

Adaptations in the Glycolytic System

Other Adaptations to Anaerobic Training
- Efficiency of Movement
- Aerobic Energetics
- Buffering Capacity
- Specificity of the Training Response

Monitoring Training Changes

Activity 6.1

Adaptations to Aerobic Training

Do this activity after reading pages 186-193 of *Physiology of Sport and Exercise.*

Aerobic training results not only in improved aerobic endurance and $\dot{V}O_2$max, but also in changed muscle physiology and improved energy production. Imagine that you are embarking on an aerobic training program—perhaps with the goal of running a 5K, swimming the 800 m, or going on a long-distance cycling tour. Fill out the table below, based on information found in your textbook, to see what types of changes your body will make as it adapts to your aerobic training regimen. The last row is completed for you as an example.

Parameter	Increase or decrease? (Use ↑ or ↓)	Further explanation for studying purposes
Ability to perform prolonged submaximal exercise		
Aerobic capacity ($\dot{V}O_2$max)		
ST fiber size		
Percentage of ST and FT fibers		
Number of capillaries supplying muscle fibers		

(continued)

(continued)

Parameter	Increase or decrease? (Use ↑ or ↓)	Further explanation for studying purposes
Muscle myoglobin content		
Number, size, and efficiency of mitochondria		
Oxidative enzyme activity		
Muscle storage of glycogen		
Muscle storage of triglyceride		
Muscle's ability to oxidize free fatty acids (FFA)		
Rate at which FFA are released from storage during prolonged exercise	↑	Elevated blood FFA levels can spare muscle glycogen, postponing exhaustion.

Activity 6.2

Evaluating an Aerobic Training Program

Do this activity after reading pages 193-195 of *Physiology of Sport and Exercise.*

The aerobic system is optimally trained through adjustments in volume and intensity. Professionals need to be able to analyze training programs and make adjustments to help athletes reach their goals. Read the following scenario and then answer the questions that follow it on a separate piece of paper.

Kari was thrilled to be preparing for RAGBRAI—The Register's Annual Great Bicycle Ride Across Iowa—where she would cycle 50 to 100 mi a day for seven days, biking with 10,000 other bicyclists across the varying, and rarely flat, terrain of Iowa. She knew the state's towns vied to be on the changing route each year and that many other would-be cyclists had not met the cutoff date for entry. Now she was training hard to be sure she could complete the 470-mi or so trek.

Kari only had two months to train for this event. She trained at the end of the day, after her classes were over, biking 15 to 20 mi continuously at a slow, steady pace. She biked four times a wk and burned about 900 kcal/day of training.

1. What was the volume of Kari's training?

2. What training method did Kari use to add intensity to her program?

3. Based on what you know about Kari's training program, how will she hold up during the long RAGBRAI rides?

4. How would you adjust Kari's training program to improve her aerobic capabilities for this event?

Activity 6.3

Adaptations to Anaerobic Training

Do this activity after reading pages 196-199 of *Physiology of Sport and Exercise.*

Anaerobic training results in adaptations in the phosphagen (ATP-PCr) and glycolytic energy systems as well as changes in fiber recruitment, aerobic capacity, and muscle buffering capacity. Imagine that you are embarking on an anaerobic training program—perhaps with the goal of improving your time in the 200-m sprint or the 100-m backstroke. Fill out the table on the next page, based on information found in your textbook, to see what types of changes your body will make as it adapts to your anaerobic training regimen. One row is completed for you as an example.

Activity 6.3 **Evaluating an Aerobic Training Program**

Parameter	Increase or decrease? (Use ↑ or ↓)	Further explanation for studying purposes
ATP-PCr enzyme activity		
Glycolytic enzyme activity	↑	Both PFK and phosphorylase are essential to the anaerobic yield of ATP, so anaerobic training might enhance glycolytic capacity and allow the muscle to develop greater tension for a longer period of time. However, not all studies confirm this finding.
Efficiency of movement		
Muscle's aerobic capacity		
Muscle's buffering capacity		

Analyzing Methods of Monitoring Training Changes

Do this activity after reading pages 199-201 of *Physiology of Sport and Exercise.*

Various methods of monitoring training adaptations have been tried, but in recent years, sports physiologists have proposed that the blood lactate level during training might provide the best gauge of aerobic fitness, including muscular and cardiorespiratory adaptations.

Find a scholarly journal article that describes a study done using either lactate threshold tests or lactate measurement during steady-state exercise. These journals are the most likely sources of articles on this subject:

International Journal of Sports Medicine

Medicine and Science in Sports and Exercise

Research Quarterly for Exercise and Sport

After reading the journal article, summarize these points on a separate sheet of paper:

- The purpose of the study
- The method of measuring blood lactate
- The results of the study
- Your analysis of how feasible this method of monitoring training changes is for coaches

For an extra challenge: How would you go about monitoring training changes in an athlete you were coaching if you did not have access to the equipment needed to measure $\dot{V}O_2$max and blood lactate?

Putting It All Together: Metabolic Adaptations to Training

Do this activity after reading chapter 6 of *Physiology of Sport and Exercise.*

Now that you have completed studying this chapter on metabolic adaptations, let's see if you can apply what you have learned to a training situation. Think of yourself as an exercise physiologist who wants to help this athlete improve his performance. Read the case study below and then answer the questions that follow it on a separate piece of paper.

Luke runs the 100 m on his high school track team. In general, his training program looks like this:

Monday: Runs 3 mi before school. After school, runs 10 intervals of 400 m with 10-s breaks in between.

Wednesday: Runs 3 to 5 mi before school. After school, runs 10 intervals of 400 m with 10-s breaks in between. Ends with a practice of the 100 m.

Friday: Runs 3 mi before school.

Although Luke feels as if he is in better shape now than he was at the beginning of the season, his time in the 100 has improved only by a fraction of a second—from 11.60 s to 11.45 s. He knows that with proper training, he should have improved much more.

1. What are some possible reasons why Luke's time has not improved much over the course of the season?

2. Based on Luke's training program, what physiological changes do you think have taken place over the course of the season?

3. In what ways have Luke's lactate threshold and $\dot{V}O_2$max probably changed because of his training program?

4. Based on the volume and intensity of Luke's training program, what type of event would he be more suited for

5. How would you have changed Luke's training program to better match his event?

6. If Luke had changed his training to better match his event, what physiological changes would you have expected his body to make?

Sample Test Questions for Chapter 6

Test yourself on your knowledge of this chapter by taking this self-test. Write the correct answers on a separate sheet of paper.

Multiple Choice

1. Aerobic training does *not* cause

   a. ST fibers to enlarge.
   b. increased myoglobin content.
   c. increased activity of oxidative enzymes.
   d. decreased number of capillaries supplying each muscle fiber.

2. $\dot{Q}O_2$ is best defined as

   a. the quotient of oxygen and carbon dioxide used in the muscle.
   b. the muscle's maximal oxidative or respiratory capacity.
   c. one's maximal aerobic capacity.
   d. the measure of an athlete's volume of training.

3. An interval training program of 20 repetitions of 400-m runs with rest periods of 10- to 15-s is designed to train the

   a. ATP-PCr energy system.
   b. glycolytic energy system.
   c. oxidative energy system.

4. Anaerobic training does *not* cause

   a. strength gains.
   b. improved efficiency of movement through optimized fiber recruitment.
   c. decreased muscle aerobic capacity.
   d. improved muscle buffering capacity.

True-False

5. Increasing the distance or time per training session will continue to improve aerobic power indefinitely.

6. Aerobic training does not change the percentage of ST and FT fibers.

7. Aerobic interval training produces greater muscular adaptations than continuous training.

8. The major value of training bouts lasting only 5 to 6 s is the improvement in the energy release from ATP and PCr.

9. Performance gains from repeated training bouts of 6 to 30 s result from improvements in strength rather than improvements in the anaerobic yield of ATP.

Fill in the Blank

10. The aerobic system is best trained by adjusting the _____ and _____ of training.

11. As one becomes better trained, blood lactate concentration is _____ [higher, lower] for the same rate of work.

Short Answer

12. Explain why repeated bouts of 30-s or more sprints increase the muscles' aerobic capacity.

13. Explain why lactate threshold can be used to gauge exercise intensity.

Essay

14. Explain the results of training-induced increases in the activities of oxidative enzymes. How does this relate to increases in $\dot{V}O_2$max?

15. How does the aerobically trained body use energy differently from one that is not aerobically trained?

16. Describe the changes in muscle buffering capacity resulting from aerobic and anaerobic training. How might these changes improve performance?

Answers to Selected Chapter 6 Activities

6.1 Adaptations to Aerobic Training

Parameter	Increase or decrease? (Use ↑ or ↓)	Further explanation for studying purposes
Ability to perform prolonged submaximal exercise	↑	Substantial interindividual variation. There is an upper limit of aerobic power for each individual.
Aerobic capacity ($\dot{V}O_2max$)	↑	Substantial interindividual variation. There is an upper limit of aerobic power for each individual.
ST fiber size	↑	Increase varies across individuals. Muscle fiber sizes in endurance athletes seem to have little relationship to the athlete's aerobic capacity or performance.
Percentage of ST and FT fibers	Stays the same	Some subtle changes in FT fibers have been reported; many years of aerobic training may cause FT_b fibers to take on characteristics of FT_a fibers.
Number of capillaries supplying muscle fibers	↑	Having more capillaries allows greater exchange of gases, heat, wastes, and nutrients between the blood and the working muscle fibers.
Muscle myoglobin content	↑	Myoglobin stores oxygen and releases it to the mitochondria when oxygen becomes limited during muscle action.
Number, size, and efficiency of mitochondria	↑	This increase results in an improved ability to use oxygen and to produce ATP via oxidation.
Oxidative enzyme activity	↑	The mitochondrial oxidative enzymes are special proteins that speed up the breakdown of nutrients to form ATP, so an increase in enzyme activity results in improved oxidative breakdown of fuels and production of ATP. Increased mitochondrial activity does not necessarily improve $\dot{V}O_2max$; however, it does seem to play a significant role in the ability to sustain a higher exercise intensity.
Muscle storage of glycogen	↑	More glycogen storage allows the athlete to better tolerate subsequent training demands because more fuel is available for use.
Muscle storage of triglyceride	↑	Fat (lipid) is stored as triglyceride in muscle. The vacuoles that contain triglyceride are distributed throughout the muscle fiber but are close to the mitochondria, making access to them for use as fuel during exercise easy.
Muscle's ability to oxidize free fatty acids (FFA)	↑	This leads to increased use of fat as an energy source, sparing glycogen.
Rate at which FFA are released from storage during prolonged exercise	↑	Elevated blood FFA levels can spare muscle glycogen, postponing exhaustion.

6.2   Evaluating an Aerobic Training Program

1. The volume of Kari's training was 15 to 20 mi, four times a wk, resulting in an expenditure for her of about 900 kcal/day.

2. There is no evidence that Kari has added intensity to her training program. The case study mentions her training only at a "slow, steady pace."

3. Because Kari did not include high-intensity workouts in her training regimen, and because she burned only about 3,600 kcal/wk in training (900 kcal/day multiplied by 4 days), she may have trouble enduring the long rides for the seven straight days of RAGBRAI. The lack of intensity in her workouts may also hinder her performance in the more hilly sections of the ride.

4. Methods may vary, but should include an increase in volume—up to 5,000 to 6,000 kcal/wk—and some type of intensity training, whether that be interval or continuous high-intensity training.

6.3   Adaptations to Anaerobic Training

Parameter	Increase or decrease? (Use ↑ or ↓)	Further explanation for studying purposes
ATP-PCr enzyme activity	Conflicting results	Maximal efforts lasting less than 6 s place the greatest demands on the ATP-PCr system. The major value of anaerobic training bouts that last only 5 to 6 s seems to be the development of muscular strength rather than an improvement in the energy release from ATP and PCr.
Glycolytic enzyme activity	↑	Both PFK and phosphorylase are essential to the anaerobic yield of ATP, so anaerobic training might enhance glycolytic capacity and allow the muscle to develop greater tension for a longer period of time. However, not all studies confirm this finding.
Efficiency of movement	↑	Anaerobic training (1) improves skill and coordination for performing at higher intensities, (2) optimizes fiber recruitment to allow more efficient movement, and (3) economizes the muscles' use of their energy supply.
Muscle's aerobic capacity	↑	Part of the energy needed for sprints of 30 seconds or more is derived from oxidative metabolism. The improvement of the muscles' oxidative potential assists the anaerobic energy system's efforts to meet muscle energy needs during anaerobic effort.
Muscle buffering capacity	↑	Buffers (bicarbonate and muscle phosphates) combine with hydrogen to reduce the fiber's acidity, thus delaying the onset of fatigue. With enhanced buffering capacity, muscles can generate energy for longer periods before a critically high concentration of H^+ inhibits the contractile process.

6.5   Putting It All Together: Metabolic Adaptations to Training

1. The 100-m sprint is primarily an anaerobic event, but Luke's training program has had an aerobic focus. All of Luke's oxidative capacities are improving through his training, but he is doing little to improve his ATP-PCr and glycolytic energy systems.

2. Despite Luke's desires to improve his anaerobic capabilities, it is really his aerobic or oxidative systems that have been improved through his training. He has likely increased his ability to perform prolonged submaximal exercise and increased his maximal aerobic capacity ($\dot{V}O_2$max), thereby improving his aerobic power. He might have experienced these additional adaptations: enlargement of ST fibers, increased capillary supply to muscle fibers, increased myoglobin content, and improved mitochondrial function, both in terms of an increased number and size of mitochondria and enhanced activity of oxidative enzymes. In addition, his muscles probably store more glycogen and triglyceride now than at the beginning of his training program. Luke's body has probably become more efficient at using fat as an energy source, allowing muscle and liver glycogen to be used at a slower rate. It is likely that Luke's $\dot{Q}O_2$—his muscles' respiratory capacity—has also improved.

3. Because Luke's training program has included long-distance runs as well as 400-m interval training, his $\dot{V}O_2$max has likely improved, and his lactate threshold is probably at a higher percentage of $\dot{V}O_2$max than it was at the outset of the season.

4. Luke's training program, which contains a lot of aerobic training, lends itself more to middle-distance events, between 800 m and 3,000 m, as well as to long-distance events.

5. Answers will vary but should include a reduction in long-distance runs, the addition of shorter intervals (e.g., 20 sets of 100-m sprints with 5-s rest periods), and perhaps the addition of resistance and plyometrics training.

6. With a training program that better matched his training goals, it is likely that Luke's performance would have improved due to increases in muscle strength from both the resistance training and the sprint training. His body might have experienced an increase in ATP-PCr and glycolytic enzyme activity. In addition, Luke might have experienced improved efficiency of movement, thereby reducing energy expenditure; increased muscle aerobic capacity; and improved muscle buffering capacity, allowing his muscles and blood to accumulate more lactate before a critically high concentration of H^+ inhibited the contractile process.

Answers to Selected Chapter 6 Test Questions

Multiple Choice

1. d;   2. b;   3. c;   4. c

True-False

5. False;   6. True;   7. False;   8. False;   9. True

Fill in the Blank

10. volume, intensity;   11. lower

Short Answer and Essay

For questions 12 to 16, check your answers against the explanations given in the textbook.

Cardiovascular Control During Exercise

concepts

- The cardiovascular system is a circulatory system made up of the heart, the blood vessels, and the blood.

- Cardiac tissue is capable of autoconduction and has its own conduction system. It initiates its own pulse without neural control. Heart rate and contraction strength can be altered by the autonomic nervous system or the endocrine system.

- Arteries always carry blood away from the heart to the arterioles and then the capillaries. Blood returns to the heart by leaving the capillaries and flowing to the venules and then the veins.

- Blood and lymph are the substances that transport materials to and from body tissues. Oxygen is transported primarily by binding to the hemoglobin in red blood cells.

- During exercise, heart rate increases; stroke volume increases; cardiac output increases; blood is redirected away from areas where it is not essential and directed to those areas that are active during exercise; and systolic blood pressure increases.

- The major changes that occur in the blood during exercise include an increase in a-$\bar{v}O_2$ diff; a decrease in plasma volume; hemoconcentration as plasma fluid is lost; and a decrease in blood pH, as the blood becomes more acidic due to increased blood lactate accumulation.

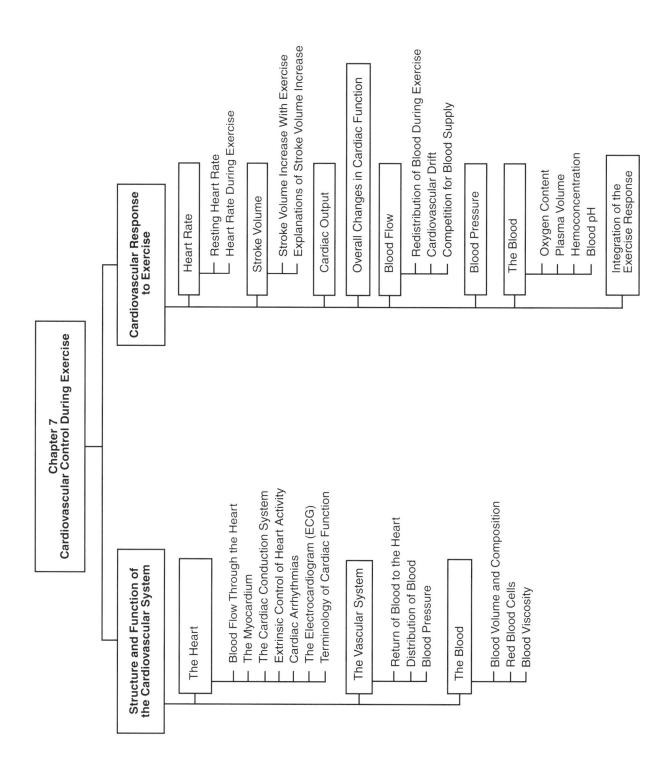

Chapter 7
Cardiovascular Control During Exercise

Structure and Function of the Cardiovascular System

The Heart
— Blood Flow Through the Heart
— The Myocardium
— The Cardiac Conduction System
— Extrinsic Control of Heart Activity
— Cardiac Arrhythmias
— The Electrocardiogram (ECG)
— Terminology of Cardiac Function

The Vascular System
— Return of Blood to the Heart
— Distribution of Blood
— Blood Pressure

The Blood
— Blood Volume and Composition
— Red Blood Cells
— Blood Viscosity

Cardiovascular Response to Exercise

Heart Rate
— Resting Heart Rate
— Heart Rate During Exercise

Stroke Volume
— Stroke Volume Increase With Exercise
— Explanations of Stroke Volume Increase

Cardiac Output

Overall Changes in Cardiac Function

Blood Flow
— Redistribution of Blood During Exercise
— Cardiovascular Drift
— Competition for Blood Supply

Blood Pressure

The Blood
— Oxygen Content
— Plasma Volume
— Hemoconcentration
— Blood pH

Integration of the Exercise Response

The Anatomy of the Heart and the Heart's Conduction System

Activity 7.1

Do this activity after reading pages 208-212 of *Physiology of Sport and Exercise.*

The heart is the primary pump that circulates blood through the entire vascular system. Below is a drawing of the anatomy of the heart. First label each part of the heart, and then on the same drawing, draw the pathway of blood flow through the heart. Answer the questions that follow on separate paper.

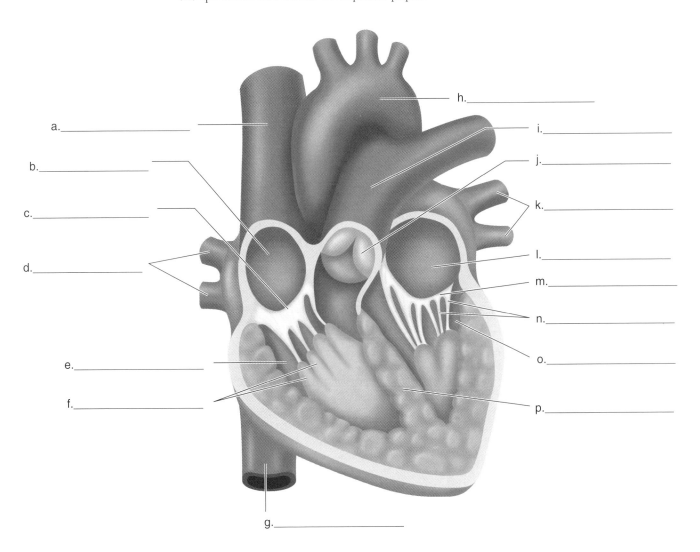

a._____

b._____

c._____

d._____

e._____

f._____

g._____

h._____

i._____

j._____

k._____

l._____

m._____

n._____

o._____

p._____

1. Why is the right side of the heart called the pulmonary side?

2. Why is the left side of the heart called the systemic side?

3. What is a heart murmur and what can it indicate?

4. Why is it important that the left ventricle is the most powerful of the four heart chambers?

5. How does the size and strength of the left ventricle change over time with more vigorous exercise?

Cardiac muscle has the unique ability to generate its own electrical signal, which allows it to contract rhythmically without neural stimulation. The figure below illustrates the components of the conduction system. First, fill in the blanks with the correct labels, and then on the same drawing, sketch the pathway of the electrical impulse through the heart.

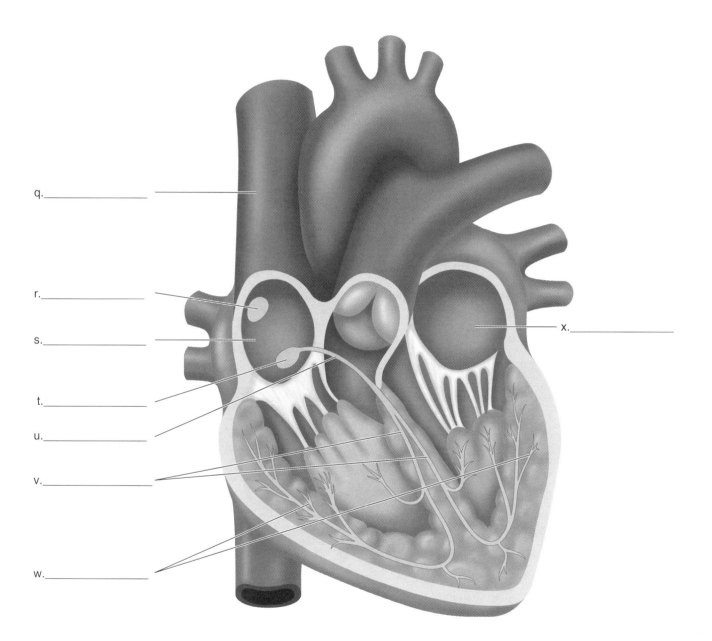

q._____

r._____

s._____

t._____

u._____

v._____

w._____

x._____

6. Explain the role of each of these components of the intrinsic conduction system:

- Sinoatrial (SA) node
- Atrioventricular (AV) node
- AV bundle
- Purkinje fibers

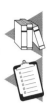

Activity 7.2

Extrinsic Control of Heart Activity

Do this activity after reading pages 212-213 of *Physiology of Sport and Exercise*.

Although the heart initiates its own electrical impulses, their timing and effects can be altered. This is primarily accomplished through the parasympathetic nervous system, the sympathetic nervous system, and the endocrine system.

Fill in the following table: Place an **X** in the column that matches the effects of each extrinsic system, and in that same column write a brief explanation of the mechanisms at work.

	Slows impulse conduction speed and heart rate	Increases impulse conduction speed and heart rate
Parasympathetic system		
Sympathetic system		
Endocrine system		

After each description below, write, on separate paper, (a) which extrinsic system is likely involved in the situation and (b) why.

1. Paul is a seasoned long-distance runner. He has run eight marathons and is training for another one. His resting heart rate is 40 beats/min.

2. Mikala just woke up. She is in a very relaxed state without a care in the world. Upon waking, her heart rate is 55 beats/min.

3. Sheila just sprinted the 50-yd dash. Gasping to catch her breath, she takes her pulse and finds her heart is beating 157 beats/min.

4. Alex is lounging in the library, about to fall asleep after studying for several hours. He doesn't hear Tony sneak up on him. The tap on his shoulder startles him, and all of his senses seem to be aroused. As he starts talking with Tony, Alex notices that his heart is beating markedly faster than it was just a few seconds ago.

Activity 7.3

The Vascular System

Do this activity after reading pages 216-220 of *Physiology of Sport and Exercise.*

The vascular system is made up of a series of vessels that transport blood from the heart to the tissues and back. When we consider that the needs of the various body tissues are constantly changing, it is remarkable that the cardiovascular system can respond so efficiently, guaranteeing an adequate blood supply to the areas where it is most needed.

This exercise will reinforce for you the role each part of the vascular system plays. Read the scenario and then match the vascular system items on the left with the roles in the story on the right.

Mr. Jones's Supply World is the lucky supplier of the biggest store in town. Mr. Jones's Supply World is so important that it is actually located right in the store! Like all good suppliers, Mr. Jones tries to keep **supplies** flowing continuously to the different **departments** throughout the store. When this big store needs supplies, Mr. Jones's Supply World loads up several **large forklifts** with supplies; the forklifts transfer the supplies to many **smaller delivery carts**; and then at each department, the supplies get transferred to **an intricate system of conveyors**, which deliver the supplies directly where they are needed. The most active departments receive the most supplies.

When the supplies reach the departments, the receiving agent in each department might return some supplies and some exchanged items to Mr. Jones's Supply World. This is done through a separate system of many **return delivery carts** and a few **return forklifts.** The store's **return clerks** are very important in forcing supplies back to the Supply World.

If there is a sale going on in a department or if a department is running low on supplies, **the department heads are very good at cooperating.** They will share supplies with each other during the time of the sale or extra need.

If the entire store is in need of extra assistance, the **regional manager** will sometimes step in with good ideas for helping Mr. Jones's Supply World or the departments deal with the problem.

Mr. Jones is a smart businessman and knows that if he doesn't keep his own staff healthy, his Supply World, and then the entire store, may fail. So, Mr. Jones's Supply World has its own **support department** to help in daily tasks so it doesn't become worn out. There have been times when **a member of the support department has become ingrown and stagnant.** That member might be replaced if his or her behavior cannot be repaired.

_____ 1. Blood

_____ 2. Heart

_____ 3. Heart's own vascular system

_____ 4. Atherosclerosis

_____ 5. Arteries

_____ 6. Arterioles

_____ 7. Capillaries

_____ 8. Venules

_____ 9. Veins

_____ 10. Tissues and organs

_____ 11. Breathing, muscle pump, and valves assisting in return of blood

_____ 12. Autoregulation

_____ 13. Extrinsic neural control

a. Mr. Jones's Supply World

b. return clerks

c. supplies

d. forklifts

e. delivery carts

f. an intricate system of conveyors

g. departments

h. return delivery carts

i. return forklifts

j. support department to the Supply World

k. departmental cooperation in times of extra work

l. regional manager

m. a member of the support department becoming ingrown or worn out

Activity 7.4

Blood Composition and Viscosity

Do this activity after reading pages 220-222 of *Physiology of Sport and Exercise.*

During exercise, blood helps with transportation, temperature regulation, and acid-base (pH) balance. In this activity, we will review blood volume and composition, the nature of red blood cells, and the effects of blood viscosity.

When you go to breakfast one day, put about a cup of milk in a bowl and then add a little less than a cup of cereal. The milk represents the plasma in your blood, and the cereal represents the formed elements, or hematocrit.

1. What percentage of whole blood is typically plasma volume? What is the plasma portion of the blood made up of?

2. What percentage of whole blood is typically made up of formed elements? What is included in those formed elements?

Eat some of the cereal—enough so that you notice the decreased amount of the "hematocrit."

3. By eating some of the cereal, you are imagining the destruction of red blood cells during exercise. Why is an adequate number of red blood cells necessary for effective exercise performance? What is one characteristic of the production of red blood cells that can help maintain an adequate balance of these cells?

Now pour in more cereal, so that your bowl contains more cereal than milk.

4. You have just increased the viscosity of your cereal/milk mixture, or of your blood. How would this increased viscosity affect the blood's ability to reach active tissues? (Imagine pouring this mixture of cereal and milk through a narrow tube; would it flow through easily?) How would this increased viscosity, then, affect oxygen delivery?

5. What would be the optimal blood composition for physical activity?

Activity 7.5

Cardiovascular Responses to Exercise

Do this activity after reading pages 222-239 of *Physiology of Sport and Exercise.*

Numerous cardiovascular changes occur during exercise. All share a common goal: to allow the system to meet the increased demands placed on it and to carry out its functions with maximum efficiency. Imagine that you are in the middle of exercising— perhaps you are roller blading, skiing, mountain biking, or rowing. Fill out the table below, based on information found in your textbook, to see what types of changes your body is making as it adapts to your bout of physical activity.

Parameter	Increase or decrease? (Use ↑, ↓, or ↔)	Further explanation for studying purposes
Heart rate		
Stroke volume		
Cardiac output		
Blood flow to active areas		
Blood pressure		

Parameter	Increase or decrease? (Use ↑, ↓, or ↔)	Further explanation for studying purposes
a-v̄O₂ diff		
Plasma volume		
Fluid portion of blood		
Blood pH		

Individual Applications of Cardiovascular Responses to Exercise

Activity 7.6

Do this activity after reading pages 222-239 of *Physiology of Sport and Exercise*.

Even when you are at rest, your cardiovascular system constantly works to meet the demands of your body's tissues. But during exercise, you place numerous and far more urgent demands on this system. Through this activity, you will learn how each component of the cardiovascular system adapts to changes in the body's internal environment that result from physical activity.

1. Estimate your maximum heart rate (HRmax) by subtracting your age in years from 220. Write your answer here. *If at any time during this activity you meet or exceed 80% of your estimated HRmax, slow your work rate or cease the activity.*

2. Take your resting heart rate when you first wake up and before you rise. Write your resting heart rate here.

   Resting heart rate: _____/min

3. Prepare to exercise. Using a treadmill is preferable for this activity; if that is impossible, walking at intentionally faster speeds will work, too. Immediately prior to exercising, take your heart rate. Write your pre-exercise heart rate here.

   Pre-exercise heart rate: _____/min

4. What differences do you see between your resting heart rate and your pre-exercise heart rate? What caused this difference? (Answer on separate paper.)

5. Start out at a slow pace on the treadmill, gradually working up to each of the speeds listed. At each speed, take your heart rate and write it in the blank provided. Continue to a speed at which you feel challenged but not uncomfortable (you do not need to fill in all the blanks below; be sure not to exceed 80% of your estimated HRmax). Once you reach the top speed of your choice for this activity, record your heart rate every 30 s at that speed until you believe you have reached your steady-state heart rate for that speed. Record that steady-state heart rate and its corresponding speed in the blanks provided.

4 km/h	HR: _____
6 km/h	HR: _____
8 km/h	HR: _____
10 km/h	HR: _____
12 km/h	HR: _____
_____ km/h	HR: _____ (< 80% HRmax)

   Steady-state HR = _____ at _____ km/h

   After you have reached a steady-state heart rate, end your exercise session by gradually slowing your work rate until you feel sufficiently cooled down.

6. What pattern appeared in your heart rate as you increased your speed? What are the physiological reasons for this pattern?

7. What factors typically influence stroke volume? As you were exercising, how did your stroke volume likely change? What are some possible explanations for this?

8. Let's say your stroke volume (SV) at rest is 60 ml/beat. Calculate your cardiac output at rest (resting HR × SV), convert this to L/min (divide previous answer by 1,000), and write your answer here:

9. What assumptions can you make about the changes that probably took place in your cardiac output while you were exercising on the treadmill? What is the purpose of the increase in cardiac output? How did changes in stroke volume and heart rate contribute to the change in cardiac output?

10. As you walked, jogged, or ran at increasing speeds on the treadmill, your blood flow pattern changed markedly. Shade the vials below to show the approximate amount of blood that goes to skeletal muscle when you are at rest and the amount of blood that goes to skeletal muscle during exhaustive exercise.

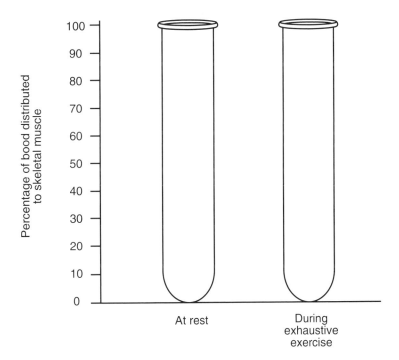

11. Why is this redistribution of blood during exercise necessary? How is it accomplished? Be specific in describing all of the mechanisms at work.

Activity 7.7

Blood Pressure Responses to Exercise

Do this activity after reading pages 234-235 of *Physiology of Sport and Exercise.*

Blood pressure also changes markedly during exercise. Systolic and diastolic blood pressure exhibit different responses to exercise, representing different changes in the cardiovascular system. And blood pressure responds differently to endurance exercise versus resistance exercise as well as to lower-body exercise versus upper-body exercise. In this activity, you will witness some of these differences firsthand.

You will need to find someone qualified to take your blood pressure or a machine that takes it automatically. (Many shopping centers, pharmacies, and grocery stores have blood pressure testing machines. Though these are not highly accurate, they will suffice for this activity.)

1. Take your resting blood pressure (BP) and record it here.

   Systolic BP: _____   Diastolic BP: _____

2. Note how your blood pressure compares to these categories. Circle the category that your blood pressure matches.

   Optimal blood pressure: < 120 systolic *and* < 80 diastolic

   Normal blood pressure: < 130 systolic *and* < 85 diastolic

   High normal blood pressure: 130-139 systolic *or* 85-89 diastolic

   High blood pressure (hypertension):   140 systolic *or*   90 diastolic

   If your resting blood pressure falls in either of the high zones or is unusually low, consult with a physician. High blood pressure is dangerous but is also usually easily controlled through diet, exercis, and, sometimes medication.

Source: The Sixth Report of the Joint National Committee on Detection, Evaluation, and Treatment of High Blood Pressure, NIH publication, 1997.

3. Cycle at a relatively fast pace on a stationary bike for 10 min. Take your blood pressure again and write it here.

   Systolic BP: _____   Diastolic BP: _____

   If your diastolic blood pressure rose by 15 or more mmHg, discontinue this activity and alert a physician.

   Take your heart rate and write it here.

4. Which pressure—systolic or diastolic—rose significantly from your resting BP? Why did one stay the same and the other rise?

   Cycling heart rate: _____/min

5. After resting for a length of time, so that your blood pressure returns to resting levels, take your resting blood pressure again and record it here.

   Systolic BP: _____   Diastolic BP: _____

6. Now, do 8 biceps curls at 50% of your 1RM. (See activity 3.2 for help in calculating your 1RM.) Take your blood pressure upon completing the biceps curls and record it here.

    Systolic BP: _____   Diastolic BP: _____

    Take your heart rate and write it here.   Biceps curl heart rate: _____/min

7. What differences do you see between doing exercise that primarily uses the lower body and exercise that primarily uses the upper body? Why is this so?

8. Calculate your double product (HR × systolic BP) for the stationary cycle and the biceps curl. Which activity worked the heart more?

    Double product for stationary cycle: _____

    Double product for biceps curl: _____

Putting It All Together: Cardiovascular Control During Exercise

Activity 7.8

Do this activity after reading chapter 7 of *Physiology of Sport and Exercise.*

As you now know from studying this chapter, the cardiovascular system is extremely complex and of the utmost importance in the proper functioning of the human body both at rest and during exercise. This activity will test your knowledge of the cardiovascular system by seeing whether you can identify how cardiovascular responses contribute to real-life situations.

After reading each scenario, explain the underlying cardiovascular mechanisms that most likely contribute to the situation. Although many other physiological responses might be at work in each case, focus on the cardiovascular responses.

1. Brandon is a 25-year-old recreational long-distance runner. He competes regularly, mostly for the fun of it and to keep himself motivated to train. Today he ran a 10K in 95 °F heat. His time was unusually slow.

2. After staying up all night to study for exams, Jan took a nap the next afternoon. She awoke suddenly to the sound of the phone ringing and immediately stood up

    to answer it. Her heart rate quickly increased from 55 beats/min while reclining to 65 beats/min while standing.

3. Amber is a swimmer on her high school swim team. Her specialty is the 800-m freestyle. After a long drive, her team finally arrived at an away meet, and Amber was very hungry. She and a few friends found a fastfood place, and Amber downed a burger, fries, and a shake 30 to 45 min before her event. She figured that the food would give her enough energy to compete. To her surprise, she finished a distant sixth instead of her usual top-three finish.

4. Ben is a competitive weightlifter at his university. He is studying exercise physiology and asked a med student to take his blood pressure immediately after performing the clean and jerk at 80% of his 1RM. Ben was shocked when the blood pressure reading was 250/120.

5. As part of a research study, Kassee's stroke volume was measured in different situations. Her resting stroke volume in a reclining position was 75 ml. After swimming five laps, Kassee's stroke volume was measured at 90 ml. Her resting stroke volume in an upright position was 55 ml. While running on a treadmill, Kassee's stroke volume was measured at 100 ml. Kassee wonders why her stroke volume increased so much, almost doubling, while running on a treadmill as compared to swimming.

6. Five minutes into a long-distance cycling race, Rhonda reached a steady-state heart rate of 130 beats/min. But 10 min into the race, she was surprised to find her heart rate gradually increasing. By the last few min of the race, Rhonda's heart rate was 164 beats/min.

7. Josh plays soccer on a park district team in his community. He's a solid offensive player, but today he just can't seem to stay focused. The sun is hot, the air is humid, and he is exhausted from playing almost the entire first half. The game is very close, and his team is anxious to score another goal before halftime. The coach gives Josh a short break with 4 min to go, but sends him back in after less than a minute's respite. Josh didn't even have a chance to find a water bottle. A few seconds later, Josh collapses.

Sample Test Questions for Chapter 7

Test yourself on your knowledge of this chapter by taking this self-test. Write the correct answers on a separate sheet of paper.

Multiple Choice

1. Which of the following is an example of external control of heart activity?

   a. The SA node initiates the impulse.
   b. The impulse enters the AV bundle, which travels along the ventricular septum and then branches into both ventricles.
   c. Norepinephrine and epinephrine are released and increase heart rate.
   d. The Purkinje fibers transmit the impulse extremely fast through the ventricles, causing all parts of the ventricle to contract at about the same time.

2. Which of the following is *not* a role the sympathetic nervous system plays in regulating distribution of blood?

   a. causes muscle cells to contract, constricting vessels so that less blood can pass through

b. under normal conditions, transmits impulses continuously to blood vessels, keeping the vessels in a state of moderate constriction to maintain adequate blood pressure

c. during a crisis and during exercise, causes vasodilation directly through sympathetic fibers that supply some blood vessels in skeletal muscles and in the heart, increasing blood flow to the muscles and the heart

d. sends CO_2, K^+, and oxygen to body tissues in response to the arteriole's autoregulatory mechanisms

3. During exercise, in addition to transporting oxygen and nutrients to active muscles and regulating temperature, blood also helps to _____.

a. lower mean arterial pressure.
b. maintain the proper pH for metabolic processes.
c. minimize swelling of active areas.
d. regulate a regular heart rate.

4. Which of the following situations is ideal for physical activity?

a. a low hematocrit with an accompanying low plasma volume
b. a low hematocrit with a decreased number of red blood cells
c. a low hematocrit with a normal or slightly elevated number of red blood cells
d. a high hematocrit with a very low plasma volume

5. Which of the following is *not* a normal response to exercise?

a. Venous return decreases.
b. Ventricular contractility increases.
c. Heart rate increases in proportion to the increase in exercise intensity, until you are near a point of exhaustion, at which point it levels off.
d. Cardiac output increases in order to meet the muscles' increased demand for oxygen.

True-False

6. Low resting heart rate in endurance athletes is uncommon and could be an indication of pathological bradycardia.

7. The electrocardiogram is a direct reflection of the heart's contractile activity.

8. The small size of the heart represents the small role it plays in the functioning of the body.

9. Arteries always carry blood away from the heart to the arterioles.

Fill in the Blank

10. Heart muscle is collectively called the _____.

11. The _____ is the most powerful of the four heart chambers.

12. One full cardiac cycle consists of all heart chambers undergoing a relaxation phase, called _____, and a contraction phase, called _____. The _____ phase is longer than the _____ phase.

Short Answer

13. Why should pre-exercise heart rates not be used as estimates of resting heart rate?

14. How does the myocardium differ from skeletal muscle? Why is this important?

15. Define stroke volume. How is it measured?

16. If the arteries carry blood away from the heart, how is it that blockage of a coronary artery can lead to myocardial infarction?

Essay

17. How does the muscle pump work? What would be the consequences of two-way valves instead of unidirectional valves in the veins?

18. What is the conflict in research about stroke volume? How could body position, training status, and exercise modality impact research findings on stroke volume?

19. Compare and contrast how blood pressure changes during endurance exercise, resistance exercise, upper-body exercise, and lower-body exercise.

Answers to Selected Chapter 7 Activities

7.1 The Anatomy of the Heart and the Heart's Conduction System

a. Superior vena cava;   b. Right atrium;   c. Tricuspid valve;   d. Right pulmonary veins; e. Right ventricle;   f. Papillary muscles;   g. Inferior vena cava;   h. Aorta;   i. Right and left pulmonary veins;   j. Pulmonary semilunar valve;   k. Left pulmonary veins;   l. Left atrium;   m. Bicuspid (mitral) valve;   n. Chordae tendineae;   o. Left ventricle;   p. Interventricular septum;

1. The right side of the heart is called the pulmonary side because it sends blood that has circulated throughout the body into the lungs for reoxygenation.

2. The left side of the heart is called the systemic side because blood from the left side is ultimately sent to all body parts and systems. It receives the oxygenated blood from the lungs and sends it out to supply all body tissues.

3. A heart murmur is a condition in which abnormal heart sounds are detected with a stethoscope; the usual clicking of a heart valve snapping shut sounds instead like a blowing noise. This can indicate the turbulent flow of blood through a narrowed or leaky valve, or it can indicate errant blood flow through a hole in the wall separating the right and left sides of the heart (septal defect).

4. The left ventricle must pump blood to the entire systemic route. When the body is sitting or standing, the left ventricle must contract with enough force to overcome the effect of gravity, which causes blood to pool in the lower extremities. With vigorous exercise, the demands on the left ventricle are very high.

5. In response to the demands of exercise, the left ventricle increases in size (hypertrophy) and strength, much like skeletal muscle.

   q. Superior vena cava;   r. SA node;   s. Right atrium;   t. AV node;   u. AV bundle;   v. Bundle branches;   w. Purkinje fibers;   x. Left atrium.

6. Sinoatrial (SA) node—Generates the impulse for heart contraction. Also known as the heart's pacemaker because of the regular rhythm it establishes (known as sinus rhythm).

Atrioventricular (AV) node—Conducts the impulse from the atria into the ventricles.

AV bundle—Is located along the ventricular septum and has right and left bundle branches that extend into both ventricles. These branches send the impulse toward the apex of the heart and then outward.

Purkinje fibers—Terminal branches of the AV bundle. They transmit the impulse through the ventricles approximately six times faster than the impulse is conducted through the rest of the cardiac conduction system, allowing all parts of the ventricle to contract at about the same time.

7.2   Extrinsic Control of Heart Activity

	Slows impulse conduction speed and heart rate	Increases impulse conduction speed and heart rate
Parasympathetic system	X Acts on heart through vagus nerve.	
Sympathetic system		X Predominates during times of physical or emotional stress.
Endocrine system		X Exerts its effects through the catecholamines, epinephrine and norepinephrine, whose release is triggered by sympathetic stiumlation. They prolong the sympathetic response.

1. Paul's very low resting heart rate is probably mainly because of a reduced intrinsic heart rate and increased parasympathetic stimulation as a result of several years of endurance training.

2. Mikala's parasympathetic system is exerting control on the heart when she initially wakes up. At rest, the vagus nerve has a depressant effect on the heart, slowing impulse conduction and thus heart rate.

3. The sympathetic system is likely exerting the most control in Sheila's situation, where she has a high heart rate upon completing the 50-yard dash. The sympathetic system predominates during times of physical or emotional stress.

4. In this stressful situation, Alex's sympathetic system triggered his endocrine system to release the catecholamines, epinephrine and norepinephrine, which, together with the sympathetic system, stimulated his heart, increasing its rate.

7.3   The Vascular System

1. c;   2. a;   3. j;   4. m;   5. d;   6. e;   7. f;   8. h;   9. i;   10. g;   11. b;   12. k;   13. l

7.4   Blood Composition and Viscosity

1. Blood is typically made up of 55% plasma, which is composed of 90% H_2O, 7% plasma proteins, and 3% other items.

2. Blood is usually about 45% formed elements, which is composed of 99% red blood cells and less than 1% white blood cells and platelets.

3. Red blood cells transport oxygen, which is primarily bound to their hemoglobin, so a destruction of red blood cells means less oxygen may reach the tissues. Red blood cells normally are continuously produced and destroyed at about equal rates.

4. The increased viscosity would limit the blood's ability to reach the active tissues. Since oxygen is transported bound to hemoglobin, less oxygen would reach the tissues.

5. For physical activity, a low hematocrit with a normal or slightly elevated number of red blood cells is desirable. This combination should facilitate oxygen transport.

7.5   Cardiovascular Responses to Exercise

Parameter	Increase or decrease? (Use ↑, ↓ or ↔)	Further explanation for studying purposes
Heart rate	↑	Increases directly in proportion to exercise intensity until you are at a point of exhaustion. As you approach that point, heart rate begins to level off. When rate of work is held constant at submaximal levels of exercise, heart rate plateaus. This is the steady-state heart rate, and it is the optimal heart rate for meeting circulatory demands at that specific rate of work.
Stroke volume	↑	SV is a major determinant of cardiorespiratory endurance capacity. Increases with increasing rates of work. Some disagreement about whether SV plateaus at 40% to 60% maximal capacity. Increase likely due to increased venous return, increased ventricular contractility, and decrease in total peripheral resistance because of vasodilation of blood vessels going to active muscles.
Cardiac output	↑	Increases in heart rate and stroke volume increases cardiac output, forcing more blood out of the heart and speeding up circulation. This ensures that adequate oxygen and nutrients reach muscles and that waste products are quickly cleared away.
Blood flow to active	↑	Blood flow to muscles increases markedly during exercise, from 15% to 20% at rest to 80% to 85% during exercise. Blood flow to kidneys, liver, stomach, and intestines is reduced.
Blood pressure	↑	Increased systolic BP results from increased cardiac output. This helps drive blood quickly through vasculature, facilitating the delivery process. With whole-body endurance exercise, systolic BP increases in direct proportion to exercise intensity and diastolic BP remains unchanged.

Parameter	Increase or decrease? (Use ↑, ↓ or ↔)	Further explanation for studying purposes
Blood pressure (cont.)		BP responses to high-intensity resistance exercise are exaggerated, increasing a great deal. Use of upper-body musculature causes greater blood pressure responses than does use of lower-body musculature.
a-v̄O₂ diff	↑	Reflects a decreasing venous oxygen content during exercise. More oxygen is required by the active muscles, so more oxygen is extracted from the blood. Arterial oxygen content remains essentially unchanged.
Plasma volume	↓	With onset of exercise, there is an almost immediate loss of blood plasma volume to the interstitial fluid space. Additional plasma volume is lost to sweating. A reduction in plasma volume can impair performance.
Fluid portion of blood	↓	Because the fluid portion of the blood decreases during exercise, the cellular and protein portions represent a larger fraction of the total blood volume. This hemoconcentration increases red blood cell concentration. As a result, the hemoglobin content is increased, thereby increasing the blood's oxygen-carryingcapacity.
Blood pH	↓	As exercise intensity increases above 50% of maximal aerobic capacity, pH starts to decrease as the blood becomes more acidic. This drop results primarily from an increased reliance on anaerobic metabolism and corresponds to increases in blood lactate observed with increasing exercise intensity.

7.8   Putting It All Together: Cardiovascular Control During Exercise

1. It is likely that Brandon's body started to overheat due to the high temperatures. More of his blood was directed to his skin to conduct heat away from the body's core to its periphery, where heat is lost to the environment. Because more blood was directed to his skin, less blood was left for his muscles, thereby hindering his performance.

2. When your body shifts from a reclining to a standing position, your stroke volume immediately drops. This is primarily because gravity causes blood to pool in your legs, which reduces the volume of blood returning to your heart. Your heart rate responds by increasing in order to maintain cardiac output.

3. Although many other factors could have contributed to Amber's disappointing time, one cardiovascular explanation is that upon her eating the big meal, more blood was immediately sent to the digestive system to benefit the activity there. This meant less blood was available to supply oxygen to her muscles during this long-distance event.

4. Blood pressure responses to heavy resistance exercise are high; one reason for this might be the use of the Valsalva maneuver, where the person tries to exhale

while the mouth, nose, and throat are closed. This causes an enormous increase in intrathoracic pressure, and much of the subsequent blood pressure increase results from the body's effort to overcome the high internal pressures. Ben might have experienced an even greater blood pressure response had he done an exercise that used only upper-body muscles.

5. When the body is in a supine position, blood does not pool in the lower extremities. This allows blood to return more easily to the heart, making for higher stroke volume. Because the resting stroke volume in a supine position is already rather high, maximal exercise in a supine position does not cause nearly the stroke-volume increase that maximal exercise in an upright position does. Stroke volume at rest in an upright position is lower than in a reclined position; yet when you are performing upright exercise, stroke volume must increase a great deal to compensate for the force of gravity.

6. Rhonda experienced a classic case of cardiovascular drift; with prolonged aerobic exercise at a constant rate of work, stroke volume gradually decreases, heart rate gradually increases, and systemic and pulmonary arterial pressures decline. Cardiovascular drift might result from an increased amount of blood being directed to the skin in an attempt to lose body heat and attenuate the rise in body core temperature. In addition, there is a small decrease in blood volume resulting from sweating and from a generalized shift of plasma across the capillary membrane into the surrounding tissues. These combine to decrease venous return to the right side of the heart. The resulting reduction in end-diastolic volume reduces stroke volume. The heart rate compensates by increasing, in an effort to maintain cardiac output.

7. While many physiological processes likely contributed to Josh's collapse, the primary cardiovascular cause is a decrease in plasma volume. As blood pressure increases, the hydrostatic pressure within the capillaries increases. The increase in blood pressure forces water from the vascular compartment to the interstitial compartment. As metabolic waste products build up in the active muscle, intramuscular osmotic pressure increases, attracting fluid to the muscle. In Josh's case, the heat and humidity likely caused sweating, resulting in additional plasma loss. All of these cardiovascular factors probably combined with other physiological processes to cause Josh to collapse from dehydration.

Answers to Selected Chapter 7 Test Questions

Multiple Choice

1. c;   2. d;   3. b;   4. c;   5. a

True-False

6. False;   7. False;   8. False;   9. True

Fill in the Blank

10. myocardium;   11. left ventricle;   12. diastole, systole, diastolic, systolic

Short Answer and Essay

For questions 13 to 19, check your answers against the explanations given in the textbook.

Respiratory Regulation During Exercise

concepts

- Pulmonary ventilation (breathing) is the process by which air is moved into and out of the lungs. It has two phases: inspiration and expiration.

- Pulmonary diffusion is the process by which gases are exchanged across the respiratory membrane in the alveoli. The amount of gas exchange that occurs across the membrane depends primarily on the partial pressure of each gas.

- Oxygen is transported in the blood primarily bound to hemoglobin, as oxyhemoglobin. Oxygen delivery to the tissues depends on the oxygen content of the blood, the amount of blood flow to the tissues, and local conditions such as tissue temperature and PO_2.

- Carbon dioxide exits the cells by simple diffusion in response to the partial pressure gradient between the tissue and the capillary blood. The majority of carbon dioxide produced by active muscle is transported back to the lungs as bicarbonate ion in the blood.

- Pulmonary ventilation is regulated by the respiratory centers in the brain stem, the central chemoreceptors in the brain, peripheral receptors, and stretch receptors in the air passages and lungs.

- Ventilation increases during exercise in direct proportion to the rate of work being performed, up to the ventilatory breakpoint. Beyond this point, ventilation increases disproportionately as the body tries to clear excess CO_2.

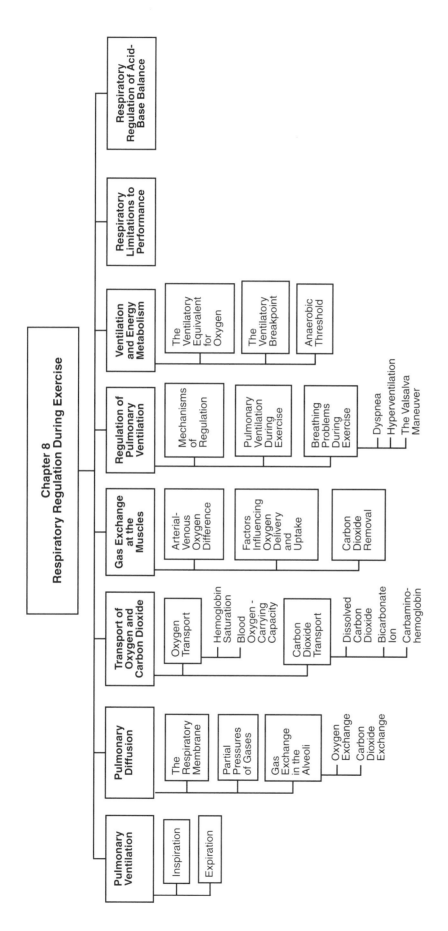

Chapter 8
Respiratory Regulation During Exercise

Pulmonary Ventilation
- Inspiration
- Expiration

Pulmonary Diffusion
- The Respiratory Membrane
- Partial Pressures of Gases
- Gas Exchange in the Alveoli
  - Oxygen Exchange
  - Carbon Dioxide Exchange

Transport of Oxygen and Carbon Dioxide
- Oxygen Transport
  - Hemoglobin Saturation
  - Blood Oxygen-Carrying Capacity
- Carbon Dioxide Transport
  - Dissolved Carbon Dioxide
  - Bicarbonate Ion
  - Carbamino-hemoglobin

Gas Exchange at the Muscles
- Arterial-Venous Oxygen Difference
- Factors Influencing Oxygen Delivery and Uptake
- Carbon Dioxide Removal

Regulation of Pulmonary Ventilation
- Mechanisms of Regulation
- Pulmonary Ventilation During Exercise
- Breathing Problems During Exercise
  - Dyspnea
  - Hyperventilation
  - The Valsalva Maneuver

Ventilation and Energy Metabolism
- The Ventilatory Equivalent for Oxygen
- The Ventilatory Breakpoint
- Anaerobic Threshold

Respiratory Limitations to Performance

Respiratory Regulation of Acid-Base Balance

Activity 8.1

Anatomy of the Respiratory System and Pathways of Pulmonary Ventilation

Do this activity after reading pages 245-249 of *Physiology of Sport and Exercise.*

Pulmonary ventilation, or breathing, is the process by which we move air into and out of our lungs. The drawing below illustrates the anatomy of the respiratory system. Without looking in your textbook, fill in the correct labels. Then draw the pathway of inspired air in the left-hand portion of the figure.

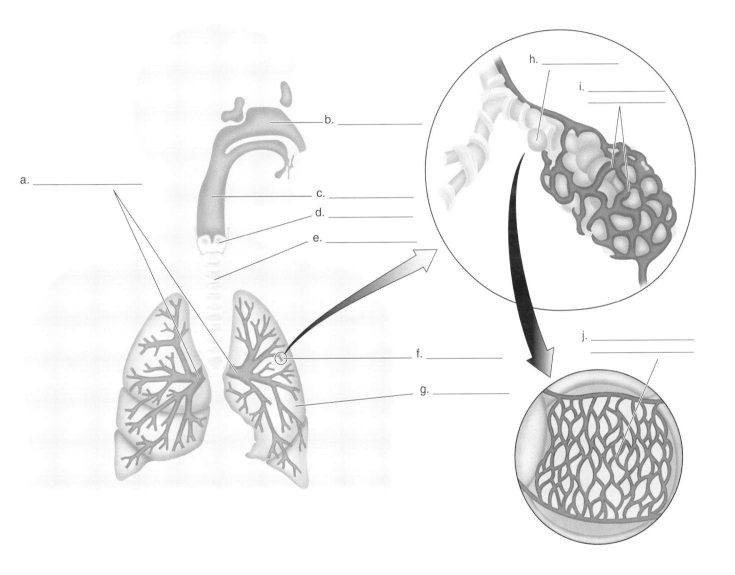

Activity 8.2

Inspiration and Expiration

Do this activity after reading pages 246-249 of *Physiology of Sport and Exercise.*

The two phases of pulmonary ventilation are inspiration and expiration. These two processes are quite different in nature. In the table on the next page, place an **X** in the correct column, depending on whether the description on the left is something that occurs during inspiration or during expiration.

Activity 8.2 **Inspiration and Expiration**

	Inspiration	Expiration
An active process involving the diaphragm and the external intercostal muscles.		
The ribs and sternum are moved by the external intercostal muscles: The ribs swing up and out, and the sternum swings up and forward.		
The diaphragm contracts, flattening down toward the abdomen.		
The lungs expand, causing lung pressure to be less than atmospheric pressure.		
Air rushes into the lungs to balance the pressure.		
During forced or labored breathing, this action is further assisted by muscles that help raise the ribs even more than during regular breathing.		
At rest, this is a passive process, involving the relaxation of the inspiratory muscles and elastic recoil of the lung tissue.		
The diaphragm relaxes, returning to its normal upward, arched position.		
The external intercostal muscles relax, and the ribs and sternum lower to their resting positions.		
The lung recoils to its resting size, increasing the pressure in the thorax.		
Air is forced out of the lungs to balance pressure.		
During forced breathing, this action becomes more active, with the internal intercostal muscles actively pulling the ribs down.		

Activity 8.3

Pulmonary Diffusion

Do this activity after reading pages 250-253 of *Physiology of Sport and Exercise.*

Gas exchange between the air in the alveoli and the blood in the pulmonary capillaries occurs across the respiratory membrane. Differences in the partial pressures of the gases in the alveoli and the gases in the blood create a pressure gradient across the respiratory membrane. This forms the basis of gas exchange during pulmonary diffusion.

To help visualize diffusion, try this simple experiment:

Fill two drinking glasses of the same size to the brim with water. Put several drops of red food coloring in one glass and several drops of blue food coloring in the other. The red water represents pulmonary capillary blood, carrying hemoglobin. The blue water represents the oxygen in an alveolus. Place a piece of cellophane over the glass with blue water, binding it tightly and securely with rubber bands. Using a toothpick or a pin, poke several holes in the cellophane covering. Now turn the blue-colored glass upside down on top of the glass filled with red water.

The blue water should slowly permeate the red water. (If it doesn't, try poking a few more holes in the cellophane.)

Although this experiment uses the force of gravity, rather than partial pressure, to permeate the membrane (cellophane), it does help us to visualize the exchange of oxygen between the alveolus and the pulmonary capillary blood.

To make sure you thoroughly understand pulmonary diffusion, answer the following questions on separate paper.

1. What structures make up the respiratory membrane?

2. What is a partial pressure?

3. What is Dalton's law?

4. How do partial pressures affect diffusion?

5. What is the oxygen diffusion capacity?

6. How does the oxygen diffusion capacity differ at rest and during exercise?

7. What causes this difference?

8. How would you have changed the experiment of the blue- and red-colored water to illustrate carbon dioxide exchange?

Transport and Exchange of Oxygen and Carbon Dioxide

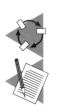

Activity 8.4

Do this activity after reading pages 253-259 (top) of *Physiology of Sport and Exercise.*

The blood is an efficient means of transportation for gases. Blood delivers oxygen to the tissues and removes carbon dioxide that the tissues produce. In this activity, we first consider oxygen and then carbon dioxide, both looking at how these gases are transported via the blood and how gas exchange at the muscles takes place.

Oxygen Transport and Exchange

The oxygen-carrying capacity of blood is determined largely by hemoglobin concentration. When oxygen leaves hemoglobin to enter active muscles, the oxygen is said to be "dissociated." The two figures on the next page show oxygen-hemoglobin dissociation curves.

1. On the graph on the left (see next page), draw a line to illustrate how the curve would change if the blood pH were to decrease. What does this indicate is happening to the oxygen in the blood?

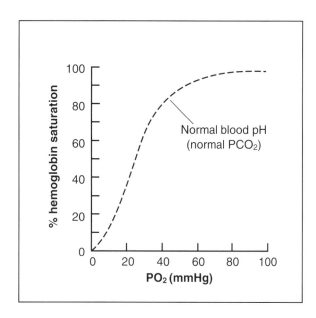

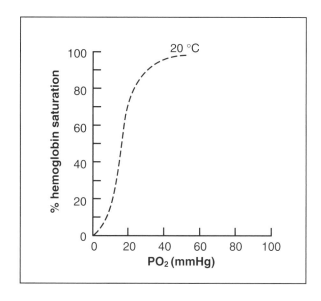

2. On the graph on the right above, draw a line to illustrate how the curve would change if the blood temperature were to increase. What does this indicate is happening to the oxygen in the blood?

3. How does exercise impact blood pH and blood temperature, and therefore the oxygen-hemoglobin dissociation curve?

4. The difference in oxygen content between arterial and venous blood is called the arterial-venous oxygen difference. It reflects the amount of oxygen taken up by the tissues. Look at the following bar graphs. What is the arterial-venous oxygen difference in each bar graph? What is the likely current activity level of the subject in each bar graph?

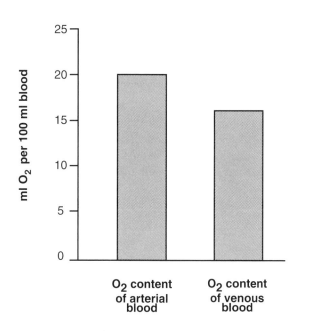

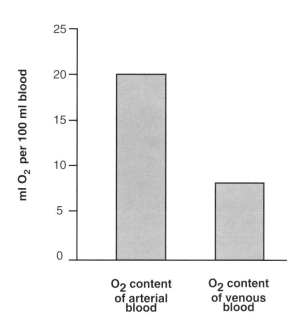

a-$\bar{v}O_2$ diff of left graph: _____

Activity level of subject in left graph: _____

a-$\bar{v}O_2$ diff of left graph: _____

Activity level of subject in right graph: _____

5. What would be the consequences of each of the following events?
   * A hemoglobin saturation of 80%

   * Increased blood flow

   * Increased muscle acidity

   * Decreased muscle temperature

Carbon Dioxide Transport and Exchange

Although some carbon dioxide is transported back to the lungs dissolved in plasma and bound to hemoglobin, the majority of carbon dioxide produced by the active muscle is transported back to the lungs in the form of bicarbonate ions.

Draw a flowchart depicting the steps of carbon dioxide exchange at the muscle and transport in the form of bicarbonate ion to the lungs. See pages 255 and 257 in *Physiology of Sport and Exercise* for help. Your flowchart should begin with the carbon dioxide diffusing out of the muscle cells and into the blood, and end with the re-formed carbon dioxide entering the alveoli and being exhaled.

Activity 8.5	# Regulation of Pulmonary Ventilation

Do this activity after reading pages 259-260 of *Physiology of Sport and Exercise*.

Maintaining homeostatic balance in blood PO_2, PCO_2, and pH requires a high degree of coordination between the respiratory and circulatory systems. Much of this coordination is accomplished by involuntary regulation of pulmonary ventilation.

Without looking in your textbook, match the respiratory regulation mechanism on the left with its action on the right.

_____ 1. Inspiratory center

_____ 2. Expiratory center

_____ 3. Central chemoreceptors (in brain)

_____ 4. Peripheral chemoreceptors (in the aortic arch and in the bifurcation of the common carotid artery)

_____ 5. Stretch receptors in the lungs

_____ 6. Cerebral motor cortex

a. Helps us to exert voluntary control over breathing although this voluntary control is very limited and can be overridden by the involuntary control mechanisms.

b. Respond to changes in carbon dioxide (PCO_2) and H^+ (pH) levels. When the levels increase, these send signals to the inspiratory center activating the neural circuitry to increase the rate and depth of inspiration, which increases the removal of carbon dioxide and H^+.

c. Located within the brain stem. Helps establish the rate and depth of breathing by sending out periodic impulses to the respiratory muscles. Contracts the intercostal and abdominal muscles, causing the thoracic volume to decrease and force air out of the lungs.

d. Located in the pleurae, bronchioles, and alveoli. When excessively stretched, they relay information to the expiratory center, which responds by shortening the duration of an inspiration, thereby decreasing the risk of overinflating the respiratory structures.

e. Located within the brain stem. Helps establish the rate and depth of breathing by sending out periodic impulses to the respiratory muscles. Stimulates the external intercostal and diaphragm muscles to contract to increase the volume of the thorax, thereby drawing ir into the lungs.

f. Sensitive primarily to blood changes in PO_2 but also respond to changes in H^+ concentration and PCO_2. Send signals to the inspiratory center to increase the rate and depth of inspiration.

▶ Activity 8.6   Pulmonary Ventilation During Exercise

Do this activity after reading pages 261-265 of *Physiology of Sport and Exercise.*

During exercise, control of pulmonary ventilation usually involves all of the mechanisms listed in Activity 8.5, with no one mechanism clearly predominant. But there are some clear patterns of pulmonary ventilation during exercise. In this activity, we will first look at pulmonary ventilation in general during exercise; then we will focus in on ventilation and energy metabolism.

1. On the graph below, draw a line showing the usual response of pulmonary ventilation to a moderate bout of exercise. Don't worry about exact data points; the purpose is simply to show general trends.

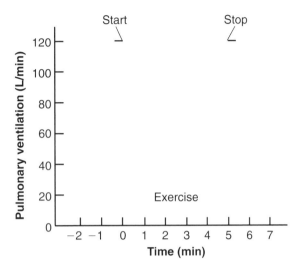

2. Your graph should have showed a two-phase adjustment in pulmonary ventilation. Explain the likely causes of each phase.

3. What is one possible reason that respiratory recovery upon the end of exercise takes several minutes, even though the muscles' energy needs drop almost immediately to resting levels following exercise?

4. Define the ventilatory equivalent for oxygen ($\dot{V}E/\dot{V}O_2$).

5. On the graphs below, draw a line that generally represents the relationship of $\dot{V}E/\dot{V}O_2$ during (a) submaximal, steady-state exercise, (b) heavy, near-maximal exercise, and (c) incremental exercise. Don't worry about exact data points; the purpose is simply to show general trends.

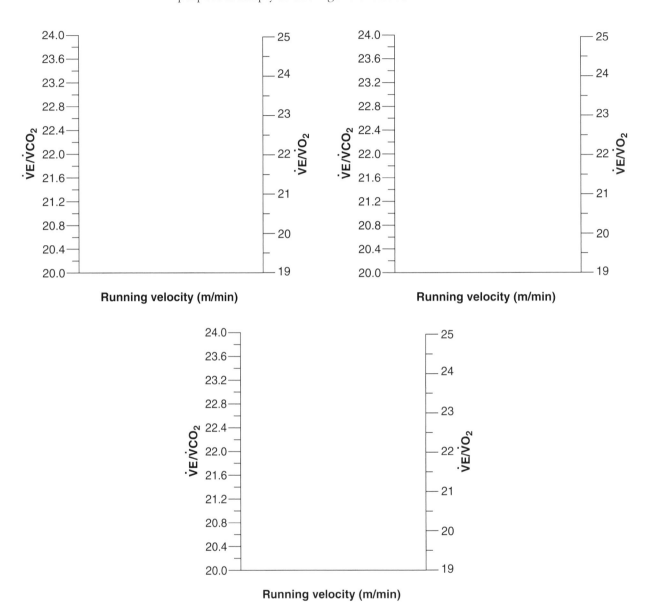

6. If the $\dot{V}E/\dot{V}O_2$ remains relatively constant, what does this indicate?

7. If the $\dot{V}E/\dot{V}O_2$ increases, what does this indicate?

8. Define ventilatory breakpoint.

9. On the open graph below, draw two lines in different colors—one to illustrate oxygen uptake and one to illustrate ventilation during increasingly intense exercise. Don't worry about exact numbers; the purpose is simply to show the general trend of each of these mechanisms. Draw an arrow pointing to the ventilatory breakpoint in your graph.

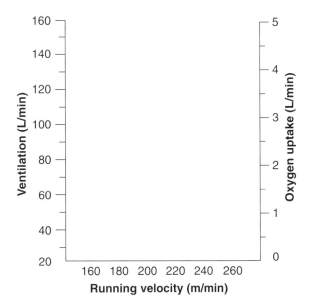

10. Why does ventilation increase disproportionately after the ventilatory breakpoint?

11. What is the most accurate way to estimate anaerobic threshold?

12. On the third (far right) graph in question 5, use a different colored pen or pencil to draw a line representing the $\dot{V}E/\dot{V}O_2$ during incremental exercise. Again, don't concern yourself with exact data points; concentrate on the general trend. Circle the point of anaerobic threshold in your graph.

13. How is the anaerobic threshold related to the lactate threshold?

Respiratory Limitations and Breathing Problems During Exercise

> **Activity 8.7**

Do this activity after reading 261-263 and 265-266 of *Physiology of Sport and Exercise*.

Both the very makeup of the respiratory system and specific breathing problems can limit our ability to exercise, or hinder our performance. First, answer the questions about respiratory limitations to performance, and then choose one of the breathing problems to research and report on.

Respiratory Limitations

Place the correct letter in the blanks below to indicate which type of athlete each respiratory limitation affects.

_____ 1. Pulmonary ventilation

_____ 2. Airway resistance

_____ 3. Gas diffusion

a. Normal, healthy individuals during submaximal exercise

b. Highly trained endurance athletes during maximal exercise

c. Both a and b

d. Neither a nor b

Respiratory Problems or Diseases

Ideally, during exercise our breathing is regulated in a way that maximizes our ability to perform. Unfortunately, this doesn't always occur. Many respiratory problems and diseases can accompany exercise and hinder performance.

Choose one of the following problems or diseases to research:

- Dyspnea

- Hyperventilation

- Valsalva maneuver

- Exercise-induced asthma

- Emphysema

Write a report that summarizes the following information:

- The definition of the problem or disease

- The causes of the problem or disease

- The symptoms of the problem or disease

- For exercise-induced asthma and emphysema, the diagnosis and treatment of the disease

- Any implications this problem or disease has for exercise

Be sure to document your sources. If your instructor requests, turn in your report or present your report orally.

Putting It All Together: Respiratory Regulation During Exercise

Activity 8.8

Do this activity after reading chapter 8 of *Physiology of Sport and Exercise*.

The respiratory system is fascinating and complex. Even more interesting is how it responds to exercise. Now that you have learned the details of this chapter, let's see how all of the respiratory mechanisms work together to regulate respiration during exercise. Read the following case study and be sure you can explain the answers to each of the subsequent questions. To save time, and if your instructor approves, you can choose not to write each answer, but instead simply to study each topic thoroughly.

Jenna is going out for a run. She spends a little time warming up and stretching, and then is off on a steady run on the country roads near her home. She loves this time alone when she can reflect on the day's events and let all her worries fade away as she concentrates on her body's physical activity. Today she runs at an easy pace for a few miles, winding her way up and down some gradual inclines, taking in the pure country air at dusk. As she rounds the corner to the road her house is on, she wonders how fast and for how long she can sprint. She sizes up the distance of the long, straight road that will take her home—she can barely see her house from here—and decides to go for it. She kicks it into high gear and runs as if there is no tomorrow. The breeze hits her briskly in the face and she enjoys a moment of pure exhilaration. She barely makes it all the way to her house, though, and gasps for air as she walks around her front yard, trying to recover from the all-out sprint. She's never run that fast for that far before, and she's thrilled with her accomplishment.

1. Before Jenna goes out for her run, while she is at rest, what are the mechanics of pulmonary ventilation (including inspiration and expiration), pulmonary diffusion, the transport of oxygen and carbon dioxide, and gas exchange at the muscles?

2. How do each of the activities in question 1 change as Jenna starts her run?

3. What factors influence the changes in respiration, gas exchange at the alveoli, oxygen and carbon dioxide transport, arterial-venous oxygen difference, oxygen delivery and uptake, and carbon dioxide removal during Jenna's steady-state run?

4. Before Jenna starts her run, how is her pulmonary ventilation being regulated? How does this change as she begins her run?

5. Describe what likely happens to Jenna's volume of air ventilated, oxygen consumed by the tissues, and amount of carbon dioxide produced during her initial few miles, where she is running at a steady pace.

6. Describe what likely happens to Jenna's volume of air ventilated, oxygen consumed by the tissues, and amount of carbon dioxide produced during her final sprint, when she is exercising at near-maximal levels.

9. In what ways did Jenna's respiratory system probably help to regulate her acid-base balance both during and immediately after exercise?

10. What are some techniques and breathing problems that could have limited Jenna's performance? Describe the physiological consequences these techniques and problems have for exercise.

Sample Test Questions for Chapter 8

Test yourself on your knowledge of this chapter by taking this self-test. Write the correct answers on a separate sheet of paper.

Multiple Choice

1. An increased PCO_2 stimulates the inspiratory center to increase respiration in order to

   a. bring in more oxygen.
   b. rid the body of excess CO_2 and minimize pH changes.
   c. increase the oxygen diffusion capacity.
   d. stabilize the arterial-venous oxygen difference.

2. Which of the following is *not* a result of increased ventilation during exercise?

   a. More air is brought into the lungs.
   b. More oxygen is supplied to help with the muscles' metabolic needs.
   c. Arterial blood PO_2 increases.
   d. Less carbon dioxide is exhaled, helping to maintain the acid-base balance of the blood.

3. As an athlete exercises,

   a. the ability to unload oxygen to the muscles decreases as the muscle pH decreases.
   b. CO_2 concentration decreases because of increased metabolism.
   c. the contact time of blood and the alveolar air increases.
   d. blood temperature rises slightly, causing hemoglobin to unload oxygen more efficiently.

4. The goal of respiration is to

   a. help to slow heart activity.
   b. decrease ventilation so that less chemical stimulation occurs.
   c. maintain appropriate levels of the blood and tissue gases and maintain proper pH for normal cellular function.
   d. reduce the rate of metabolism.

True-False

5. As the rate of oxygen use decreases, the arterial-venous oxygen difference (a-$\bar{v}O_2$ diff) increases.

6. Gases move from an area of low partial pressure to an area of high partial pressure.

7. Oxygen diffusion capacity increases as you move from rest to exercise.

8. During exercise, the initial immediate rise in ventilation is caused by the mechanics of body movement and not chemical stimulation.

9. Pulmonary ventilation is often a limiting factor for performance in moderately trained people.

Fill in the Blank

10. Pulmonary diffusion replenishes _____ and removes _____.

11. The arterial-venous oxygen difference reflects an increased extraction of oxygen from _____ blood by active muscle, thus decreasing the oxygen content of the _____ blood.

12. When the lungs' stretch receptors sense an excessive stretch, that information is relayed to _____, which responds by _____ the duration of an inspiration, thereby decreasing the risk of _____.

13. About 15% of the body's total oxygen consumption during heavy exercise can occur in the _____ muscles.

Short Answer

14. What are the advantages of breathing through the nose as opposed to breathing through the mouth?

15. How is it that carbon dioxide binding to hemoglobin and oxygen binding to hemoglobin do not compete with each other?

16. Describe the role of lung pressure and atmospheric pressure during inspiration and expiration.

17. Where does pulmonary diffusion occur?

18. Why is hyperventilation not recommended before a dive?

Essay

19. How is the majority of carbon dioxide transported in the blood? Why is this so? What process takes place so that the carbon dioxide can enter the alveoli and be exhaled?

20. Describe the relationships among the ventilatory breakpoint, the anaerobic threshold, and the lactate threshold. Why would an athlete be interested in knowing his or her anaerobic threshold for a given intensity of activity?

Answers to Selected Chapter 8 Activities

8.1 Anatomy of Respiratory System and Pathway of Pulmonary Ventilation

a. Primary bronchii; b. Nasal cavity; c. Pharynx; d. Larynx; e. Trachea; f. Bronchiole; g. Lung; h. Alveolus; i. Pulmonary capillaries; j. Capillary network on surface of alveolus

8.2   Inspiration and Expiration

	Inspiration	Expiration
An active process involving the diaphragm and the external intercostal muscles.	X	
The ribs and sternum are moved by the external intercostal muscles: The ribs swing up and out, and the sternum swings up and forward.	X	
The diaphragm contracts, flattening down toward the abdomen.	X	
The lungs expand, causing lung pressure to be less than atmospheric pressure.	X	
Air rushes into the lungs to balance the pressure.	X	
During forced or labored breathing, this action is further assisted by muscles that help raise the ribs even more than during regular breathing.	X	
At rest, a passive process, involving the relaxation of the inspiratory muscles and elastic recoil of the lung tissue.		X
The diaphragm relaxes, returning to its normal upward, arched position.		X
The external intercostal muscles relax, and the ribs and sternum lower to heir resting positions.		X
The lung recoils to its resting size, increasing the pressure in the thorax.		X
Air is forced out of the lungs to balance pressure.		X
During forced breathing, this action becomes more active, with the internal intercostal muscles actively pulling the ribs down.		X

8.3   Pulmonary Diffusion

1. The alveolar wall, the capillary wall, and their membrane structures make up the respiratory membrane.

2. A partial pressure is the individual pressure of a gas in a mixture of several gases.

3. Dalton's law states that the total pressure of a mixture of gases equals the sum of the partial pressures of the individual gases in that mixture.

4. Differences in the partial pressures of the gases in the alveoli and the gases in the blood create a pressure gradient across the respiratory membrane. Gases diffuse along a pressure gradient, moving from an area of higher pressure to one of lower

pressure. At the respiratory membrane, oxygen *enters* the blood because the alveolar oxygen has a higher partial pressure than the oxygen in the returning blood, and carbon dioxide *leaves* the blood because carbon dioxide's partial pressure in the venous blood is greater than the pressure of the carbon dioxide in alveolar air.

5. The oxygen diffusion capacity is the rate at which oxygen diffuses from the alveoli into the blood.

6. At rest, about 23 ml of oxygen diffuse into the pulmonary blood each minute for each mmHg of pressure difference between the alveoli and pulmonary capillary blood. During maximal exercise, the oxygen diffusion capacity may increase to 50 ml/minute or higher, up to two to three times the resting rate.

7. At rest, the circulation through the lungs is relatively inefficient and sluggish, primarily due to limited perfusion of the upper regions of the lungs because gravity. During maximal exercise, however, blood flow through the lungs is greater, primarily due to elevated blood pressure, thereby increasing lung perfusion.

8. Answers may vary. One possibility is to cover the glass with red water with cellophane and to cut very large holes in the cellophane. The red water would represent the carbon dioxide returning in the blood to the lungs, whereas the blue water would still represent the alveolar air. When the glass with red water is turned upside down on top of the glass with blue water, the large holes will allow for a faster exchange, symbolizing carbon dioxide's high membrane solubility.

8.4 Transport and Exchange of Oxygen and Carbon Dioxide

1. A decrease in pH, meaning the blood is becoming more acidic, causes the dissociation curve to shift to the right. This indicates that more oxygen is being unloaded from the hemoglobin at the tissue level, thereby supplying needed oxygen to tissues, as could be needed during exercise.

2. Increased blood temperature also shifts the dissociation curve to the right, indicating that oxygen is unloaded more efficiently at higher temperatures.

3. With exercise, the temperature in the exercising muscle increases and the pH decreases, due to increased hydrogen ion concentration. This causes more oxygen to be unloaded to supply the active muscle, meaning the oxygen-hemoglobin dissociation curve shifts to the right.

4. The bar graph on the left, with only slightly higher oxygen content of arterial blood is typical of a subject at rest; only 4 to 5 ml of oxygen per 100 ml of blood is being taken up by the tissues. On the other hand, the bar graph on the right is likely of a subject who is exercising; about 12 ml of oxygen per 100 ml of blood is being taken up by the tissues.

5.

- An 80% hemoglobin saturation is substantially lower than the usual 98% saturation. This low hemoglobin saturation would hinder oxygen delivery and reduce cellular uptake of oxygen.

- Increased blood flow would improve oxygen delivery and uptake.

- Increased muscle acidity would increase oxygen unloading from the hemoglobin molecule, facilitating oxygen delivery and uptake by the muscles.

- Decreased muscle temperature would decrease oxygen unloading from the hemoglobin molecule, hindering oxygen delivery and uptake by the muscles.

8.5 Regulation of Pulmonary Ventilation

1. e;   2. c;   3. b;   4. f;   5. d;   6. a

8.6 Pulmonary Ventilation During Exercise

1. See page 261 of *Physiology of Sport and Exercise* for an example of the general trend this graph should show.

2. The first phase shows an almost immediate, marked increase in pulmonary ventilation. This is likely caused by the mechanics of body movement, because it occurs before the results of any chemical stimulation can be seen. The second phase shows a more gradual increase in pulmonary ventilation and is produced by changes in the temperature and chemical status of the arterial blood. (See page 261 of *Physiology of Sport and Exercise* for more details.)

3. If the rate of breathing perfectly matched the metabolic demands of tissues, respiration would drop to the resting level within seconds after exercise. Because respiratory recovery takes several minutes, it is likely that postexercise breathing is regulated primarily by acid-base balance, PCO_2, and blood temperature.

4. The ventilatory equivalent for oxygen, or $\dot{V}E/\dot{V}O_2$, is the ratio between the volume of air ventilated ($\dot{V}E$) and the amount of oxygen consumed by the tissues ($\dot{V}O_2$) in a given amount of time. It is usually measured in liters of air breathed per liter of oxygen consumed per minute.

5. The graph for submaximal, steady-state exercise should show $\dot{V}E/\dot{V}O_2$ to be relatively stable or constant. The graph for heavy, near-maximal exercise should show a $\dot{V}E/\dot{V}O_2$ that increases rather sharply. The graph for incremental exercise should show a $\dot{V}E/\dot{V}O_2$ that remains relatively stable for quite a while and then, at the ventilatory breakpoint, rises markedly.

6. If the $\dot{V}E/\dot{V}O_2$ remains relatively constant, the control systems for breathing are properly matched to the body's need for oxygen.

7. If the $\dot{V}E/\dot{V}O_2$ increases, oxygen delivery to the muscles is no longer supporting the oxygen requirements of oxidation, and respiration is increasing to help remove excess carbon dioxide produced through glycolysis.

8. The ventilatory breakpoint is the point at which ventilation abruptly increases, even though oxygen consumption does not.

9. The lines on your graph should look similar to those shown in figure 8.10 on page 264 of *Physiology of Sport and Exercise*. The arrow should be pointing to the point on the "ventilation" line where ventilation starts to increase disproportionately as compared to the "oxygen uptake" line.

10. At the ventilatory breakpoint, oxygen delivery to the muscles can no longer support the oxygen requirements of oxidation. To compensate, more energy is derived from glycolysis, which results in increased carbon dioxide levels. The excess carbon dioxide stimulates the chemoreceptors that signal the inspiratory center to increase ventilation. Ventilation increases in order to remove excess carbon dioxide. (See page 264 of *Physiology of Sport and Exercise* for more details.)

11. The most accurate way to estimate anaerobic threshold is to identify the point at which there is a systematic increase in $\dot{V}E/\dot{V}O_2$ without a concomitant increase in $\dot{V}E/\dot{V}CO_2$.

12. The line representing $\dot{V}E/\dot{V}CO_2$ during incremental exercise should be relatively stable, though some decrease may occur. The point where the $\dot{V}E/\dot{V}O_2$ starts to increase sharply, when the $\dot{V}E/\dot{V}CO_2$ is remaining relatively constant, is the anaerobic threshold.

13. Though the relationship is not always exact, the anaerobic threshold reflects the lactate threshold under most conditions. Recall that the lactate threshold is the point at which blood lactate begins to accumulate above resting levels during a graded exercise test.

8.7   Respiratory Limitations and Breathing Problems During Exercise

1. b;   2. d;   3. b

Answers to Selected Chapter 8 Test Questions

Multiple Choice

1. b;   2. d;   3. d;   4. c

True-False

5. False;   6. False;   7. True;   8. True;   9. False

Fill in the Blank

10. the blood's oxygen supply, carbon dioxide from returning venous blood

11. arterial, venous

12. expiratory center, decreasing/shortening; overinflating the respiratory structures

13. respiratory

Short Answer and Essay

For questions 14 to 20, check your answers against the explanations given in the textbook.

Cardiorespiratory Adaptations to Training

concepts

- Cardiorespiratory endurance is the ability of the whole body to sustain prolonged exercise. It is highly related to aerobic development and should be the foundation of any athlete's general conditioning program.

- $\dot{V}O_2$max—the highest rate of oxygen consumption obtainable during maximal or exhaustive exercise—increases substantially following training. Most sport scientists regard $\dot{V}O_2$max to be the best indicator of cardiorespiratory endurance.

- The cardiovascular system responds to training with general improvements in heart size, stroke volume, heart rate, cardiac output, blood flow, blood pressure, and blood volume.

- Because the respiratory system is already quite adept at bringing adequate amounts of oxygen into the body, the major respiratory system training adaptations are apparent only during maximal exercise, when all systems are being maximally stressed.

- Endurance training increases lactate threshold, allowing performance at higher rates of work and levels of oxygen consumption without increasing blood lactate above resting levels.

- A significant response to aerobic training is more likely with an initial low level of conditioning, high genetic $\dot{V}O_2$max boundary and response level, younger age, male sex, specificity of training, and appropriate cross-training.

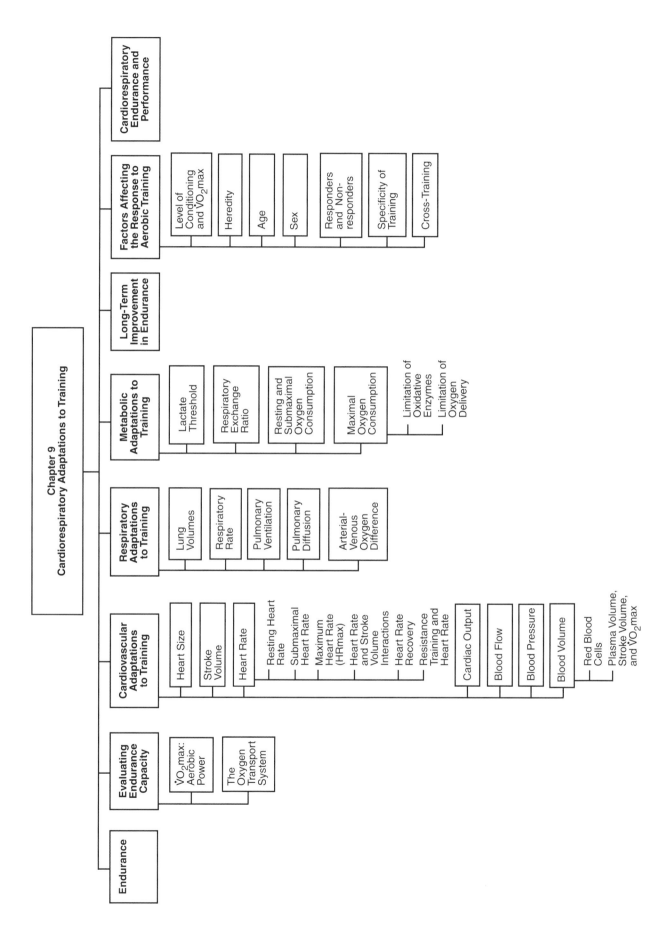

Chapter 9
Cardiorespiratory Adaptations to Training

Endurance

Evaluating Endurance Capacity
- $\dot{V}O_2$max: Aerobic Power
- The Oxygen Transport System

Cardiovascular Adaptations to Training
- Heart Size
- Stroke Volume
- Heart Rate
  - Resting Heart Rate
  - Submaximal Heart Rate
  - Maximum Heart Rate (HRmax)
  - Heart Rate and Stroke Volume Interactions
  - Heart Rate Recovery
  - Resistance Training and Heart Rate
- Cardiac Output
- Blood Flow
- Blood Pressure
- Blood Volume
  - Red Blood Cells
  - Plasma Volume, Stroke Volume, and $\dot{V}O_2$max

Respiratory Adaptations to Training
- Lung Volumes
- Respiratory Rate
- Pulmonary Ventilation
- Pulmonary Diffusion
- Arterial-Venous Oxygen Difference

Metabolic Adaptations to Training
- Lactate Threshold
- Respiratory Exchange Ratio
- Resting and Submaximal Oxygen Consumption
- Maximal Oxygen Consumption
  - Limitation of Oxidative Enzymes
  - Limitation of Oxygen Delivery

Long-Term Improvement in Endurance

Factors Affecting the Response to Aerobic Training
- Level of Conditioning and $\dot{V}O_2$max
- Heredity
- Age
- Sex
- Responders and Non-responders
- Specificity of Training
- Cross-Training

Cardiorespiratory Endurance and Performance

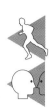

Activity 9.1

What Is Endurance?

Do this activity after reading pages 276-278 of *Physiology of Sport and Exercise*.

Endurance is actually a reflection of both muscular endurance and cardiorespiratory endurance. Do the following activities to learn the difference between these two aspects of endurance.

Muscular Endurance

Take the time to do as many outer thigh lifts as you can. Be sure to use correct form: Lie on your side, with your lower arm outstretched and your head resting on this arm. Place the other arm across your torso, and put that hand flat on the floor to stabilize you. Both legs are outstretched so that your body forms a straight line. Slowly raise the top leg. You do not need to raise it very high; focus on control rather than height. Slowly lower the top leg. Raise and lower this leg as many times as you can until you can no longer perform the exercise.

What caused you to have to stop doing the thigh lifts? More than likely, it was fatigue of a particular muscle group—probably the vastus lateralis in your outer thigh—that kept you from performing any more thigh lifts. Had this particular muscle group not worn out, you could have continued with the exercise. This is a good example of pushing your *muscular endurance* to its limits.

Cardiorespiratory Endurance

This chapter concentrates on cardiorespiratory endurance, which is the ability of the whole body to sustain prolonged exercise. Think back to a time when you performed an activity at a fairly fast pace over a long distance and ended up feeling fatigued all over. It wasn't just one muscle group that ran out of steam—your whole body felt exhausted. Perhaps you cycled a lengthy bicycle trail, mountain biked a challenging course, ran a competitive road race, swam across a lake at a camp, went cross-country skiing or inline skating, or something of that nature.

Write notes about that experience on a separate piece of paper, commenting especially on how your body felt upon reaching the state of overall fatigue. This is an example of pushing your *cardiorespiratory endurance* to its limits. Chapter 9 of *Physiology of Sport and Exercise* focuses entirely on this aspect of endurance.

Cardiovascular Adaptations to Training

Activity 9.2

Do this activity after reading pages 278-291 of *Physiology of Sport and Exercise*.

Cardiorespiratory endurance is the ability of the whole body to sustain prolonged exercise. The cardiovascular system plays a key role in oxygen transport and adapts quite remarkably to endurance training. Fill out the table on the next three pages, based on information found in your textbook, to see what types of changes your cardiovascular system makes in response to endurance training.

Activity 9.2 **Cardiovascular Adaptations to Training**

Parameter	Increase or decrease? (Use ↑, ↓ or ↔)	Notes for studying purposes
Heart's weight		
Heart volume		
Myocardial wall thickness, especially of the left ventricle		
Stroke volume		
Resting heart rate		
Heart rate during submaximal exercise		

Parameter	Increase or decrease? (Use ↑, ↓ or ↔)	Notes for studying purposes
Maximum heart rate (HRmax)		
Heart rate recovery period		
Cardiac output at rest and during submaximal exercise		
Cardiac output during maximal exercise		
Blood flow to muscles		List the four reasons for increased blood flow:

(continued)

(continued)

Parameter	Increase or decrease? decrease? (Use ↑, ↓ or ↔)	Notes for studying purposes
Blood pressure during submaximal and maximal exercise		
Blood pressure at rest, if borderline or moderately hypertensive before training		
Blood volume		
Red blood cell volume		
Blood plasma volume		

For an extra challenge . . . See the discussion of heart rate and stroke volume interactions on page 285 of *Physiology of Sport and Exercise*. An unanswered question for exercise physiologists is, Which comes first—does increased stroke volume allow a decreased heart rate, or does decreased heart rate allow an increased stroke volume?

Spend some time researching this in scholarly journals, and then prepare to debate this with your classmates, backing up your assertions with reasoned and documented arguments.

Activity 9.3

Respiratory Adaptations to Training

Do this activity after reading pages 291-293 of *Physiology of Sport and Exercise*.

No matter how efficient the cardiovascular system is at supplying adequate amounts of blood to the tissues, endurance would be hindered if the respiratory system didn't bring in enough oxygen to meet oxygen demands. Because it is already quite adept at bringing adequate amounts of oxygen into the body, it shows quite different responses to endurance training than does the cardiovascular system. Fill out the table below, based on information found in your textbook, to see what types of changes your respiratory system makes in response to endurance training.

Parameter	Increase or decrease? (Use ↑, ↓ or ↔)	Notes for studying purposes
Vital capacity		
Residual volume		
Total lung capacity		
Tidal volume at rest and during submaximal exercise		
Tidal volume at rest and during submaximal exercise		
Respiratory rate at rest and during submaximal exercise.		
Respiratory rate during maximal exercise		

(continued)

(*continued*)

Parameter	Increase or decrease? (Use ↑, ↓ or ↔)	Notes for studying purposes
Pulmonary ventilation at rest and during sub-maximal exercise		
Pulmonary ventilation during maximal exercise		
Pulmonary diffusion at rest and during submaximal exercise		
Pulmonary diffusion during maximal exercise		
Oxygen content of arterial blood		
a-$\bar{v}O_2$diff		

Activity 9.4

Metabolic Adaptations to Training

Do this activity after reading pages 293-297 of *Physiology of Sport and Exercise*.

The cardiovascular and respiratory systems integrate with metabolism in the active tissues to improve the delivery and use of oxygen. Fill out the table below, based on information found in your textbook, to see what types of metabolic changes your body makes in response to endurance training.

Parameter	Increase or decrease? (Use ↑, ↓ or ↔)	Notes for studying purposes
Lactate threshold		
RER during submaximal exercise		
RER during maximal exercise		
Oxygen consumption ($\dot{V}O_2$) at rest		
Oxygen consumption ($\dot{V}O_2$) during submaximal exercise		
Maximal oxygen consumption $\dot{V}O_2$max		

For an extra challenge . . . Research the arguments of the utilization theory and the presentation theory (see page 295 of *Physiology of Sport and Exercise*). Listed below are some possible sources. Explain why researchers came to view the presentation theory as more accurate.

Clausen, J.P. (1977). Effect of physical training on cardiovascular adjustments to exercise in man. *Physiological Reviews, 57,* 779-816.

Coyle, E.F. (1995). Integration of the physiological factors determining endurance performance ability. *Exercise and Sport Science Reviews, 23,* 25-63.

Holloszy, J.O., & Coyle, E.F. (1984). Adaptations of skeletal muscle to endurance exercise and their metabolic consequences. *Journal of Applied Physiology, 56,* 831-838.

Saltin, B., & Rowell, L.B. (1980). Functional adaptations to physical activity and inactivity. *Federation Proceedings, 39,* 1506-1513.

Factors Affecting the Response to Aerobic Training

Activity 9.5

Do this activity after reading pages 297-303 of *Physiology of Sport and Exercise*.

Even though many generalizations hold true in how the body adapts to endurance training, not everyone responds in the same way. Several factors can affect individual response to aerobic training. Read each of the case studies and answer the questions that follow them on a separate piece of paper.

> Debra, age 19, and her father, Jack, age 41, are training to run a 5K together. The race is in early September, and they began training together in early June, at the beginning of Debra's summer break from college. Jack has been running in road races for 10 years, and he's thrilled that his daughter is taking an interest in his avocation. He finds the training easy and always has. He distinctly remembers how quickly he improved his race times in the first year and a half of competing. Debra, on the other hand, finds the training a challenge, although she can tell that she is quickly improving in her ability to run longer and at a faster pace.

1. During the training period for this particular race, who do you think will show the most improvement in $\dot{V}O_2$max? Why?

2. a. It is unlikely that most recreational runners reach their highest attainable $\dot{V}O_2$max. But when do you believe Jack reached a peak $\dot{V}O_2$max?

    b. Why did you select the answer you did?

    c. If Jack's performances continued to improve for several years without a concurrent improvement in $\dot{V}O_2$max, what would account for his improved race times?

3. a. What factors will likely benefit Debra's response to aerobic training?

    b. What factors might hinder her response?

    c. Given these positive and negative factors, summarize how you think Debra will respond overall to the training.

Josh is a recreational triathlete. He finds several minitriathlons in which to compete in his region of the country each summer and fall. Although the lengths of each portion of the triathlons vary from event to event, Josh looks for mini-triathlons with 0.25- to 1-mi swims, 10- to 15-mi bikes, and 4- to 8-mi runs. Josh trains three times a week, working in the training sessions around his busy work schedule. In a typical training session, Josh bikes 5 to 10 mi and runs 2 to 4 mi. Because he doesn't have access to a pool, Josh doesn't get in any actual swimming training. To compensate for this, he trains with weights three times a week, focusing on upper body strength, thinking that this will at least help him have strong enough arm and shoulder muscles for the swim.

4. Given Josh's training program, which portions of the minitriathlons will Josh be most successful at? Least successful? Why?

5. Focus for a moment on Josh's resistance training. What philosophies need to be considered before including resistance training in an overall endurance training program? Why might Josh not get the full benefit (muscular strength) from his resistance training?

6. How would you modify Josh's training program to optimize his performance?

Activity 9.6

The Consequences of Not Training for Endurance

Do this activity after reading pages 303-305 of *Physiology of Sport and Exercise.*

Many people consider cardiorespiratory endurance to be the most important component of physical fitness. Yet many athletes and coaches of sports that seem nonendurance in nature fail to recognize the benefits of endurance training.

On a separate sheet of paper, explain how not training adequately for endurance could impact people participating in the following activities.

1. An offensive player on a soccer team

2. A defensive lineman in American football

3. A golfer

4. A mountain biker

5. The personal trainer at a fitness club

For each situation, be sure to comment on

- muscular strength,
- reaction and movement times,
- agility and neuromuscular coordination,
- whole-body movement speed, and
- concentration and alertness.

Putting It All Together: Cardiorespiratory Adaptations to Training

Do this activity after reading chapter 9 of *Physiology of Sport and Exercise.*

With repeated bouts of endurance training, the cardiorespiratory system adapts to improve the body's performance of endurance activities. Perhaps improved endurance capacity is a goal of yours. Even if not, endurance training produces tremendous health benefits. In answering these questions on a separate piece of paper, you will not only design an endurance training program for yourself, but you will be challenged to recall what you have learned in this chapter about how the body responds to endurance training.

1. Which rating best describes your current level of cardiorespiratory endurance: High; medium; low?

2. Briefly design a training program to improve your cardiorespiratory endurance in order to help you improve your performance in your favorite sport or endurance activity.

3. Given your heredity, age, sex, current level of conditioning, and whether you believe you are a responder or a nonresponder, how quickly do you think your body will respond and what level of improvement in cardiorespiratory endurance would you expect to gain with the training program you have outlined?

4. Briefly note the changes you would expect in these areas if you followed your training program (even if you do not write notes for all of these, for studying purposes make sure you know all of the responses your body would make to endurance training):

Cardiovascular adaptations

Heart size

Stroke volume

Heart rate

Cardiac output

Blood flow

Blood pressure

Blood volume

Metabolic adaptations

Lactate threshold

Respiratory exchange ratio

Oxygen consumption

    At rest

    Submaximal

    Maximal

Respiratory adaptations

Lung volume

Respiratory rate

Pulmonary ventilation

Pulmonary diffusion

Arterial-venous oxygen difference

Sample Test Questions for Chapter 9

Test yourself on your knowledge of this chapter by taking this self-test. Write the correct answers on a separate sheet of paper.

Multiple Choice

1. If you increase your exercise intensity beyond the point at which you reach $\dot{V}O_2$max,

   a. you will continue to be able to exercise effectively, because your body will continue to meet the oxygen demands of your muscles.
   b. your coordination will improve because the increased oxygen will stimulate efficient functioning of the muscles.
   c. the end of your exercise bout is near because your oxygen consumption will either plateau or decrease, meaning you can't deliver oxygen as quickly as needed to reach your muscles' demands.
   d. your blood pressure will plummet drastically, causing dizziness and fatigue.

2. Megan is an avid cross-country skier. She trains several days a week year-round, skiing outdoors in the winter months and using a cross-country skiing machine in the off-season. Megan's cardiovascular system has probably adapted in these ways:

   a. Increased stroke volume, increased resting heart rate, an increased heart rate recovery period upon finishing exercising, and increased blood flow to the muscles.
   b. Decreased heart weight and volume, decreased resting heart rate, and increased blood flow to the muscles.
   c. Increased cardiac output at rest, decreased red blood cell volume, a decreased heart rate recovery period, and decreased blood flow to the muscles.
   d. Increased stroke volume, decreased resting heart rate, a decreased heart rate recovery period after finishing exercising, and increased blood flow to the muscles.

3. A person with bradycardia likely has

   a. abnormal cardiac function or a diseased heart.
   b. a highly conditioned heart.
   c. an extremely high resting heart rate.
   d. Either a or c.

4. Craig is a long-distance cyclist who trains year round. He has probably experienced these respiratory adaptations due to his training:

   a. Decreases in tidal volume, pulmonary ventilation, pulmonary diffusion, and respiratory rate at maximal levels of exercise.
   b. Increases in tidal volume, pulmonary ventilation, pulmonary diffusion, and respiratory rate at maximal levels of exercise.
   c. Decreases in tidal volume, pulmonary ventilation, pulmonary diffusion, and respiratory rate at submaximal levels of exercise.
   d. None of the above.

5. Four people enter the same training program, having the following conditions. Which one will likely experience the greatest cardiorespiratory responses to training?

   a. Subject A, who has an initial high level of conditioning, is the second youngest of the subjects, is male, and whose immediate family has a high $\dot{V}O_2$max.
   b. Subject B, who has an initial low level of conditioning, is the youngest of the subjects, is male, and whose immediate family has a high $\dot{V}O_2$max.
   c. Subject C, who has an initial low level of conditioning, is the oldest of the subjects, is female, and whose immediate family has a low $\dot{V}O_2$max.
   d. Subject D, who has an initial high level of conditioning, is the second oldest of the subjects, is male, and whose immediate family has a low $\dot{V}O_2$max.

6. Which would be the best activity during which to test the $\dot{V}O_2$max of a competitive cyclist?

a. Running uphill on a treadmill.

b. Stair stepping.

c. Rowing on a rowing machine.

d. Pedaling a cycle ergometer.

True-False

7. Cardiorespiratory endurance is the ability of one muscle group to sustain prolonged exercise.

8. The left ventricular wall becomes thicker only with resistance training.

9. Resting and submaximal oxygen consumption greatly increases following endurance training.

10. Maximal oxygen consumption ($\dot{V}O_2$max) is limited primarily by the oxygen transport to the working muscles, not the available mitochondria and oxidative enzymes.

11. The higher the initial state of conditioning, the smaller the relative improvement in $\dot{V}O_2$max for the same program of training.

Fill in the Blank

12. If a person's stroke volume is 83 ml, heart rate is 72, and a-$\bar{v}O_2$ diff is 8 ml O_2 per 100 ml blood, that person's $\dot{V}O_2$ is _____. The resulting value tells us the rate at which _____ is being consumed by the body tissues.

13. Training may cause a(n) _____ [increase, decrease] in the number of red blood cells and a(n) _____ [increase, decrease] in the ratio of red blood cell volume to total blood volume. This reduces the blood's _____, thereby enhancing _____ delivery to the active muscles.

14. After endurance training, a person's lactate threshold will occur at a _____ [higher, lower] speed than it did prior to training.

Short Answer

15. Define $\dot{V}O_2$max.

16. List the four factors that account for enhanced blood flow to muscles following training. Why is this one of the most important cardiorespiratory adaptations to endurance training?

17. What is the most likely cause of improved performance if an athlete continues to improve his or her performance without experiencing an increase in $\dot{V}O_2$max?

Essay

18. Explain the mechanisms that lead to the overall increase of stroke volume as a result of endurance training.

19. Describe the interaction between heart rate and stroke volume in providing an appropriate cardiac output for a given rate of work. What is the ultimate purpose of changes in heart rate and stroke volume in response to training?

20. Present three examples of respiratory responses that take place only at maximal exercise levels, and explain why each of these responses occurs only at maximal exercise levels.

21. Given what you have learned in this chapter, how would your cardiorespiratory system respond to detraining?

Answers to Selected Chapter 9 Activities

9.2 Cardiovascular Adaptations to Training

Parameter	Increase or decrease? (Use ↑, ↓ or ↔)	Notes for studying purposes
Heart's weight	↑	
Heart volume	↑	
Myocardial wall thickness, especially of the left ventricle	↑	
Stroke volume	↑	
Resting heart rate	↓	
Heart rate during submaximal exercise	↓	
Maximum heart rate (HRmax)	↔ or ↓	
Heart rate recovery period	↓	
Cardiac output at rest and during sub-maximal exercise	↔ or ↓	
Cardiac output during maximal exercise	↑	
Blood flow to muscles	↑	List the four reasons for increased blood flow: 1. Increase capillarization of trained muscles 2. Greater opening of existing capillaries in trained muscles 3. More effective blood redistribution (diverted to active muscles) 4. Increased blood volume
Blood pressure during submaximal and maximal exercise	↔	
Blood pressure at rest, if borderline or moderately hyper-tensive before training	↓	
Blood volume	↑	
Red blood cell volume	↑	
Blood plasma volume	↑	

9.3 Respiratory Adaptations to Training

Parameter	Increase or decrease? (Use ↑, ↓ or ↔)	Notes for studying purposes
Vital capacity	↑	
Residual volume	↓	
Total lung capacity	↔	
Tidal volume at rest submaximal exercise	↔	
Tidal volume during maximal exercise	↑	
Respiratory rate at rest and during sub-maximal exercise	↓	
Respiratory rate during maximal exercise	↑	
Pulmonary ventilation at rest and during sub-maximal exercise	↔ or ↓	
Pulmonary ventilation during maximal exercise	↑	
Pulmonary diffusion at rest and during sub-maximal exercise	↔	
Pulmonary diffusion during maximal exercise	↑	
Oxygen content of arterial blood	↔	
a-$\bar{v}O_2$ diff	↑	

9.4   Metabolic Adaptations to Training

Parameter	Increase or decrease? (Use ↑, ↓ or ↔)	Notes for studying purposes
Lactate threshold	↑	
Respiratory exchange ratio during submaximal exercise	↓	
Respiratory exchange ratio during maximal exercise	↑	
Oxygen consumption ($\dot{V}O_2$) at rest	↑ or ↔	
Oxygen consumption ($\dot{V}O_2$) during submaximal exercise	↔ or ↓	
Maximal oxygen consumption ($\dot{V}O_2$max)	↑	

Answers to Selected Chapter 9 Test Questions

Multiple Choice

1. c;   2. d;   3. d;   4. b;   5. b;   6. d

True-False

7. False;   8. False;   9. False;   10. True;   11. True

Fill in the Blank

12. 4.78 L, oxygen; see the Fick equation on page 278 of *Physiology of Sport and Exercise*.

13. increase, decrease, viscosity, oxygen

14. higher

Short Answer and Essay

For questions 15 to 21, check your answers against the explanations given in the textbook.

Thermoregulation and Exercise

concepts

- Body heat is transferred by conduction, convection, radiation, and evaporation. At rest, most heat is lost via radiation, but during exercise, evaporation becomes the most important avenue of heat loss.

- When body temperature fluctuates, normal temperature can usually be restored by the actions of the sweat glands, the smooth muscle around the arterioles, the skeletal muscles, and several endocrine glands.

- During exercise in the heat, the heat loss mechanisms compete with the active muscles for more of the limited blood volume. Thus, neither area is adequately supplied under extreme conditions.

- Air temperature alone is not an accurate index of the total physiological stress imposed on the body in a hot environment. Humidity, air velocity, and amount of thermal radiation also contribute to the total heat stress of exercising in the heat.

- Heat cramps, heat exhaustion, and heat stroke can result from the combination of external heat stress and the inability to dissipate metabolically generated heat. Repeated exposure to heat stress causes heat acclimatization—a gradual improvement in the ability to lose excess heat.

- The primary means by which our bodies avoid excessive cooling are shivering, nonshivering thermogenesis, and peripheral vasoconstriction. Because these mechanisms are often inadequate, we must also rely on clothing, muscles, and subcutaneous fat to help insulate our deep body tissues from the environment.

- Hypothermia and frostbite can result from cold stress. Repeated exposure to the cold may alter peripheral blood flow and skin temperatures, allowing greater cold tolerance.

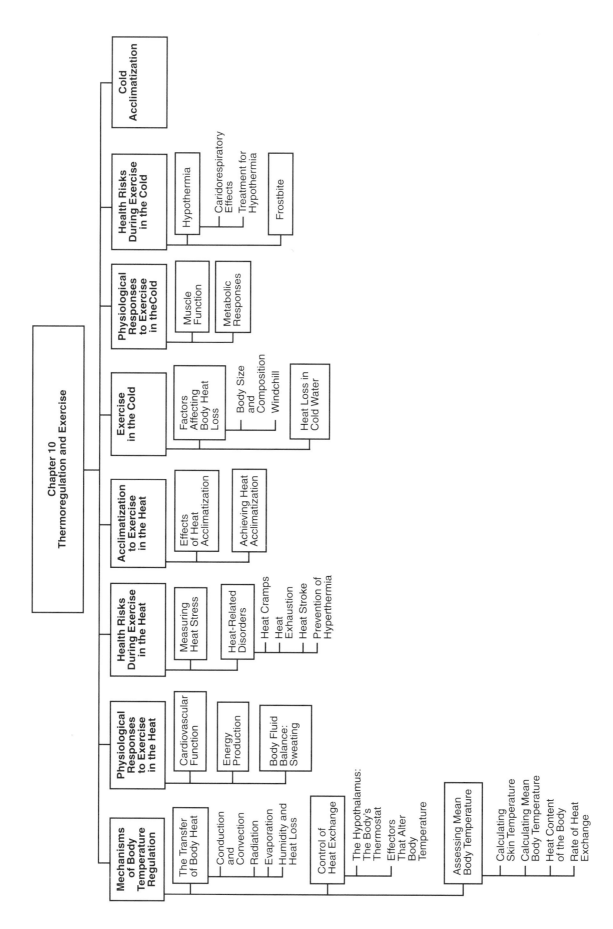

Chapter 10
Thermoregulation and Exercise

Mechanisms of Body Temperature Regulation

The Transfer of Body Heat
└─ Conduction and Convection
└─ Radiation
└─ Evaporation
└─ Humidity and Heat Loss

Control of Heat Exchange
└─ The Hypothalamus: The Body's Thermostat
└─ Effectors That Alter Body Temperature

Assessing Mean Body Temperature
└─ Calculating Skin Temperature
└─ Calculating Mean Body Temperature
└─ Heat Content of the Body
└─ Rate of Heat Exchange

Physiological Responses to Exercise in the Heat

Cardiovascular Function

Energy Production

Body Fluid Balance: Sweating

Health Risks During Exercise in the Heat

Measuring Heat Stress

Heat-Related Disorders
└─ Heat Cramps
└─ Heat Exhaustion
└─ Heat Stroke
└─ Prevention of Hyperthermia

Acclimatization to Exercise in the Heat

Effects of Heat Acclimatization

Achieving Heat Acclimatization

Exercise in the Cold

Factors Affecting Body Heat Loss
└─ Body Size and Composition
└─ Windchill

Heat Loss in Cold Water

Physiological Responses to Exercise in theCold

Muscle Function

Metabolic Responses

Health Risks During Exercise in the Cold

Hypothermia
└─ Caridorespiratory Effects
└─ Treatment for Hypothermia

Frostbite

Cold Acclimatization

Transfer of Body Heat to the Environment

Activity 10.1

Do this activity after reading pages 312-316 of *Physiology of Sport and Exercise*.

For your body to transfer heat to the environment, the heat produced in your body must have access to the outside world. The heat from deep in your body is moved by the blood to your skin. Once heat nears your skin, it can be transferred to the environment through conduction, convection, radiation, or evaporation.

In this activity, you will conduct experiments that create situations of conduction, convection, radiation, and evaporation. Do the activities as directed, and, on separate paper, answer the questions interspersed between experiments.

Conduction

Get an ice cube from the freezer, or, if you don't have access to an ice cube, get some crushed ice from a soda dispenser or fast-food restaurant. Place the ice cube or crushed ice directly on your hand.

1. What happens to the ice?

2. What caused the ice to melt?

3. At the same time that the temperature of the ice changed, how did the temperature of your hand change? What caused this change?

Conduction is the exchange of heat between two substances that are in contact with each other; the heat always moves from the body of higher energy to the body of lower energy. Without taking all of the physiological variables into account, this causes the warmer body to cool and the cooler body to warm until they reach a common equilibrium (Kenneth L. Knight, *Cryotherapy in Sport Injury Management,* Human Kinetics: 1995, p. 64).

Convection

For this experiment, you will need a fan. A fan of any sort will work—you can use a ceiling fan, a pedestal fan, a small personal fan, or even a handmade paper fan.

First, stand still in a room with no fan running. Then turn on the fan (or start fanning yourself with the paper fan). If your mechanical fan has speed settings on it, start it on a low speed, leave it there for a couple of minutes, and then turn it to the highest speed. If you are using a handmade fan, start by fanning yourself slowly for a couple of minutes, and then change to fanning yourself at a faster rate.

4. What difference did you sense in your body or skin temperature when you first turned on the fan?

5. What difference in temperature did you feel when you turned your fan to a higher speed? What principle of convection does this prove?

6. The differences you felt in body temperature were likely the result of convection. Explain what convection is and how it caused your body to cool in this experiment.

7. Explain how conduction and convection can actually cause the body to *gain* heat in a very hot environment, when the surroundings are hotter than the skin.

Radiation

Place the palm of your hand about a quarter inch from your face. There should be some, but not much, air between your hand and your face. Hold this position for a minute or so. You should feel warmth between the two. You might also want to try this with another person, holding the palm of your hand close to, but not touching, the hand of another person.

8. What caused you to feel warmth when you put your hand close to your face?

9. Give an example of the body *receiving* heat from radiation.

Evaporation

Think back to (1) a time when you exercised and barely noticed your sweat and (2) a time when you exercised and were dripping with sweat. Jot some notes about those situations here. What type of exercise were you doing? What was the environment or weather like in each situation?

10. In which instance did you likely lose more body heat through evaporation? In this instance, what environmental conditions probably contributed to your body being able to lose heat through evaporation?

11. In your second example—the one in which you were dripping in sweat—did you feel any cooling effect of the sweat? What environmental conditions likely caused the dripping sweat and prevented evaporation?

12. At rest, through which method of heat transfer is most heat lost?

13. During exercise, through which method of heat transfer is most heat lost?

Control of Heat Exchange

Do this activity after reading pages 316-318 of *Physiology of Sport and Exercise*.

Internal body temperature (measured rectally) at rest is kept at approximately 37 °C (98.6 °F). When the body becomes overheated or when the temperature of the blood and body tissues falls below normal, the body works to bring its temperature back to normal. Read the following scenarios and answer the questions in order to learn how the body regulates its internal temperature.

Chris is going cross-country skiing. Even though it is chilly outside, she dresses in light layers, knowing that her body will heat up quickly and start to sweat in this high-energy activity.

1. List the steps Chris's body will take in order to try to maintain normal body temperature. Be sure to include the roles of both sets of thermoreceptors, the thermoregulatory center, the hypothalamus, the sweat glands, the smooth muscles around the arterioles, the skeletal muscles, and the endocrine glands. Draw a small picture that depicts each step.

2. How will most of Chris's heat be lost?

Mark is going ice fishing, a relatively sedentary outdoor activity. It is very cold outside, and even though Mark dresses as warmly as he can, he knows he will still be quite cold from time to time.

3. List the steps Mark's body will take in order to try to maintain normal body temperature. Be sure to include the roles of both sets of thermoreceptors, the thermoregulatory center, the hypothalamus, the sweat glands, the smooth muscles around the arterioles, the skeletal muscles, and the endocrine glands. Draw a small picture that depicts each step.

4. From what you have learned so far in this chapter, what steps can Mark take to stay warm throughout the day?

Activity 10.3

Assessing Body Temperature

Do this activity after reading pages 318-320 of *Physiology of Sport and Exercise.*

By assessing mean body temperature and the heat content of the body, we can estimate the body's rate of heat exchange. In this activity, you will practice calculating these data, and then you will apply your knowledge by discerning which of two subjects has a higher rate of heat exchange.

Skin Temperature

1. Calculate the average skin temperature, assuming these temperature readings were gained from placing temperature sensors on the skin:

   Arm temperature = 31.7 °C

   Trunk temperature = 32.7 °C

   Leg temperature = 32.3 °C

   Head temperature = 31.5 °C

Mean Body Temperature

2. Define mean body temperature.

3. Using the answer from the previous question and given an average rectal temperature of 37 °C, calculate the mean body temperature of the subject.

Heat Content of the Body

4. Define heat content.

5. Using the average specific heat of body tissues (see page 319 in your textbook), a body weight of 70 kg, and a mean body temperature of 35.2 °C, calculate the heat content of this subject's body.

Rate of Heat Exchange

6. Assume two subjects are exercising.

   Subject A is experiencing these variables in an hour's time:

   Specific heat = 0.83 kcal $\cdot$ kg^{-1} $\cdot$ °C^{-1}

   Body weight = 70 kg

   Temperature change = 2 °C

   Subject B is experiencing these variables in an hour's time:

   Specific heat = 0.98 kcal $\cdot$ kg^{-1} $\cdot$ °C^{-1}

   Body weight = 70 kg

   Temperature change = 7 °C

   Calculate the heat gain of each subject.

7. How is each subject's body doing at dissipating heat? What factors might be affecting each subject's ability to dissipate body heat?

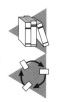

Physiological Responses to Exercise in the Heat

Do this activity after reading pages 320-324 of *Physiology of Sport and Exercise.*

When you exercise in a thermally neutral environment or in a hot environment, the metabolic heat load places a considerable burden on the mechanisms that control body temperature. In this activity, you will explore some of the physiological changes that occur in response to exercise while the body is exposed to heat stress.

First, fill out the table below, based on information found in your textbook, to see what types of changes your cardiovascular and energy production systems make in response to exercising under conditions of heat stress. Then draw a flowchart showing how the body tries to maintain fluid balance when the demands for sweating increase.

> **Activity 10.4**

Parameter	Increase or decrease? (Use ↑, ↓, or ↔)	Notes for studying purposes
Demand for blood flow and oxygen to muscles		
Demand for blood flow to skin		
Volume of blood returning to the heart		
End-diastolic volume		

Parameter	Increase or decrease? (Use ↑, ↓, or ↔)	Notes for studying purposes
Cardiac output		
Stroke volume		
Heart rate		
Body temperature		
Oxygen uptake		
Use of glycogen		

(continued)

(continued)

Parameter	Increase or decrease? (Use ↑, ↓, or ↔)	Notes for studying purposes
Production of muscle lactate		
Sweating		

The mechanisms of sweating and maintaining fluid balance are quite complex. Read pages 322-324 in *Physiology of Sport and Exercise* and then, on a separate piece of paper, construct a flowchart that shows the process of sweating and fluid balance. Start with the temperature of the environment approaching or exceeding skin and deep body temperature, and end with steps related to hormone release and water retention.

Activity 10.5   Heat-Related Disorders

Do this activity after reading pages 324-329 of *Physiology of Sport and Exercise*.

Despite the body's defenses against overheating, certain conditions may elevate the internal body temperature to levels that impair normal cellular functions. Such conditions include excessive heat production by active muscles, heat gained from the environment, and conditions that prevent the dissipation of excess body heat. Exposure to the combination of external heat stress and the inability to dissipate metabolically generated heat can lead to three heat-related disorders: heat cramps, heat exhaustion, and heat stroke.

Read the following case studies. Identify the heat-related disorder the person is suffering from and the appropriate treatment that should be taken.

Valerie is race walking in her first 5K today. After not being physically active for many years, she is glad to be exercising again and really notices the difference it makes in both her physical and emotional well-being. It's a hot summer day, and as the starting gun fires, Valerie wonders if she should have carried a water bottle with her instead of relying only on the water stops along the course. By the midway mark,

Valerie chastises herself for doubting her abilities. Even though she's sweating quite a bit more than usual, she is doing fine and feeling as if she'll set a good race time for herself. But by the 4K mark, Valerie begins to fear she's set too fast a pace. She feels slightly dizzy and is tiring quickly. These sensations progress quite rapidly, and soon Valerie feels as if she's going to faint. She can barely move her body, she's terribly out of breath, and she pauses to lower her head in order to stop the dizziness. She notices that her skin is cold and clammy. A volunteer at the nearby water station notices Valerie's distress and leads her off the course.

1. What heat-related disorder is Valerie experiencing? What are the symptoms of this disorder?

2. What causes this heat-related disorder?

3. What should the volunteer do when he or she notices that Valerie is having problems? How should this disorder be treated?

José is a running back on his college football team in Georgia. He grew up in New York and enjoyed great success on his high school football team. The training for his college team has been tough, but José has stayed with it and is making it off the bench more than he expected. In fact, in today's game, his team's offense has dominated the game, and José hasn't had many breaks at all. He has tried to get some water during the timeouts, but that just hasn't seemed to be enough to satisfy his thirst. The sun is blazing hot, and he is sweating profusely. Late in the third quarter, José's leg muscles started tightening up. At first he ignores it, thinking he is just nervous. But soon he can hardly make his body move the way he wants, his muscles are so tense. His legs hurt so much, he doesn't know whether he can keep playing.

4. What heat-related disorder is José experiencing? What are the symptoms of this disorder?

5. What causes this heat-related disorder?

6. What should José's coach or athletic trainer do when he or she notices that José is having problems? How should this disorder be treated?

Shaquita, a young professional just a few years out of college, is running in her fourth marathon today. She took up running in college, when she and her roommate began an exercise routine to lose a few pounds. Now she finds running an excellent way to release the day's tension and clear her head. Shaquita is really proud that she has been able to compete in marathons and finish in the middle of the pack. Not bad for a girl who never looked forward to gym class for fear of what uncoordinated move she would make that day. The day of the marathon is turning out to be hot and humid—more so than it was during her previous three marathons. Resigned to making a slower time than usual due to the humidity, Shaquita sets a slightly slower pace for herself. The first miles go relatively well, but by mile 20, Shaquita is really struggling to maintain focus. By mile 22, she feels a little dizzy and surprisingly chilled; she has even stopped sweating. And then it hits. She can hardly see straight and feels like she's going to throw up. Her head is throbbing. Her heart seems to be beating a mile a minute. She collapses somewhere to the side of the course, barely conscious and still thinking she can go on if only she could have some water.

7. What heat-related disorder is Shaquita experiencing? What are the symptoms of this disorder?

8. What causes this heat-related disorder?

9. How should the event physician treat Shaquita's disorder?

| Activity 10.6 | Heat Acclimatization |

Do this activity after reading pages 329-331 of *Physiology of Sport and Exercise.*

Many studies have shown that repeated exercise in the heat causes a gradual adjustment that enables us to perform better in hot conditions. In this activity, we will look at the physiological responses to heat acclimatization and the best ways to achieve it.

How Does the Body Respond to Heat Acclimatization?

After studying pages 329-331 in *Physiology of Sport and Exercise,* jot notes below about each physiological parameter, noting how each responds to heat acclimatization. That is, after a person has acclimated to working out in the heat, how do these systems respond differently than they would have before the person was heat acclimated?

Sweating

Rate of

When starts

Mineral content of

Skin temperature

Heart rate

Stroke volume

Muscle glycogen use

Body temperature

Amount of work that can be done before exhaustion

How Can I Achieve Heat Acclimatization?

How can we prepare for prolonged activity in the heat? Does training in the heat make us more tolerant of thermal stress? After studying pages 329-331 in *Physiology of Sport and Exercise,* write notes below about each of the items listed, noting how to optimize training in order to achieve heat acclimatization.

Rest in heat versus training in heat

Temperature of training environment

Time of day of training

Workout intensity for first few days of exercise in heat

Applying Your Knowledge of Heat Acclimatization

Recall our example of José, the football running back in Activity 10.5. Note that he goes to college in Georgia, which is generally more hot and humid during football season than his home state of New York is.

Design a heat acclimatization program for José to prevent him from experiencing heat cramps, or an even more serious heat-related disorder, in the future. Be sure to comment on the appropriate temperature of the training environment, time of day of training, and workout intensity.

Activity 10.7

Factors Affecting Heat Loss

Do this activity after reading pages 331-334 of *Physiology of Sport and Exercise.*

The body's ability to meet the demands of thermoregulation is limited when exposed to extreme cold. Too much heat loss can occur. But what factors can affect the rate of heat loss? And how does the body try to avoid excessive cooling? This activity will help you to answer these questions.

For questions 1 to 5, identify (1) which subject will lose the most heat and (2) why.

1. Subject A with 28% body fat OR Subject B with 17% body fat.

2. Subject C, an 8-year-old boy who weighs 22 kg OR Subject D, a 25-year-old female who weighs 50 kg.

3. Subject E, who is exercising outdoors with a temperature of –1.1 °C and a wind speed of 40.2 km/h OR Subject F, who is exercising outdoors with a temperature of –23.3 °C and a wind speed of 16.1 km/h.

4. Subject G, who is standing still and is fully immersed in 20 °C water OR Subject H, who is swimming in the same 20 °C water.

5. Subject I, who is standing still and fully immersed in a fast-moving river of 20 °C water OR Subject J, who is standing still and fully immersed in a swimming pool of 20 °C water.

6. List and define the three mechanisms that these people's bodies will use to avoid excessive cooling.

Physiological Responses to Exercise in the Cold

Activity 10.8

Do this activity after reading pages 335-336 of *Physiology of Sport and Exercise.*

The body must struggle to maintain its internal temperature when exposed to a cold environment. But what happens when you add the demands of physical activity to that struggle? In this activity, you will explore some of the physiological changes that occur in response to exercise while the body is exposed to cold stress.

Fill out the table on the following two pages, based on information found in your textbook, to see what types of muscle function and metabolic changes your body makes in response to exercising under conditions of cold stress. In the third column, be sure to make notes about the reasons for these responses and the resulting consequences.

Parameter	Increase or decrease? (Use ↑, ↓, or ↔)	Notes for studying purposes
Muscle shortening velocity		
Muscle power		
Body heat production		
Fatigue, if you try to perform at the same muscle velocity and power as in warmer weather		
Body heat production, once fatigue sets in		

(continued)

(continued)

Parameter	Increase or decrease? (Use ↑, ↓, or ↔)	Notes for studying purposes
Epinephrine and nore-pinephrine release		
Vasoconstriction in vessels supplying the skin and subcutaneous tissues		
Blood glucose level		
Muscle glycogen usage		

Cold-Related Health Risks

Do this activity after reading pages 336-338 of *Physiology of Sport and Exercise*.

Despite the efforts of the body's thermoregulatory system, once the body temperature falls below 34.5 °C (94.1 °F), the hypothalamus begins to lose its ability to regulate body temperature. And exposed skin can freeze when its temperature is lowered just a few degrees below the freezing point. These conditions can result in hypothermia and frostbite, respectively.

Read the following case studies. Identify the cold-related health risk the person is suffering from and the appropriate treatment that should be taken.

Heather has been downhill skiing all day long. She lost her gloves earlier in the day and borrowed a pair of light knit gloves from the lost-and-found box in the ski lodge. It has been a bitterly cold and windy day, but Heather has hardly noticed, she loves skiing so much. Around noon, Heather takes a short break and notices that her fingers are red; she can barely feel her fingertips, although she feels a burning sensation of some sort. She has fallen a few times, and her gloves are soaking wet. But soon she is back on the slopes, challenging herself to some runs with moguls, ignoring the lack of feeling in her fingertips. On what seems like her 30th ride up the ski lift, Heather takes off a glove to adjust her coat. To her dismay, she sees that the skin on her fingertips has turned white and hard, and she has no feeling in her fingertips.

1. What cold-related problem is Heather experiencing?

2. What are the physiological causes of this cold-related health concern?

3. How should Heather treat her condition?

Tyrone is leading a group of teenagers on an outdoor adventure week in the Rocky Mountains of Colorado. Earlier in the day, they donned backpacks and hiking shoes and started up a mountain. After six h of hiking, they have reached the area where they will be camping—just below the tundra line. As evening approaches, it begins to snow lightly. Tyrone assures the group that this is typical—the weather changes often at this altitude. He gets the group busy setting up camp. But Tyrone does begin to worry as he sizes up the clouds; to this experienced camper, it just doesn't feel right. Sure enough, the light snow becomes a blizzard that lasts for two days. The group is stuck in the tents with little ability to move around to keep warm. Tyrone keeps an eye on all of the young people, making sure they are all staying warm and getting enough to eat. Early on the second day, Tyrone notices that Rick, age 16, is shivering and Tyrone cannot seem to get him warm. Rick can hardly stay awake, looks pale, and seems confused.

4. What cold-related problem is Rick suffering from?

5. What are the physiological causes of this cold-related health concern?

6. How should Tyrone approach the treatment of Rick's health problem?

7. How is Rick's cardiorespiratory system probably being affected by his hypothermia?

Putting It All Together: Thermoregulation and Exercise

Activity 10.10

Do this activity after reading chapter 10 of *Physiology of Sport and Exercise*.

In this chapter, we looked at the effects of extreme heat and cold and the body's responses to them, especially during physical activity. We considered the health risks associated with these temperature extremes and how the body tries to adapt to these conditions through acclimatization.

In this closing activity, you are challenged to discern which of two subjects will better tolerate heat and which of the two will better tolerate cold. Answer the following questions on a separate piece of paper.

Heat Tolerance

Coralee, age 23, is a competitive cyclist, who is just starting to compete on the amateur circuit. Today she is competing in a 20-mi race. The temperature is 32.2 °C (90 °F) and the humidity is 80%. There is a light 5- to 10-mph breeze. In preparation for today's event, Coralee trained four times a week for 60 min, but in much cooler weather, since she is from Maine. In each training session, she cycled the first 50 minutes at an easy, comfortable pace and then sprinted for the last 10 min. She usually trained after work, in the early evening hours. Coralee added an extra water bottle to her bike for this event, knowing she might need it.

Jeremy, age 45, is a recreational cyclist. As part of his extended vacation, Jeremy and his family drove out to see the Grand Canyon. He found a bike trail near their campground that he wants to try out. The temperature is 35 °C (95 °F) and the humidity is 15%. There is no breeze. Jeremy hasn't officially prepared for riding this 20-mi bike trail, but in his travels around the nation, he often brings his bike with him. Twenty times in the past six wk, Jeremy has cycled long stints in the southwest United States, generally in very hot and relatively dry conditions and in the heat of the day. He and his oldest son have raced the last 5 mi of every bike tour, pedaling as hard and as fast as they could, and Jeremy is looking forward to the friendly competition today. As usual, he packed plenty of water for him and his son to drink.

1. Given the events they are cycling in today and what you know about each cyclist, which cyclist is likely to tolerate the heat better? Why?

2. What symptoms might the person who isn't as able to dissipate body heat experience? What physiological events might take place as this person becomes overheated?

3. Contrast the probable physiological responses to exercising in the heat of the person who is heat acclimated versus the one who is not.

Cold Tolerance

Travis, age 19, is a fullback on his college intramural soccer team. Travis is 6 ft 3 in. tall and weighs 175 lb. The weather is awful, but the referee is still allowing the game to go on. It has been raining torrentially for 30 min, and Travis's T-shirt, sweatshirt, and shorts are soaking wet. It is 10 °C (50 °F), cloudy, and very windy. Travis is not having to move around much, because his team has been on the other half of the field working on scoring a goal for a long time now.

Amy, age 16, is a fullback on her park district soccer team. Amy is 5 ft 6 in. tall and weighs 130 lb. It is 0 °C (32 °F) with a slight breeze. The sky is clear and it is sunny. Amy's team is not strong offensively, and Amy is spending a lot of time running to defend her team's goal.

4. Which soccer player is likely to better tolerate the cold in the games they are currently playing? Why?

5. What symptoms might the person who isn't as able to retain body heat experience? What physiological events might take place as this person becomes hypothermic?

Sample Test Questions for Chapter 10

Test yourself on your knowledge of this chapter by taking this self-test. Write the correct answers on a separate sheet of paper.

Multiple Choice

1. The transfer of heat from one material to another through direct molecular contact is

   a. radiation.   b. evaporation.   c. conduction.   d. convection.

2. The conversion of sweat into vapor, and the primary avenue for heat dissipation during exercise, is

   a. radiation.   b. evaporation.   c. conduction.   d. convection.

3. Which of the following is *not* true of peripheral vasoconstriction?

   a. It occurs as a result of sympathetic stimulation to the smooth muscles surrounding the arterioles in the skin.
   b. It reduces blood flow to the shell of the body.
   c. It allows for additional heat loss.
   d. It is the constriction of the arterioles in the skin.

4. Which of the following would most likely lead to a state of hypothermia?

   a. Running for an hour on a 15 °C (59 °F) day with 80% humidity.
   b. Running for an hour during a rain shower on a 21 °C (70 °F) day.
   c. Immersion in 15 °C (59 °F) water for an hour.
   d. Swimming in 15 °C (59 °F) water for an hour.

5. Which of the following is *not* a response to hypothermia?

   a. The hypothalamus completely loses its ability to regulate body temperature when the internal temperature falls to about 29.5 °C (85.1 °F).
   b. Metabolic reactions slow to one-half their normal rates for each 10 °C (18 °F) decline in cellular temperature.
   c. Cooling primarily influences the heart's SA node, causing a decline in heart rate.
   d. Exposure to extreme cold increases respiratory rate and volume.

True-False

6. Frostbite occurs as a consequence of the body's attempts to prevent heat loss.

7. Breathing cold air can freeze the respiratory passages or lungs when ventilation is low.

8. A lesser blood flow to the muscles during exercise in the heat leads to a lesser use of muscle glycogen and production of less lactic acid, thereby contributing to the sensations of fatigue and exhaustion.

9. Although most individuals must be exposed to the heat to gain full heat acclimatization, they can gain partial heat tolerance simply by training, even in a cooler environment.

10. Sitting in a hot environment for long periods each day will prepare an individual for physical exertion in the heat.

Fill in the Blank

11. Your body's thermostat, which houses the thermoregulatory center and monitors temperature, accelerating heat loss and heat production as needed, is better known to exercise physiologists as the _____.

12. The four environmental variables that must be taken into account when assessing the total physiological stress imposed on the body in a hot environment are _____, _____, _____, and _____.

13. _____ is a rapid, involuntary cycle of contraction and relaxation of skeletal muscles and can cause a fourfold to fivefold increase in the body's resting rate of heat production.

14. During exercise in the cold, _____ causes free fatty acid (FFA) levels not to increase as much as one would think, given the elevated levels of epinephrine and norepinephrine.

Short Answer

15. Two 5K runs with the same number of runners are held on the same day, one in Chicago and one in Phoenix. In Chicago, the temperature is 32.2 °C (90 °F) and the humidity is 85%. In Phoenix, the temperature is 32.2 °C (90 °F) and the humidity is 12%. Which race is likely to see the most runners with heat-related disorders? Why?

16. Why might the sodium and chloride content of sweat be considerably higher with a high sweat rate than with a low sweat rate? How does training impact this?

17. During exercise in the heat, in what ways do your heat loss mechanisms compete with active muscles?

18. Describe the cycle of fatigue, muscle activity, and body heat production when exercising in the cold, and how this cycle can lead to hypothermia.

Essay

19. Explain the interactions of the sweat glands, smooth muscles around the arterioles, skeletal muscles, and endocrine glands, both when the body is too hot and when it is too cold.

20. Explain the roles of aldosterone and antidiuretic hormone (ADH) when exercising in the heat.

21. List as many steps as you can for preventing hyperthermia.

22. Describe the three changes in sweating that can result from heat acclimatization and, as applicable, how these relate to blood flow.

Answers to Selected Chapter 10 Activities

10.1 Transfer of Body Heat to the Environment

1. The ice melts.

2. The heat from the body is transferred to the ice through conduction, which causes the ice to melt.

3. The hand probably got colder, due to conduction of heat from the skin to the ice and conduction of cold from the ice to the skin.

4. Once the fan was turned on, the body probably felt cooler.

5. As the air speed gets faster, the body feels cooler. This illustrates the principle that the greater the movement of the air or liquid, the greater the rate of heat removal by convection.

6. Convection is movement of heat from one place to another by the motion of a gas or a liquid across the heated surface. In this experiment, the moving air swept away air molecules that had been warmed by their contact with the skin.

7. In an environment that is warmer than the skin, conduction can cause the skin, and therefore the body, to gain heat. The heat transfers from the warmer object, in this case the air, to the cooler one, in this case the skin. And since the environment is warmer, convection brings warmer molecules in contact with the skin instead of sweeping warm molecules away.

8. The warmth you felt was due to the heat radiating from your body.

9. Answers will vary. Your body receives heat via radiation from the sun and any other objects that are warmer than the body.

10. You likely lost more heat through evaporation in the situation in which you barely noticed your sweat. Low humidity probably contributed to your body's being able to lose heat through evaporation.

11. You likely did not feel any cooling effect in your second example, due to high humidity.

12. Radiation.

13. Evaporation.

10.2 Control of Heat Exchange

2. Most of Chris's heat will be lost through evaporation of sweat.

4. In addition to wearing warm layers so that radiation from his body helps to warm the air between the layers, Mark could also try to move his body parts, as the increased skeletal muscle activity will increase his temperature by increasing metabolic heat production.

10.3 Assessing Body Temperature

1. T_{skin} = (0.1 × 31.7 °C) + (0.6 × 32.7 °C) + (0.2 × 32.3 °C) + (0.1 × 31.5 °C) = 32.4 °C

2. The mean body temperature takes into account temperature variations throughout the body and is a weighted average of skin and internal body temperatures.

3. T_{body} = (0.4 × 32.4 °C) + (0.6 × 37.0 °C) = 35.16 °C

4. The heat content of the body is the total calories of heat contained in body tissues.

5. HC = 0.83 (70 kg × 35.2 °C) = 2,045.12 kcal

6. Subject A: Heat gain = 0.83 kcal · kg^{-1} · °C^{-1} × 70 kg × 2 °C = 116.2 kcal/hour

   Subject B: Heat gain = 0.98 kcal · kg^{-1} · °C^{-1} × 70 kg × 7 °C = 480.2 kcal/hour

7. Subject B's body is not doing as well at dissipating heat. Subject B might be exercising in a more hot or humid environment that is allowing for less evaporation of sweat than Subject A.

10.4 Physiological Responses to Exercise in the Heat

Parameter	Increase or decrease? (Use ↑, ↓, or ↔)	Notes for studying purposes
Demand for blood flow and oxygen to muscles	↑	
Demand for blood flow to skin		The circulatory system transports heat generated in the muscles to the surface of the body, where the heat can be transferred to the environment.
Volume of blood returning to the heart	↓	
End-diastolic volume	↓	
Cardiac output	↔	
Stroke volume	↓	
Heart rate	↑	A gradual upward drift in heart rate compensates for the drop in stroke volume, as a way to maintain cardiac output.
Body temperature	↑	
Oxygen uptake	↑	The two mechanisms related to exercising in the heat that cause the need for this changed oxygen uptake are increased sweat production and increased respiration, both of which demand more energy.
Use of glycogen	↑	
Production of muscle lactate	↑	Both glycogen depletion and increased muscle lactate contribute to the sensations of fatigue and exhaustion.
Sweating	↑	Because radiation, convection, and conduction are less effective as environmental temperature rises, evaporation becomes the most important method of heat loss. Increased dependence on evaporation means an increased demand for sweating.

10.5 Heat-Related Disorders

1. Valerie is suffering from heat exhaustion. While she has some telltale signs—extreme fatigue, breathlessness, dizziness, and cold and clammy skin—other symptoms can include vomiting, fainting, hot and dry skin, hypotension, and a weak, rapid pulse.

2. Heat exhaustion results when the simultaneous demands of the thermoregulatory system and the active muscles are not met. The blood volume decreases, by either excessive fluid loss or mineral loss from sweating. The thermoregulatory mechanisms are functioning but cannot dissipate heat quickly enough, because there is insufficient blood volume to allow adequate distribution to the skin.

3. The volunteer should get Valerie to a cooler location—under a shade tree or in an air-conditioned race vehicle—and have Valerie elevate her feet. Since Valerie is conscious, the volunteer could give her salt water, but if Valerie were to become unconscious, medically supervised intravenous administration of saline solution would be recommended.

4. José is experiencing heat cramps. Muscle cramps are the key symptoms of this disorder.

5. Heat cramps are probably brought on by the mineral losses and dehydration that accompany high rates of sweating.

6. José's coach or athletic trainer should pull him from the game, move him to a cool location like the locker room, and give José plenty to drink. They might also decide to administer a saline solution.

7. Shaquita is experiencing heat stroke, which is characterized by a rise in internal body temperature to a value exceeding 40 °C (104 °F), cessation of sweating, hot and dry skin, rapid pulse and respiration, usually hypertension, confusion, and unconsciousness.

8. Heat stroke is caused by failure of the body's thermoregulatory mechanisms.

9. The physician should rapidly cool Shaquita's body either by placing her in a bath of cold water or ice or by wrapping her in wet sheets and fanning her.

10.7 Factors Affecting Heat Loss

1. Subject B   2. Subject C   3. Subject F;   4. Subject G   5. Subject I

6. Shivering—a rapid, involuntary cycle of contraction and relaxation of skeletal muscles.

Nonshivering thermogenesis—stimulation of metabolism by the sympathetic nervous system.

Peripheral vasoconstriction—constriction of arterioles in the skin, caused by sympathetic stimulation of the smooth muscle surrounding them, which reduces the blood flow to the shell of the body.

10.8   Physiological Responses to Exercise in the Cold

Parameter	Increase or decrease? (Use ↑, ↓, or ↔)	Notes for studying purposes
Muscle shortening velocity	↓	
Muscle power	↓	
Body heat production	↓	
Fatigue, if you try to perform at same muscle velocity and power as in warmer weather	↑	
Body heat production, once fatigue sets in	↓	
Epinephrine and nore-pinephrine release	↑	
Vasoconstriction in vessels supplying the skin and subcutaneous tissues	↑	The subcutaneous tissue is the major storage site for lipids, so this vasoconstriction reduces the blood flow to the area from which the FFA would be mobilized. Thus, FFA levels do not increase as much as the elevated levels of epinephrine and norepinephrine would indicate.
Blood glucose level	↔	
Muscle glycogen usage	↑	

10.9   Cold-Related Health Risks

1. Heather is experiencing frostbite.

2. Peripheral vasoconstriction helps the body retain heat. But during exposure to extreme cold, the circulation in the skin can decrease to the point that the tissue dies from the lack of oxygen and nutrients.

3. Totally frostbitten parts should be left untreated until they can be thawed in a hospital without risk of refreezing. Note: You shouldn't massage the frozen parts or rewarm them by an open fire.

4. Rick is suffering from hypothermia.

5. Once the body temperature falls below 34.5 °C (94.1 °F), the hypothalamus begins to lose its ability to regulate body temperature. This ability is completely lost when the internal temperature falls to about 29.5 °C (85.1 °F). This loss of function is associated with slowing metabolic reactions to "one half" their normal rates for each 10 °C (18 °F) decline in cellular temperature. This can cause drowsiness or even coma.

6. Mild cases of hypothermia can be treated by protecting the affected person from the cold and providing dry clothing and warm beverages. Rick's case is more serious, though. If possible, Rick should be airlifted to a hospital to be slowly rewarmed there. Rick needs to be handled gently to avoid causing cardiac arrhythmia.

7. Hypothermia primarily affects the heart's SA node, causing the heart rate to drop, which in turn reduces cardiac output. Exposure to extreme cold decreases respiratory rate and volume.

10.10 Putting It All Together: Thermoregulation and Exercise

1. Surprisingly, Jeremy will probably tolerate the heat better. Even though he is a recreational cyclist, Jeremy is probably more acclimated than Coralee is to exercising in the heat: His exercise sessions have been rather long; they were done in the heat of the day in conditions similar to today's ride; and he cycled the last 5 miles of each session at a high level of intensity, increasing his internal heat production and helping his body to acclimate. Although Coralee will have a slight breeze to help whisk off her sweat molecules, the combination of the heat, high humidity, and lack of training in the heat will probably work against her.

4. Even though Travis has the higher ratio of body surface area to body mass, the environmental conditions in his game will challenge his body's thermoregulatory system much more than those in Amy's situation. For Travis, the torrential rain makes for a very cold situation, as water is a much better conductor of heat than air is. To complicate things, Travis isn't moving around very much, so his metabolic system isn't being called on to generate much heat.

Answers to Selected Chapter 10 Test Questions

Multiple Choice

1. c;   2. b;   3. c;   4. c;   5. d

True-False

6. True;   7. False;   8. False;   9. True;   10. False

Fill in the Blank

11. hypothalamus;   12. air temperature, humidity, air velocity, and thermal radiation; 13. shivering;   14. vasoconstriction in the vessels supplying the subcutaneous tissue

Short Answer and Essay

For questions 15 to 22, check your answers against the explanations given in the textbook.

Exercise in Hypobaric, Hyperbaric, and Microgravity Environments

concepts

- Altitude presents a hypobaric environment, one in which the atmospheric pressure is reduced. Altitudes of 1,500 m (4,921 ft) or more have a notable physiological impact on the human body.

- Though the percentages of the gases in the air we breathe remain constant regardless of altitude, the partial pressures of each of these gases vary with atmospheric pressure. The reduced PO_2 at altitude leads to decreased performance, due to a reduced pressure gradient that hinders oxygen transport to the tissues.

- Submersion in water exposes the human body to a hyperbaric environment, one in which the external pressure is greater than at sea level.

- Breathing gases under pressure, as when using scuba gear, can cause gases to accumulate in the body in toxic levels, so precautions must be taken when diving with pressurized gases.

- Most physiological changes that occur as a result of extended exposure to microgravity (reduced gravity) conditions during spaceflight are similar to those seen with detraining in athletes and with reduced activity in older people.

- Exposure to microgravity results in muscle strength losses, a decrease in cross-sectional areas of ST and FT muscle fibers, bone mineral losses, and reduced plasma volume, all of which pose health risks upon return to Earth. In-flight exercise training, bouts of maximal exercise, and resistance training might be important in preparing astronauts for return to a 1.0-g environment.

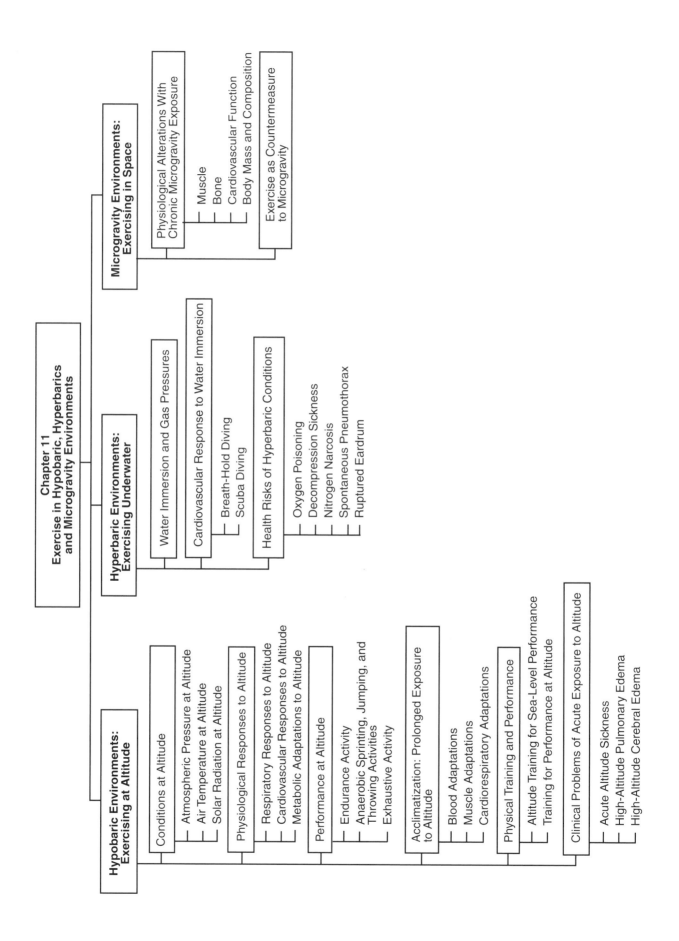

Chapter 11

Exercise in Hypobaric, Hyperbarics and Microgravity Environments

Hypobaric Environments: Exercising at Altitude

Conditions at Altitude
- Atmospheric Pressure at Altitude
- Air Temperature at Altitude
- Solar Radiation at Altitude

Physiological Responses to Altitude
- Respiratory Responses to Altitude
- Cardiovascular Responses to Altitude
- Metabolic Adaptations to Altitude

Performance at Altitude
- Endurance Activity
- Anaerobic Sprinting, Jumping, and Throwing Activities
- Exhaustive Activity

Acclimatization: Prolonged Exposure to Altitude
- Blood Adaptations
- Muscle Adaptations
- Cardiorespiratory Adaptations

Physical Training and Performance
- Altitude Training for Sea-Level Performance
- Training for Performance at Altitude

Clinical Problems of Acute Exposure to Altitude
- Acute Altitude Sickness
- High-Altitude Pulmonary Edema
- High-Altitude Cerebral Edema

Hyperbaric Environments: Exercising Underwater

Water Immersion and Gas Pressures

Cardiovascular Response to Water Immersion
- Breath-Hold Diving
- Scuba Diving

Health Risks of Hyperbaric Conditions
- Oxygen Poisoning
- Decompression Sickness
- Nitrogen Narcosis
- Spontaneous Pneumothorax
- Ruptured Eardrum

Microgravity Environments: Exercising in Space

Physiological Alterations With Chronic Microgravity Exposure
- Muscle
- Bone
- Cardiovascular Function
- Body Mass and Composition

Exercise as Countermeasure to Microgravity

186

Hypobaric, Hyperbaric, and Microgravity Environments

Do this activity after reading pages 344-346 of *Physiology of Sport and Exercise.*

> **Activity 11.1**

Previous chapters have focused on how the body responds to exercise at or near sea level. But what happens when athletes compete at high altitudes, when divers descend underwater, or when astronauts venture into space? Before we can understand how the body responds to these conditions, we must examine the differences inherent in these environments.

For each environmental condition listed on this and the next page, first conduct the brief experiment, then write the letters from the list below that match the conditions of this type of environment. (You may need to briefly skim pages 358 and 367 in *Physiology of Sport and Exercise.*)

Hypobaric

It is virtually impossible to simulate a high-altitude environment at a much lower elevation. So, let's take a brief look at one way in which your body responds to altitude. In a hypobaric environment, the atmospheric pressure is low, meaning the PO_2 is also lower, which limits pulmonary diffusion and oxygen transport to the tissues. This reduces oxygen delivery to the body tissues, resulting in hypoxia, or oxygen deficiency. Your body responds quickly to the thinner oxygen and reduced atmospheric pressure by breathing faster.

If you are able, run in place until you are winded. Note that you are breathing faster and deeper. Of course, you are doing so for different reasons than if you were at altitude. But the reaction is the same: Your body needs more oxygen, so it responds by taking more frequent breaths.

1. In the blank, write the letters from the list "Conditions to Match With Corresponding Environment" on page 188 that match a hypobaric environment: _____

_____

Hyperbaric

Recreational scuba diving and snorkeling present a unique challenge to human physiology. In addition to the thermal effects of water, which you learned about in chapter 10, the body must endure the effects of a hyperbaric environment. One of those effects is the increased pressure of gases. In addition, water is denser than air, multiplying the pressure exponentially. For years, people who freeze vegetables have used this principle to ensure a tight seal. Conduct this brief experiment in order to see the principle of pressure in action.

Find a plastic sandwich bag—preferably the kind with a zipper-lock type of seal, though any small sandwich bag will work. Put something of loose density in the plastic bag. Vegetables, a heavy cereal, beads, a handful of paper clips, or something along those lines will work well. Do not seal the bag yet. Notice that without using your hands to squeeze the air out of the bag, much air remains in it. Place the open bag in water. Submerge the bag until just the opening is showing. (Be careful not to let any water go into the bag!) Close the bag while it is still in the water. Notice that the water pressure, being greater than the air pressure, forced the air from the bag.

In this same way, when you dive, water exerts increased pressure on the gases in your paranasal sinuses, respiratory tract, and gastrointestinal tract, as well as on the gases dissolved in bodily fluids.

2. In the blank, write the letters from the list "Conditions to Match With Corresponding Environment" on that match a hyperbaric environment: _____

_____

Microgravity

In a microgravity environment, an object's weight, which reflects the strength of the gravity pulling on it, decreases as the object moves away from the Earth's surface. As in the previous two conditions, we cannot recreate microgravity on Earth, but we can conduct an experiment to help visualize it.

Pick up a heavy shoe that has laces. Hold the shoe in your hand (or, if you have a scale, place the shoe on the scale). If the shoe doesn't feel heavy to you, place something heavy in it—a paperweight, rock, or small book will work. Note the weight of the shoe—either by how much force your arm has to exert to hold the shoe or, if you have a scale, by the reading on the scale.

Now tie the shoe to something so that the shoe hangs in midair. You might tie it to a door knob, curtain rod, or the rail of a loft in your dorm room. Now place your hand or hold the scale underneath the shoe, close enough so that your hand (or scale) is touching the shoe, but do not use any force to support the shoe. If your hand is simply touching but not supporting the shoe, note the lack of force the shoe exerts on your hand—it is, in our simulation, "weightless."

3. In the blank, write the letters from the list "Conditions to Match With Corresponding Environment" that match a microgravity environment: _____

_____

For an extra challenge: If you have time, check out NASA's Microgravity Science Division's home page at **http://zeta.lerc.nasa.gov/sedhome.htm** for more information about microgravity science. Click on "Educational Information" and then "Microgravity Activities" for additional microgravity experiments you can do.

Conditions to Match With Corresponding Environment

a. Reduced gravitational force, where gravitational force is less than 1 *g*

b. Drier air, which can lead to dehydration

c. Low atmospheric pressure

d. High atmospheric pressure

e. Decreased body weight

f. Decreased partial pressures of gases; the reduced PO_2 leads to tissue hypoxia (reduced oxygen supply)

g. Increased partial pressures of gases

h. Decreased air temperature

i. Increased intensity of solar radiation

Activity 11.2

Physiological Responses to a Hypobaric Environment

Do this activity after reading pages 344-350 of *Physiology of Sport and Exercise.*

A hypobaric environment, or one with low atmospheric pressure, is usually experienced at altitude, which in this book refers to elevations above 1,500 m (4,921 ft). Mountain climbers, competitive athletes participating at high altitudes, and even tourists vacationing at sites of high altitude must contend with the conditions of a hypobaric environment.

In this activity we will look closely at how our bodies respond when presented with such an environment. Fill out the table below based on information found on pages 344-350 of *Physiology of Sport and Exercise*.

Parameter	Increase or decrease? (Use ↑ or ↓)	Why? What causes this response?	Notes for studying purposes
Pulmonary ventilation			
Hemoglobin saturation			
Exchange of oxygen from the blood to the tissues			
Maximal oxygen up-take ($\dot{V}O_2$max)			
Blood volume after initially arriving at altitude			

(continued)

(continued)

Parameter	Increase or decrease? (Use ↑ or ↓)	Why? What causes this response?	Notes for studying purposes
Blood volume after continued exposure to high altitude			
Cardiac output during submaximal work upon initial ascent to altitude			
Cardiac output during maximal work at altitude			
Blood pressure in pulmonary arteries			
Lactic acid production at sub-maximal levels of exercise			
Lactic acid production at maximal levels of exercise			

For an extra challenge: Few studies on the effects of altitude have included women and children. Given what you have learned thus far in this text, hypothesize how altitude might affect women and children differently than men.

Activity 11.3

Acclimatization at Altitude

Do this activity after reading pages 352-354 of *Physiology of Sport and Exercise.*

When people are exposed to altitude for days and weeks, their bodies gradually adjust to the lower oxygen tension in the air. Circle or highlight the items below that are true of *prolonged* exposure to altitude. Cross out the items that are *not true* of prolonged exposure to altitude and rewrite the sentence to make it true.

a. Total blood volume increases.

b. Erythrocyte production is inhibited by the lack of oxygen.

c. The blood's hemoglobin content increases.

d. The increased blood hemoglobin content improves the oxygen-carrying capacity of a fixed volume of blood.

e. Plasma volume decreases over long-term exposure to altitude.

f. ST and FT muscle fiber areas increase.

g. Total muscle area decreases.

h. The glycolytic enzyme activity of the leg muscles increases.

i. Muscles increase in their capacity to perform oxidative phosphorylation.

j. Capillary density (capillaries per mm^2) decreases.

k. Pulmonary ventilation increases, both at rest and during exercise.

l. There is no significant improvement in aerobic endurance with acclimatization.

m. Increased ventilation promotes the unloading of CO_2 and the alkalization of blood. Therefore, in order to prevent the blood from becoming abnormally alkaline, the amount of blood bicarbonate increases rapidly during the first few days at altitude and remains depressed with prolonged exposure to altitude.

For an extra challenge: Living for generations at elevations of 3,660 to 4,270 m (12,000 to 14,000 ft), highland Indians in the Andean mountains of Peru have developed extra-large lungs and hearts.

1. Based on the information presented in *Physiology of Sport and Exercise*, why might their hearts and lungs be larger than those of lowland residents?

2. Although we know the size of their hearts and lungs increases, no muscle biopsy data have been obtained from residents at high altitudes to determine whether these individuals experience any muscular adaptations as a consequence of living at these elevations. (The muscle adaptations we know of are based on studies of mountain climbers who experience hypoxia for only four to six wk.) Hypothesize how the muscle structure and function of the Andean Indians might be different from that of lowland residents.

Activity 11.4

Training and Performance at Altitude

Do this activity after reading pages 351 and 354-356 of *Physiology of Sport and Exercise.*

The effects of altitude on performance might be obvious when watching a film of climbers ascending Mount Everest. But how does it affect the performance of athletes and recreational exercisers at less extreme altitudes, yet well above sea level, and how can these people train to perform well at altitude? Read the following brief scenarios and, on separate paper, answer the questions posed by each situation.

Eric, who lives near sea level in Florida, is visiting his brother in Denver, Colorado, which has an approximate elevation of 1,600 m (5,249 ft). The local running club is hosting a 5K during Eric's stay, and Eric's brother challenges him to join him in running in the event.

1. What problems is Eric likely to have as he runs in this race? Why?

2. Keep in mind that Eric is not an elite athlete. Had Eric known he would be running a 5K at altitude, what could he have done to train for the event?

At the 1968 Olympics in Mexico City, altitude 2,240 m (7,350 ft), Bob Beamon soared almost 0.6 m (2 ft) farther than the previous world record in the long jump. This record stood for almost 20 years.

3. What characteristic of the high-altitude environment of Mexico City likely contributed to Beamon's success?

Jessie throws the discus for her secondary school track team, which is located at the foothills of the Canadian Rockies in the province of Alberta. Last weekend she and her team competed at a secondary school in the mountains, at an elevation of 1,800 m (5,904 ft). Jessie expected her discus to fly farther than usual but it didn't.

4. Why didn't Jessie's discus throw improve at altitude?

Jessie's teammate, Rachel, runs the 400 m sprint. Before their meet at altitude, Rachel overhears her coach discussing altitude training with the distance runners. She wonders if she should do anything special to prepare to run her event at altitude. She knows the team will be driving to the secondary school in the mountains on Saturday morning, competing during the day, and driving back that same night.

5. Should Rachel do anything in particular to train for running the 400 m at altitude? Why or why not?

After Eric, from our first case study, finishes running the 5K with his brother, he recognizes how much harder his body had to work to complete the race, even at a pace that was slower than his usual time. He wonders if training in the mountains would improve his times once he is back at home near sea level in Florida.

6. Will training at altitude improve Eric's performance at sea level? Why or why not?

The year is 2024 and the Olympic Games are to be held in Erzurum, Turkey, elevation 1,950 m (6,396 ft).

7. What are the training options for endurance athletes who will be competing in these Olympics but who are not accustomed to competing at such altitudes?

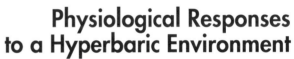

Physiological Responses to a Hyperbaric Environment

Activity 11.5

Do this activity after reading pages 358-362 of *Physiology of Sport and Exercise.*

In activity 11.1, you conducted an experiment illustrating the increased pressure your body experiences when underwater. But how does this increased pressure affect the gases in your body and the functioning of your cardiovascular system?

Read pages 358-362 carefully and, on separate paper, design a list of at least five (preferably more) safety guidelines for diving in a hyperbaric environment. For your own studying purposes, make sure you know the physiological reasons for these safety statements. An example of a safety guideline, with brief study notes in parentheses, is provided for you below.

Safety Guidelines

1. Divers should always exhale as they ascend to the surface.

(As pressure increases, volume decreases; conversely, air taken into the lungs will expand as divers near the surface. If divers don't exhale on ascent, their lungs could overdistend, rupturing the alveoli and causing pulmonary hemorrhage and lung collapse. Air bubbles could enter the circulatory system and lead to extensive damage. See page 359.)

List at least five more safety guidelines.

Activity 11.6

Do this activity after reading 356-357and 362-366 of *Physiology of Sport and Exercise.*

The conditions inherent at altitude and underwater pose health risks for even the most seasoned mountain climber or scuba diver. In the table below, fill in the blank spaces with the health risk, symptom, cause, or treatment of each hypobaric or hyperbaric health risk.

Health risk	Symptoms	Causes	Treatment
Acute altitude sickness		Not fully understood, though reduced ventilation in some people allows carbon dioxide to accumulate in the tissues, and this may induce most of the symptoms.	
	Shortness of breath, excessive fatigue, blueness in lips and fingernails, mental confusion, loss of consciousness.		Administration of supplemental oxygen and moving the victim to a lower altitude.
High altitude cerebral edema (HACE)		The cause of this accumulation of fluid in the cranial cavity is unknown.	
	Visual distortion, rapid and shallow breathing, convulsions, and in some cases penumonia.		Treatment is not discussed in the textbook.
	Symptoms are similar to alcohol intoxication: impaired judgment, perhaps without being able to recognize it.		
	Death.	Not exhaling during ascent. This can overdistend the lungs, rupturing the alveoli, and allowing gas to enter the pleural space and in turn collapse the lung. At the same time, small air bubbles can enter the pulmonary blood and form air emboli, which can become trapped in the vessels of other tissues, blocking circulation to those tissues.	
	Severe ear pain.		Prevention includes blowing with moderate pressure against the closed nostrils. Upper respiratory infections and sinusitis interfere with one's ability to do so; diving should be avoided if these symptoms exist. Treatment is not discussed in the textbook.

Physiological Responses to a Microgravity Environment

Activity 11.7

Do this activity after reading pages 367-373 of *Physiology of Sport and Exercise.*

A microgravity environment, in which the body nears weightlessness or becomes weightless, is usually experienced by astronauts—and few of us will get the opportunity to explore space. But many of the conditions experienced by astronauts also have implications for athletes who break a bone and must immobilize a limb, recreational exercisers who simply stop exercising for a while, or older people whose activity may be reduced for any number of reasons.

In this activity we will look closely at how our bodies respond when presented with such an environment. Fill out the table below based on information found on pages 367-373 of *Physiology of Sport and Exercise.*

Parameter	Increase or decrease? (Use ↑ or ↓)	Why? What causes this response?	Notes for studying purposes
Cross-sectional areas of ST and FT muscle fibers			
Muscle strength			
Percentage of bone minerals			
Plasma volume			

(continued)

(continued)

Parameter	Increase or decrease? (Use ↑ or ↓)	Why? What causes this response?	Notes for studying purposes
Cardiac output and arterial blood pressure			
Arterial pressure in the kidneys			
Body mass			

For an extra challenge: What are the implications of microgravity research for (a) a team athlete during the off-season and (b) an older person recovering from hip replacement surgery?

Activity 11.8

Putting It All Together: Exercise in Hypobaric, Hyperbaric, and Microgravity Environments

Do this activity after reading chapter 11 of *Physiology of Sport and Exercise.*

In this chapter, we examined the conditions of the hypobaric, hyperbaric, and microgravity environments; how these conditions affect our bodies; and how they affect performance. We have discussed how others have prepared for these environments and what researchers have found effective, but how would you prepare to exercise in these environments?

Think about what your favorite physical activity is (e.g., walking, playing football, playing tennis, rock climbing, cross-country skiing, weight lifting). Write that activity and answer the following questions on a separate piece of paper.

1. Imagine that you are going to compete in that activity at an altitude of 1,600 m (5,248 ft) in six wk. Briefly outline the training program that you would embark on in preparation for that competition. (We won't ask you to write the physiological reasons for the program here, but do be sure you know those in preparation for your test.)

2. Imagine that you are going to spend 15 days in a space station.

   a. In what physiological ways might this time in space affect your ability to perform your favorite activity upon your return to Earth?

   b. Briefly outline a training program you would use during your time in space in order to be able to resume your favorite physical activity as soon as possible after returning to Earth.

3. Using your preferred Internet search engine, do a search on "scuba safety."

   a. How many sites are listed? _____ Why do you suppose so many sites are listed?

   b. Quickly scan a few of these Web sites. Which health risk seems to be of most concern to dive instructors? From what you have learned in this chapter, why might this be so?

   c. Visit **http://www.diversalertnetwork.org/**. What is the purpose of this organization? Why is there a need for such an organization?

   d. If you were to get certified in scuba diving, what qualifications would you look for in an instructor?

Sample Test Questions for Chapter 11

Test yourself on your knowledge of this chapter by taking this self-test. Write the correct answers on a separate sheet of paper.

Multiple Choice

1. Which of these factors does *not* contribute to dehydration at altitude:

   a. Decreased air temperature.
   b. Decreased water vapor in the air.
   c. Decreased respiration rate.
   d. Increased insensible water loss.

2. Whose performance is most likely to decrease at altitude?

   a. The participants in a 400-m relay.
   b. The shot putter.
   c. The swimmer in the 100-yd front crawl.
   d. The 10,000-m runner.

3. In which of the following situations would a person experience reduced heart rate and an overall reduction in the cardiovascular system's work?

   a. Cycling at high altitude.
   b. Scuba diving in cold water.
   c. Living on a space station for three months.
   d. Hiking at a moderate pace at sea level.

4. Based on microgravity research, bed rest might result in

   a. Increased muscle strength.
   b. Higher percentage of bone minerals.
   c. Increased blood plasma volume.
   d. Reduced muscle size.

5. Assuming these were performed with equipment designed for microgravity exercise, which of the following seems to be the best exercise program for in-flight astronauts at this point in time?

   a. Running on a treadmill at maximal intensity.
   b. Total body resistance training.
   c. Total body resistance training combined with running on a treadmill at maximal intensity.
   d. Running on a treadmill at submaximal intensity.

6. A diver complains of severe aching in the elbows, shoulders, and knees shortly after returning to the surface. This diver is experiencing

   a. decompression sickness, due to ascending too rapidly.
   b. oxygen poisoning, due to breathing oxygen with a PO_2 of 318 mmHg or more.
   c. nitrogen narcosis, due to breathing nitrogen at very high pressures.
   d. spontaneous pneumothorax, due to not keeping the mouth open and exhaling during ascent.

True-False

7. At altitude, atmospheric pressure decreases and partial pressures of gases increase.

8. In a hyperbaric environment, the gases in the body are compressible, but the water and body fluids are noncompressible and thus are not measurably affected by either water depth or increased pressure.

9. Most physiological changes that occur as a result of extended exposure to microgravity are similar to those observed as a result of detraining in athletes.

10. People with small total lung volumes and large residual volumes can descend to great depths without risk to their health.

11. Pulmonary ventilation usually decreases both at rest and during exercise at altitude.

Fill in the Blank

12. Air that is in the body before it goes underwater _____ [is compressed, expands] when the body is submerged. The air taken in at depth _____ [is compressed, expands] during ascent.

13. Plasma volume decreases within a few hours of arrival at altitude as a result of _____ and _____.

14. After four to six weeks of chronic hypoxia, muscle fiber areas _____ [decrease, increase] and capillary density in the muscles _____ [decreases, increases].

Short Answer

15. Who will probably perform better in running a 5K at altitude?

   • Subject A, who trained at high intensities at sea level for six wk and whose $\dot{V}O_2$max is 75 ml · kg^{-1} · min^{-1}; or

- Subject B, who trained at high intensities at 1,000 m (3,280 ft) for six wk and whose $\dot{V}O_2$max is 65 ml · kg^{-1} · min^{-1}.

Why?

16. What causes reduced blood volume in astronauts, and how does this work to their advantage in a microgravity environment?

17. What physiological response causes some people to experience acute altitude sickness, and how does this response induce the symptoms of this syndrome?

Essay

18. Describe how the low PO_2 at altitude affects pulmonary ventilation, pulmonary diffusion, oxygen transport, gas exchange at the muscles, and maximal oxygen uptake, as well as how the cardiovascular system responds to these changes.

19. Explain the theoretical advantages and disadvantages of training at altitude for endurance events.

Answers to Selected Chapter 11 Activities

11.1 Hypobaric, Hyperbaric, and Microgravity Environments

1. b, c, f, h, i;   2. d, g;   3. a, e

11.2 Physiological Responses to a Hypobaric Environment

Parameter	Increase or decrease? (Use ↑ or ↓)	Why? What causes this response?
Pulmonary ventilation	↑	Because the number of oxygen molecules in a given volume of air is less at higher altitudes, more air must be inspired to supply as much oxygen as during normal breathing at sea level.
Hemoglobin saturation	↓	The PO_2 drops in direct proportion to the increase in altitude. As a result, the PO_2 within the alveoli and the pulmonary capillaries also decreases. Consequently, hemoglobin saturation drops from about 98% at sea level to about 92% at an elevation of 2,439 m (8,000 ft).
Exchange of oxygen from the blood to the tissues	↓	The reduced arterial PO_2 at altitude causes the difference, or pressure gradient, between arterial PO_2 and tissue PO_2 to decline. Because the diffusion gradient is responsible for driving the oxygen from your blood into your tissues, this lower diffusion gradient results in less oxygen reaching the tissues.
Maximal oxygen uptake ($\dot{V}O_2$max)	↓	This reduction in $\dot{V}O_2$max is the result of low arterial PO_2 that accompanies the drop in barometric pressure at altitude.

(continued)

(continued)

Parameter	Increase or decrease? (Use ↑ or ↓)	Why? What causes this response?
Blood volume after initially arriving at altitude	↓	Plasma volume initially decreases, because of an increase in the number of red blood cells per unit of blood, allowing more oxygen to be delivered to the muscles for a given cardiac output.
Blood volume after continued exposure to high altitude	↑	The diminished plasma volume eventually returns to normal levels. In addition, continued exposure to high altitude triggers increased red blood cell production. These adaptations ultimately result in a greater total blood volume, which allows the person to partially compensate for the lower PO_2 experienced at altitude.
Cardiac output during submaximal work upon initial ascent to altitude	↑	The heart rate increases to compensate for the decrease in the pressure gradient that drives oxygen exchange. This heart rate increase results in increased cardiac output.
Cardiac output during maximal work at altitude	↓	At maximal work levels at altitude, stroke volume and heart rate are both lower, resulting in reduced cardiac output. Stroke volume decreases due to the lower plasma volume. The heart rate reduction at maximal work levels may be a consequence of a decrease in the response to sympathetic nervous system activity, possibly because of a reduction in beta receptors.
Blood pressure in pulmonary arteries	↑	The cause for this is not fully understood. It could indicate some structural changes in the pulmonary arteries in addition to hypoxic vasoconstriction.
Lactic acid production at submaximal levels of exercise	↑	Because of the hypoxic conditions at altitude, oxidation is limited, so anaerobic metaboism increases to meet the body's energy demands. Anaerobic metabolism results in increased lactic acid production.
Lactic acid production at maximal levels of exercise	↓	No conclusive explanation exists. See page 350 of *Physiology of Sport and Exercise* for full discussion.

11.3 Acclimatization at Altitude

a. True; b. Change to "Erythrocyte production is stimulated by the lack of oxygen;" c. True; d. True; e. Change to "Plasma volume initially decreases within a few hours of arrival at altitude as a result of fluid shifts and respiratory water loss. But the diminished plasma volume eventually returns to normal levels;" f. Change to "ST and FT muscle fiber areas decrease;" g. True; h. Change to "The glycolytic enzyme activity of the leg muscles decreases;" i. Change to "Muscles lose some of their capacity to perform oxidative phosphorylation;" j. Change to "Capillary density increases;" k. True; l. True; m. Change to "Therefore . . . the amount of blood bicarbonate decreases rapidly . . ."

11.4 Training and Performance at Altitude

1. Because long duration events place considerable demands on oxygen transport and the aerobic energy system, Eric's performance will be negatively affected by the hypobaric conditions at altitude. His $\dot{V}O_2$max will be reduced, and it will take more perceived effort for Eric to run at his usual pace. In fact, he probably will not be able to compete at his usual level of exertion during this 5K.

2. Given that Eric is not an elite athlete and is rather a recreational runner, he had two options. (1) He could have prepared himself for the high-altitude event through high-intensity endurance training at sea level for the purpose of increasing his $\dot{V}O_2$max. Then upon arriving in Denver, he could run the 5K at a lower percentage of his $\dot{V}O_2$max. (2) He could have timed his arrival in Denver to be within 24 h of the start of the race, in the hopes of competing before the symptoms of altitude sickness started.

3. The thinner air at altitude provides less aerodynamic resistance to athletes' movements.

4. Events that require the thrown object to gain lift from the air will likely not improve at altitude because the air is thinner and provides less lift.

5. No. Whereas endurance events are impaired at altitude, anaerobic sprint activities that last less than a minute place minimal demands on the oxygen transport system and aerobic metabolism, and are therefore not usually impaired by moderate altitude.

6. There is no evidence that training at altitude will improve performance at sea level any more than sea-level training does, but the reasons for this are not clear.

7. Several options exist: (1) Compete within 24 h of arrival at the higher altitude. This does not provide acclimatization, but it does allow the athlete to compete before altitude sickness sets in. (2) Train at higher altitudes for several weeks before competing. (3) Train at a higher intensity at sea level for several weeks to increase $\dot{V}O_2$max levels, thereby letting them compete at a lower relative intensity than those who haven't prepared in this same manner. (4) In the year prior to the Olympics, live at a moderate altitude but train at lower elevations to maximize training intensity.

11.5 Physiological Responses to a Hyperbaric Environment

Answers will vary, but possible safety guidelines include these:

1. Divers should always exhale as they ascend to the surface.

2. When diving in cold water, wearing a wetsuit is highly recommended.

3. Holding your breath for as long as you possibly can is not recommended.

4. A breath-hold diver might want to hold the nose closed and blow air into the middle ear and sinuses.

5. A breath-hold diver should not descend below a depth that causes the ratio between the diver's total lung volume (TLV) and residual volume (RV), called the TLV:RV ratio, to be 1:1.

6. Wear goggles that trap only a very small air volume or that can be pressure equalized with air from the nose or the mouth.

7. When diving for long periods of time, use scuba equipment. (Scuba equipment allows you to breathe pressurized air to equal water pressure; a one-way breathing valve allows the pressurized air to be drawn into the lungs and to be expired into the water.)

11.6   Health Risks of Hypobaric and Hyperbaric Environments

Health risk	Symptoms	Causes	Treatment
Acute altitude sickness	Headache, nausea, vomiting, dyspnea (difficulty breathing), insomnia despite marked fatigue.	**Not fully understood, though reduced ventilation in some people allows carbon dioxide to accumulate in the tissues, and this may induce most of the symptoms.**	Can be prevented by gradual ascent. Can be treated with two prescription drugs or, of course, by retreating to a lower altitude.
High-altitude pulmonary edema (HAPE)	**Shortness of breath, excessive fatigue, blueness in lips and fingernails, mental confusion, loss of consciousness.**	Unknown. Accumulation of fluid in lungs interferes with air movement into and out of the lungs.	**Administration of supplemental oxygen and moving the victim to a lower altitude.**
High altitude cerebral edema (HACE)	Mental confusion, progressing to coma and death.	**The cause of this accumulation of fluid in the cranial cavity is unknown.**	Administration of supplemental oxygen and descent to a lower altitude.
Oxygen poisoning	**Visual distortion, rapid and shallow breathing, convulsions, and in some cases pneumonia.**	Excessive oxygen. High hemoglobin oxygen saturation level, which impairs carbon dioxide elimination via hemoglobin. In addition, breathing oxygen at a PO_2 greater than 318 mmHg causes cerebral blood vessels to constrict, restricting circulation to the nervous sytem.	**Treatment is not discussed in the textbook.**
Nitrogen narcosis	**Symptoms are similar to alcohol intoxication: impaired judgment, perhaps without being able to recognize it.**	At high pressures, during deep dives, nitrogen can act like an anesthetic gas.	This condition is prevented by breathing a specialized gas mixture containing mostly helium during deep dives (below 30 m). Treatment is not discussed in the textbook.

Health risk	Symptoms	Causes	Treatment
Spontaneous pneumothorax	**Death.**	**Not exhaling during ascent. This can over-distend the lungs, rupturing the alveoli, and allowing gas to enter the pleural space and in turn collapse the lung. At the same time, small air bubbles can enter the pulmonary blood and form air emboli, which can become trapped in the vessels of other tissues, blocking circulation to those tissues.**	Prevention is to exhale during ascent. Treatment is not discussed in the textbook.
Ruptured eardrum	**Severe ear pain.**	Failure to equalize the air pressure in the sinuses and middle ear during ascent and descent can rupture the small blood vessels and membranes in these cavities.	**Prevention includes blowing with moderate pressure against the closed nostrils. Upper respiratory infections and sinusitis interfere with one's ability to do so; diving should be avoided if these symptoms exist. Treatment is not discussed in the textbook.**

11.7   Physiological Responses to a Microgravity Environment

Parameter	Increase or decrease? (Use ↑ or ↓)	Why? What causes this response?	Notes for studying purposes
Cross-sectional areas of ST and FT muscle fibers	↓	This results primarily from decreased protein synthesis.	
Muscle strength	↓	The decreased cross-sectional areas of the muscle fibers leads to decreased muscle strength.	

(continued)

(continued)

Parameter	Increase or decrease? (Use ↑ or ↓)	Why? What causes this response?	Notes for studying purposes
Percentage of bone minerals	↓	The exact causes of this are not clear, but are likely in Isome way to be related to the mechanical unloading of bone when the bone is no llonger exposed to the normal gravitational or muscular forces experienced on Earth.	The magnitude of the loss depends on the length of exposure to microgravity.
Plasma volume	↓	Microgravity removes most of the effects of hydrostatic pressure experienced in a 1-*g* environment, resulting in the body dumping a large percentage of its plasma volume, which helps control blood pressure in space.	
Cardiac output and arterial blood pressure	↑	Because there is a reduced hydrostatic pressure, blood no longer pools in the lower extremities. Therefore, more blood returns to the heart, causing increases in these areas.	
Arterial pressure in the kidneys	↑	This increase helps the kidneys to excrete the excess volume in an effort to help control blood pressure.	
Body mass	↓	The loss of mass in flights of 1 to 3 days appears to be largely due to fluids loss. Longer flights of 12 days or more result in weight loss that is 50% from fluid loss and 50% from fat and protein.	

Answers to Selected Chapter 11 Test Questions

Multiple Choice

1. c; 2. d; 3. b; 4. d; 5. c; 6. a

True-False

7. False; 8. True; 9. True; 10. False; 11. False

Fill in the Blank

12. is compressed, expands; 13. fluid shifts, respiratory water loss; 14. decrease, increases

Short Answer and Essay

15. Subject A. Any given rate of work at altitude will be performed at a lower percentage of $\dot{V}O_2$max. Subject A has a higher $\dot{V}O_2$max, so the decrease at altitude will still likely result in work being performed at a higher $\dot{V}O_2$ than Subject B.

For questions 16 to 19, check your answers against the explanations given in the textbook.

Quantifying Sports Training

concepts

- Excessive training refers to training that is done with an unnecessarily high volume, intensity, or both. It leads to no additional improvements in conditioning or performance and can lead to chronic fatigue and decreased performance because of muscle glycogen depletion.

- Overtraining is attempting to do more work than you are physically capable of doing. Overtraining leads to decreased performance capacity.

- Possible explanations for overtraining syndrome include changes in the functioning of the divisions of the autonomic nervous system, altered endocrine responses, and suppressed immune function.

- Tapering—decreasing training intensity and volume before a competition—allows time for the muscles to repair any damage incurred during intense training and for the energy reserves (muscle and liver glycogen) to be restored.

- The effects from detraining, or the cessation of regular physical training, are quite minor compared to those from immobilization. However, in general, the greater the gains during training, the greater the losses during detraining.

- Retraining, or the recovery of conditioning after a period of inactivity, is affected by a person's fitness level and the duration and extent of the inactivity. Compared with less-trained individuals, more highly trained individuals experience a greater loss of conditioning from detraining, and therefore take considerably longer to regain their initial fitness levels.

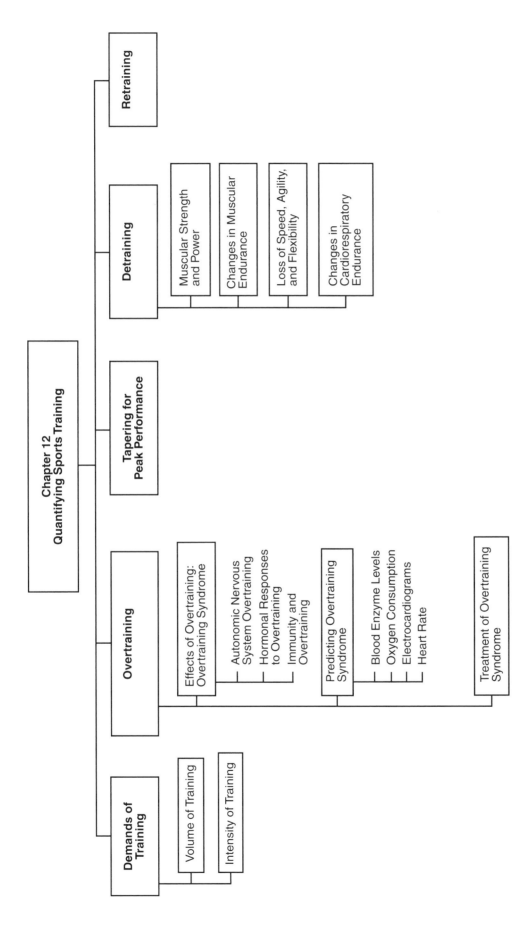

Chapter 12
Quantifying Sports Training

Demands of Training
- Volume of Training
- Intensity of Training

Overtraining
- Effects of Overtraining: Overtraining Syndrome
  - Autonomic Nervous System Overtraining
  - Hormonal Responses to Overtraining
  - Immunity and Overtraining
- Predicting Overtraining Syndrome
  - Blood Enzyme Levels
  - Oxygen Consumption
  - Electrocardiograms
  - Heart Rate
- Treatment of Overtraining Syndrome

Tapering for Peak Performance

Detraining
- Muscular Strength and Power
- Changes in Muscular Endurance
- Loss of Speed, Agility, and Flexibility
- Changes in Cardiorespiratory Endurance

Retraining

Determining an Optimal Training Load

Activity 12.1

Do this activity after reading pages 384-388 of *Physiology of Sport and Exercise.*

A well-designed training program will incorporate the principle of progressive overload, adjusting the training volume and intensity in order to achieve optimal adaptations. But how does this play out in a real training program? What you will do here is overly simplified, but it will help you see how volume and intensity can be easily adjusted and how excessive training can be avoided. Read the "base program" and then manipulate it as directed.

Base program: Roger cycles 60 min per day, three days a wk, at 40% $\dot{V}O_2$max.

For all questions, be sure you start with the "base program" as the foundation. That is, for question 3, refer back to these initial parameters, not to what you came up with in question 2.

1. Rewrite the base program so that you increase the volume of Roger's training by increasing the duration:

   Roger cycles _____ min per day, _____ days a wk, at _____ $\dot{V}O_2$max.

2. Rewrite the base program so that you increase the volume of Roger's training by increasing the frequency:

   Roger cycles _____ min per day, _____ days a wk, at _____ $\dot{V}O_2$max.

3. Rewrite the base program so that you increase the intensity of Roger's training:

   Roger cycles _____ min per day, _____ days a wk, at _____ $\dot{V}O_2$max.

4. Now adjust either the volume, or the intensity, or both in order to increase Roger's training adaptations without risking excessive training.

   Roger cycles _____ min per day, _____ days a wk, at _____ $\dot{V}O_2$max.

5. Finally, with what you know from reading these first few pages of chapter 12, design a four-week training program that shows progressive overload without excessive training. Focus only on cycling training—there's no need to add other types of training (e.g., resistance or plyometric) to this program for this activity. You can do this as briefly as rewriting our "base" sentence four different ways to show progressive overload.

Activity 12.2   Predicting Overtraining Syndrome

**Do this activity after
reading pages 389-395
of *Physiology of Sport
and Exercise*.**

Overtraining, or an unexplained decline in performance, is of serious concern to athletes. Should overtraining occur, performance is jeopardized and, in severe cases, athletes question their desire to continue in the sport and sometimes discontinue competing altogether. How can coaches and athletes prevent overtraining, and what can they do once overtraining has occurred?

First, read the case study and answer the questions that follow.

Frances and Allison are both 800-m freestyle swimmers. Frances trains twice a day, five days a wk, swimming for 2 h each session, for a combined total of 4 h of training each day. Her training intensity is consistently high—usually at or near race pace.

Allison trains once a day, five times a wk, for one and 1.5 h. She trains hard the first two days, then at a moderate intensity for two days, then at a light intensity for one day; then she begins the cycle all over again.

1. Which swimmer is most likely to experience overtraining syndrome? Why?

2. What are the symptoms Frances might exhibit if she experiences overtraining syndrome? Put a capital **S** by the items that reflect sympathetic overtraining and a **P** by the items that reflect parasympathetic overtraining.

3. Which symptom might her coach most be likely to notice?

4. Assuming Frances succumbs to overtraining syndrome, what should she do to recover?

5. After Frances recovers from overtraining and modifies her training to be more cyclic in nature, what dietary issue should she pay attention to? Why?

Finding the right balance between volume and intensity is difficult and varies from athlete to athlete. So researchers and coaches have searched for scientific ways to predict the onset of overtraining. Four of these methods are listed in the table below. For each method listed, fill in the relationship it has to overtraining and its advantages and disadvantages. One row is completed for you as an example.

Method	Relationship to overtraining	Advantages	Disadvantages
Measuring blood enzyme levels			
Measuring oxygen consumption during standardized exercise			
Taking a resting electrocardiogram	Athletes who show sudden decrements in performance often exhibit T wave inversions.	None.	This is not a reliable predictor: Some athlets who clearly have overtraining syndrome do not have T wave inversions.
Monitoring heart rate during standardized exercise			

| **Activity 12.3** | **Tapering for Peak Performance** |

Do this activity after reading pages 396-397 of *Physiology of Sport and Exercise*.

Failure to understand the value of tapering can undermine all of the hard work you have put into your training program. Consider these two athletes:

Will and Russ are both runners with similar personal records in the 5K. They challenge each other to a duel in the upcoming All-City 5K. They both run about 40 mi per wk. Two weeks before the All-City, Will gets swamped at work *and* he has to study for finals. Between studying and working overtime, Will gets in only about 15 mi of training each wk.

Russ, on the other hand, is not going to college and has no extra work demands. He is able to sustain his 40-mi-per-wk training program until the day of the All-City 5K and even takes the opportunity to increase the intensity of his training a bit, figuring he will do all he can to get the edge over Will.

1. Which runner is most likely to better his personal record in the All-City 5K? Why?

2. Describe the effects the taper period likely had on Will's

   a. muscle strength, including

      contractile mechanisms

      repair of muscle damage

   b. energy reserves

   c. $\dot{V}O_2max$

For an extra challenge: The tapering phase of training has traditionally meant a straight reduction in volume and intensity of training prior to competition—for instance, swimmers might reduce their training from 9,000 to 3,500 yd per day and swim at 60% of their usual intensity for all 14 days prior to a competition. A second method, though, is beginning to receive some research attention. In this method, the taper is gradual— for instance, the swimmers might reduce the volume and/or intensity of their training by 20% for 2 days, then by 40% for 2 days, and so on, perhaps swimming a decreasing number of intervals at a specified pace, until the competition occurs.

Research the results of these two methods and write a brief summary, on separate paper, of your findings. From your research, which taper method seems to result in the greatest performance increases?

Examining Physiological Responses to Detraining

Activity 12.4

Do this activity after reading pages 397-403 of *Physiology of Sport and Exercise.*

Have you ever practiced hard while playing on a sports team and then discontinued practicing altogether once the season ended? Or have you embarked on a 12-week aerobics class and then stopped exercising after the 12 weeks ended? Or maybe your activities are climate driven, so you cycle, ski, or kayak for several months and then do not have an alternate activity for when the weather changes. If so, you have experienced detraining—the cessation of regular physical training.

Researchers have found that while the physiological effects of detraining are similar to those experienced during total inactivity or bed rest, the extent of those physiological effects differs greatly between the two.

In the table, use arrows to indicate whether the physiological parameter increases or decreases during detraining, explain the mechanism that causes this increase or decrease (if the text discusses the mechanisms), and jot notes to yourself for studying purposes. One row is filled in for you as an example.

Parameter	Increase or decrease? (Use ↑ or ↓)	Mechanism that causes change	Notes for studying purposes
Muscular strength and power—total inactivity	↓	Atrophy causes decrease in muscle mass and water content, which could account for loss in development of maximal muscle fiber tension. Part of strength loss could result from inability to activate some muscle fibers. Muscle requires minimal stimulation to retain the strength, power, and size gained during training.	Total inactivity leads to rapid losses.
Muscular strength and power—cessation of training			

(continued)

(continued)

Parameter	Increase or decrease? (Use ↑ or ↓)	Mechanism that causes change	Notes for studying purposes
Muscular endurance—total inactivity			
Muscular endurance—cessation of training			
Speed			
Agility			
Flexibility			
Cardiovascular endurance			
Submaximal heart rate			

Parameter	Increase or decrease? (Use ↑ or ↓)	Mechanism that causes change	Notes for studying purposes
Submaximal stroke volume			
Cardiac output			
Maximal oxygen uptake ($\dot{V}O_2$max)			

Maintaining Aerobic Power During Detraining

Cardiorespiratory endurance capacity is rapidly lost following the cessation of formal endurance training, even if the athlete is not completely immobilized. How can athletes keep from losing their endurance capacity even during the off-season?

Examining Physiological Responses to Retraining

Activity 12.5

Do this activity after reading page 404 of *Physiology of Sport and Exercise*.

If you have ever had to recondition your body at the start of a sport season or tried to go for a jog after your leg has been in a cast for 6 wk, you are familiar with retraining. At some time or another, most athletes will experience detraining or immobilization. Regaining initial fitness levels is critical, especially for competitive athletes.

First read page 404 in *Physiology of Sport and Exercise*. Then, without looking in your textbook, fill in the blanks to make sure you know the material. Finally, design a retraining program as requested in question 6.

1. Recovery of conditioning after a period of inactivity is known as _____.

2. The length of time it takes to recover initial conditioning levels is affected by two factors: _____ and _____.

3. More highly trained individuals take _____ [less time, more time] to regain their initial fitness levels than subjects who are less trained.

4. After immobilization, regaining the range of joint motion is a relatively _____ [slow, fast] process.

5. A muscle that has been completely immobilized will recover _____ [more slowly, faster] than one that has been partially movable.

6. Design a retraining program for Shane, a tennis player whose lower leg has been in a cast for the last six wk due to a broken ankle. Now that his cast is off, what should he do?

Putting It All Together: Quantifying Sports Training

Activity 12.6

Do this activity after reading chapter 12 of *Physiology of Sport and Exercise*.

Coaches and athletes do not have it easy! Too much training can actually impair your performance, yet too little training can lead to decrements in many of the gains achieved during regular training. Finding the right balance is both a science and an art; one has to know the physiological responses the body will make as well as the unique ways in which each individual might respond to training changes.

Assuming we do not know the psychological makeup of the following subject nor the unique ways in which her body might respond to training changes, see if you can keep her from overtraining; then help her train properly during the off-season; and finally help her to retrain after she has failed to stick with your training program. Write your answers on a separate piece of paper.

Lisa, a collegiate 1,650-m swimmer, trains five days per wk, swimming 10,000 m per day, with 8,000 of those m at her 1,650-m race pace. She trains this way year-round, nonstop.

1. Given the high volume and high intensity of her training program, Lisa is destined for overtraining. Briefly outline an alternate training program that would prevent her from succumbing to overtraining syndrome.

2. Now, assume that Lisa needs to take a break from daily training during the off-season. Although she is a competitive collegiate swimmer, in the off-season, she wants to concentrate more fully on her studies and enjoy a social life. Briefly outline a training program that would help Lisa maintain her fitness level during this period of detraining.

3. Despite her best intentions, Lisa did not stick entirely to the off-season training program you designed for her. The new swimming season is about to start. What physiological changes might have resulted from Lisa's lack of training?

4. Briefly outline a training program that will help Lisa retrain in order to regain her initial fitness levels.

Sample Test Questions for Chapter 12

Test yourself on your knowledge of this chapter by taking this self-test. Write the correct answers on a separate sheet of paper.

Multiple Choice

1. Which of the following is *not* a sign of overtraining?

    a. Decreased immunity.
    b. Increased appetite.
    c. Increased resting heart rate.
    d. Decreased body mass.

2. With two weeks of detraining, which athlete is most likely to experience performance deficits?

    a. 100-m hurdler.
    b. 400-m sprinter.
    c. Long jumper.
    d. 5,000-m distance runner.

3. Taking both accuracy and ease of assessment into account, which method presents the best possibility of predicting overtraining?

    a. Measuring blood enzyme levels.
    b. Measuring oxygen consumption during standardized exercise.
    c. Measuring heart rate response during standardized exercise.
    d. Taking an electrocardiogram.

4. Which of the following is accomplished during the taper period?

    a. Increased muscular strength.
    b. Reduction in FT fibers' maximal shortening velocity.
    c. Reduction in muscle and liver glycogen stores.
    d. Reduction in $\dot{V}O_2$max.

True-False

5. Muscle requires only minimal stimulation to retain the strength, power, and size gained during training.

6. Several hours of daily training will provide the adaptations needed for athletes who participate in events of short duration.

7. $\dot{V}O_2$max gains can be maintained even when training frequency is reduced by two thirds.

8. With detraining, the muscles' capacity for aerobic performance is maintained longer than their capacity for anaerobic performance.

9. Both the intensity and volume of training must be very high for adaptations to occur.

10. The body responds exactly the same to total inactivity as to periods of reduced activity.

Fill in the Blank

11. A training program that progressively increases the training stimulus as the body adapts to the current stimulus is incorporating the concept of _____.

12. Pushing the body beyond its ability to adapt, with too high a volume or intensity, is termed _____.

13. Training volume can be increased by increasing either the _____ or the _____ of training bouts.

14. If training intensity is reduced, training _____ must be increased to achieve adaptation.

15. _____ is often the first indication and a tell-tale sign of overtraining syndrome. _____

Short Answer

16. Why is it important for endurance athletes to pay particular attention to their carbohydrate intake?

17. List the possible physiological mechanisms responsible for the loss of muscular strength that occurs with either immobilization or inactivity.

18. Present two possible methods of reducing the time needed for retraining while a limb is immobilized in a cast.

Essay

19. Explain in detail the physiological mechanisms that may lead to a decrease in muscular endurance during periods of detraining.

20. Why is it particularly important for highly trained endurance athletes to maintain cardiorespiratory fitness during the off-season? How can this be best accomplished?

Answers to Selected Chapter 12 Activities

12.1   Determining an Optimal Training Load

> **Base program:** Roger cycles 60 min per day, 3 days a wk, at 40% $\dot{V}O_2$max.

1. The number in the first blank should be greater than in the base program. The second blank should have remained at 3 and third blank at 40%.

2. The number in the second blank should be greater than in the base program. The first blank should have remained at 60 and the third at 40%.

3. The number in the third blank should be greater than in the base program. The first blank should have remained at 60 and the second at 3.

4. Answers will vary. Certainly the 40% $\dot{V}O_2$max should be increased to somewhere between 50% and 90%. Volume should be adjusted accordingly—the greater the increase in intensity, the lesser the increase in volume and vice versa.

5. Answers will vary.

12.2   Predicting Overtraining Syndrome

1. Frances is most likely to experience overtraining syndrome. Her high-volume, high-intensity training program offers her body no chance for recovery, and likely experiences more catabolism than anabolism.

2. Decreased physical performance; loss in muscular strength, coordination, and maximal working capacity; decreased appetite (S); decreased body mass or loss of weight (S); muscle tenderness; head colds, allergic reactions, or both; occasional nausea; increased resting heart rate (S); increased blood pressure (S); sleep disturbances (S); emotional instability (S); elevated basal metabolic rate (S); early onset of fatigue (P); decreased resting heart rate (P); rapid heart rate recovery after exercise (P); decreased resting blood pressure (P).

3. An unexplained decline in performance.

4. In order to recover from overtraining, Frances should rest completely for 3 to 5 days or change to low-intensity exercise.

5. Frances, and Allison, too, for that matter, should pay particular attention to her carbohydrate intake. Repeated days of hard training cause a gradual reduction of muscle glycogen. These swimmers need to consume extra carbohydrate during those periods, so that their muscle and liver glycogen reserves are not depleted.

Predicting Overtraining Syndrome

Method	Relationship to overtraining	Advantages	Disadvantages
Measuring blood enzyme levels	The presence of large amounts of certain enzymes in the blood suggests that muscle cell membranes have suffered some damage, allowing the enzymes to escape.	None.	No evidence links this to overtraining syndrome. Measuring blood enzyme levels is difficult and expensive.
Measuring oxygen consumption during standardized exercise	As athletes become overtrained, they often show a loss of skill, which decreases their performance efficiency. As their movements become less efficient, their oxygen consumption typically increases.	Provides a clear indication of oxygen consumption increase, which might indicate less efficient movements—a sign of overtraining syndrome.	These tests are too complex, time consuming, and impractical for field use.
Taking a resting electrocardiogram	Athletes who show sudden decrements in performance often exhibit T wave inversions.	None.	This is not a reliable predictor: Some athletes who clearly have overtraining syndrome do not have T wave inversions.
Monitoring heart rate during standardized exercise	Heart rate is higher when the runner is in the overtrained state than when the runner is responding well to training.	Provides easily obtained, objective measurement. Provides immediate information. Correlates closely to blood lactate measurements.	None.

12.3   Tapering for Peak Performance

1. Will is most likely to set a new personal record because, without knowing it, he used a taper period, which allowed his muscles to repair damage from training and his energy reserves to be restored.

2. Will's muscle strength likely increased during the taper period.

   a. During intensified training, FT fibers exhibit a significant reduction in their maximal shortening capacity, so it could be that during Will's taper period, his FT fibers recovered and improved their contractile properties.

      The taper period likely allowed the muscle damage done during intense training to be repaired.

   b. Will's muscle and liver glycogen was probably restored to optimal levels during his taper period.

   c. Developing optimal $\dot{V}O_2$max initially requires a lot of training, but once it has been developed, much less training is needed to maintain it at its highest level. Because Will still trained above one-third of his usual amount during his taper period, his $\dot{V}O_2$max probably remained the same.

12.4 Examining Physiological Responses to Detraining

Parameter	Increase or decrease? (Use ↑ or ↓)	Mechanism that causes change	Notes for studying purposes
Muscular strength and power—total inactivity	↓	Atrophy causes decrease in muscle mass and water content, which could account for loss in development of maximal muscle fiber tension. Part of strength loss could result from inability to activate some muscle fibers. Muscle requires minimal stimulation to retain the strength, power, and size gained during training.	Total inactivity leads to rapid losses.
Muscular strength and power—cessation of training	↓	Same as above.	These reductions are relatively small during the first few months, as compared with drastic reductions experienced with total inactivity. Changes can be largely prevented by continuation of training at a greatly reduced level.
Muscular endurance—total inactivity	↓	Activities of oxidative enzymes decrease drastically within the first week or two of immobilization. Dramatic shift in percentages of ST and FT fibers, with shift toward more FT fibers.	Drastic changes will occur within first 2 weeks of immobilization.
Muscular endurance—cessation of training	↓	Activities of glycolytic enzymes change little, but muscle glycogen content decreases. Blood lactate levels increase, leading to disturbed acid-base balance, reflecting a rise in blood lactate levels and a drop in bicarbonate levels. Muscle fiber composition does not appear to change. Some evidence that muscle capillary supply decreases, impairing oxygen delivery to muscles.	Muscle oxidative and anaerobic energy systems are unaffected by only a few days of rest. Only during complete inactivity (immobilization) do such changes impair performance in the first week or two.
Speed	↓	Not commented on in text.	Training produces less improvement in speed and agility than in many other parameters, so losses of speed and agility that occur with inactivity are relatively small. Peak levels of both can be maintained with limited training.

(continued)

Parameter	Increase or decrease? (Use ↑ or ↓)	Mechanism that causes change	Notes for studying purposes
Agility	↓	Not commented on in text.	Same as above.
Flexibility	↓	Not commented on in text.	Lost quickly during inactivity; also can be reestablished in less time.
Cardiovascular endurance	↓	Largely caused by a reduction in plasma volume, which in turn diminishes stroke volume.	Reduction in cardiovascular endurance is much greater than the reductions of strength, power, and muscular endurance.
Submaximal heart rate	↑	Not commented on in text.	
Submaximal stroke volume	↓	Not commented on in text.	
Cardiac output	↓	Results from reduced stroke volume, which is caused by a decrease in heart volume, total blood volume, plasma volume, and ventricular contractility.	
Maximal oxygen uptake ($\dot{V}O_2$max)	↓	Same as above.	Highly conditioned athletes experience greater decreases in $\dot{V}O_2$max and need longer to regain their initial level of conditioning than less-fit people.

Losses of aerobic capacity are significant only when the frequency and duration are reduced by two-thirds of the regular training load. But training intensity plays a more crucial role in maintaining aerobic power during periods of reduced training. Research indicates that at least three training sessions per week at an intensity of at least 70% $\dot{V}O_2$max are needed to maintain aerobic conditioning.

12.5 Retraining

1. retraining

2. initial fitness level, duration and extent of inactivity

3. more time

4. slow

5. more slowly

6. Answers will vary, but should include a discussion of combined strength training and aerobic training in order to improve muscle aerobic capacity and flexibility.

Answers to Selected Chapter 12 Test Questions

Multiple Choice

1. b; 2. d; 3. c; 4. a

True-False

5. True; 6. False; 7. True; 8. False; 9. False; 10. False

Fill in the Blank

11. progressive overload
12. excessive training
13. duration, frequency
14. volume
15. An unexplained decline in physical performance

Short Answer and Essay

For questions 16 to 20, check your answers against the explanations given in the text-book.

13

Ergogenic Aids and Performance

concepts

- An ergogenic aid is any substance or phenomenon that enhances performance. An ergolytic substance is one that has a detrimental effect on performance. Some substances generally thought to be ergogenic are actually ergolytic.

- Establishing the ergogenic effect of a substance requires careful research that includes both laboratory and field studies and controls for possible placebo effects.

- Some pharmacological agents, or drugs, are thought to have ergogenic properties. Of interest are alcohol, amphetamines, beta blockers, caffeine, cocaine, diuretics, marijuana, and nicotine.

- Some hormonal agents are thought to have ergogenic properties. Both anabolic steroids and human growth hormone are banned from all sports, and the medical risks associated with their use are high.

- Many physiological agents have been proposed as ergogenic aids. The goal of using these agents is to improve the body's physiological response to exercise. With these agents, the athlete typically adds something that occurs naturally in smaller quantities in the body to try to improve performance. Using certain physiological agents in this way carries some risk.

- Many nutritional agents—including amino acids, L-carnitine, creatine, and chromium—have been proposed to have specific ergogenic properties, but most of these nutritional agents have not been adequately researched.

- All athletes must recognize the legal, ethical, moral, and medical consequences of using any ergogenic agent. Athletes who use banned substances risk disqualification from a particular competition, being banned from competition in their sport for a year or more, and serious health risks.

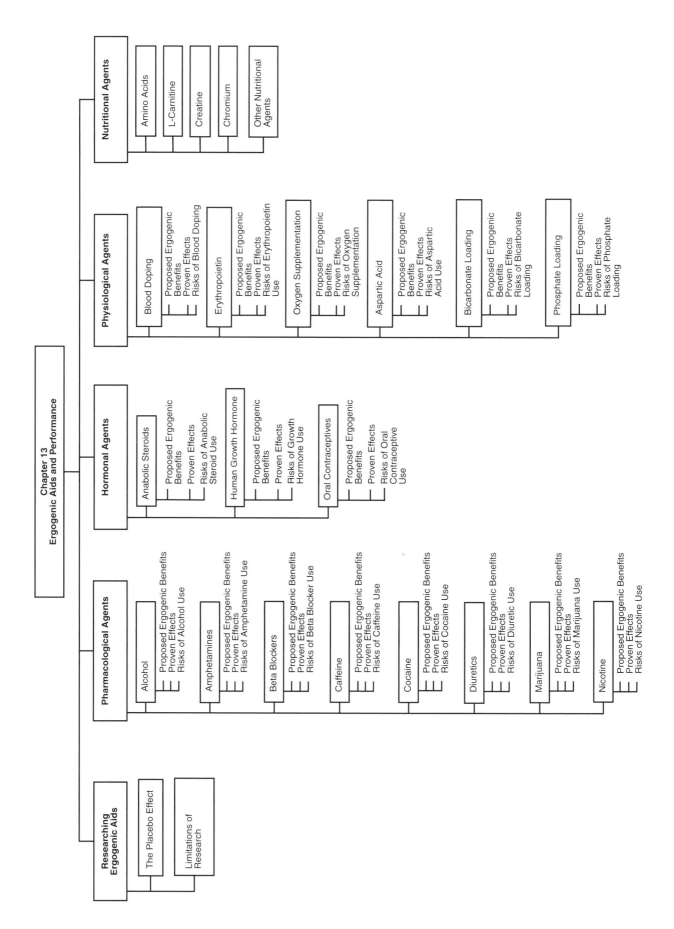

Chapter 13
Ergogenic Aids and Performance

Researching Ergogenic Aids
- The Placebo Effect
- Limitations of Research

Pharmacological Agents
- Alcohol
  - Proposed Ergogenic Benefits
  - Proven Effects
  - Risks of Alcohol Use
- Amphetamines
  - Proposed Ergogenic Benefits
  - Proven Effects
  - Risks of Amphetamine Use
- Beta Blockers
  - Proposed Ergogenic Benefits
  - Proven Effects
  - Risks of Beta Blocker Use
- Caffeine
  - Proposed Ergogenic Benefits
  - Proven Effects
  - Risks of Caffeine Use
- Cocaine
  - Proposed Ergogenic Benefits
  - Proven Effects
  - Risks of Cocaine Use
- Diuretics
  - Proposed Ergogenic Benefits
  - Proven Effects
  - Risks of Diuretic Use
- Marijuana
  - Proposed Ergogenic Benefits
  - Proven Effects
  - Risks of Marijuana Use
- Nicotine
  - Proposed Ergogenic Benefits
  - Proven Effects
  - Risks of Nicotine Use

Hormonal Agents
- Anabolic Steroids
  - Proposed Ergogenic Benefits
  - Proven Effects
  - Risks of Anabolic Steroid Use
- Human Growth Hormone
  - Proposed Ergogenic Benefits
  - Proven Effects
  - Risks of Growth Hormone Use
- Oral Contraceptives
  - Proposed Ergogenic Benefits
  - Proven Effects
  - Risks of Oral Contraceptive Use

Physiological Agents
- Blood Doping
  - Proposed Ergogenic Benefits
  - Proven Effects
  - Risks of Blood Doping
- Erythropoietin
  - Proposed Ergogenic Benefits
  - Proven Effects
  - Risks of Erythropoietin Use
- Oxygen Supplementation
  - Proposed Ergogenic Benefits
  - Proven Effects
  - Risks of Oxygen Supplementation
- Aspartic Acid
  - Proposed Ergogenic Benefits
  - Proven Effects
  - Risks of Aspartic Acid Use
- Bicarbonate Loading
  - Proposed Ergogenic Benefits
  - Proven Effects
  - Risks of Bicarbonate Loading
- Phosphate Loading
  - Proposed Ergogenic Benefits
  - Proven Effects
  - Risks of Phosphate Loading

Nutritional Agents
- Amino Acids
- L-Carnitine
- Creatine
- Chromium
- Other Nutritional Agents

226

| Activity 13.1 | # The Placebo Effect and Limitations of Research |

Do this activity after reading pages 410-414 of *Physiology of Sport and Exercise.*

Establishing the ergogenic effect of a substance requires careful research that includes both laboratory and field studies and controls for possible placebo effects. First, conduct the experiment below to study the placebo effect; then answer the questions about laboratory and field testing.

The Placebo Effect

Though the placebo effect has a psychological origin, the body's physical response to a placebo is not merely imagined; it is quite real. This clearly illustrates how effective our mental state can be in altering our physical state.

Try this experiment. You will need a decaffeinated beverage of some sort (decaffeinated soda or coffee will work well). You will also need a willing participant. Tell your participant that you are doing an experiment on the effects of caffeine to see if caffeine really does improve performance. Choose an activity for this participant to perform. You might choose running until exhaustion or doing as many sit-ups as possible. Try to choose an activity that will not take much time to perform. Whatever activity you choose, have the participant perform this event one time (run as far as possible, or do as many sit-ups as possible). Record the results. After a long recovery time, give the participant the decaffeinated beverage, but tell him or her that it is caffeinated and that performance might improve because of the stimulating effects of caffeine. Have the participant perform the same activity again and record the results. Did the performance improve? If so, to what do you attribute this?

(You could also try this experiment with yourself as the participant. After recording your baseline result in the activity, ask one of your friends to give you a beverage without telling you whether it is caffeinated or decaffeinated. Perform the activity again and record the results. Now ask the friend which type of beverage it was—was it caffeinated or not? If it was not caffeinated and your performance improved, to what do you attribute this?)

Record your observations from this experiment here:

Laboratory and Field Testing

Science is limited in its ability to determine the efficacy of ergogenic aids, and one of the difficulties in researching these is the test setting. Both laboratory testing and field testing have distinct advantages and disadvantages. What are they?

Laboratory setting

Advantages:

Disadvantages:

Field setting

Advantages:

Disadvantages:

| Activity 13.2 | Pharmacological Agents |

Do this activity after reading pages 415-426 of *Physiology of Sport and Exercise*.

Pharmacological agents are a group of drugs believed by some athletes to have ergogenic properties. While some of these drugs can actually improve some performance parameters, others have no effect on performance, and still others have an ergolytic effect, causing decrements in performance. In addition, some of these drugs carry serious health risks.

Read pages 415-426 in *Physiology of Sport and Exercise* to learn the proven effects of each pharmacological agent as well as the risks of using the drug. Then, without looking in your textbook, try to match the pharmacological agents with their proven effects and risks. You will use more than one letter in some blanks.

Pharmacological agent

1. Alcohol   Proven effects: _____   Risks: _____
2. Amphetamines   Proven effects: _____   Risks: _____
3. Beta blockers Proven effects: _____   Risks: _____
4. Caffeine   Proven effects: _____   Risks: _____
5. Cocaine   Proven effects: _____   Risks: _____
6. Diuretics   Proven effects: _____   Risks: _____
7. Marijuana   Proven effects: _____   Risks: _____
8. Nicotine   Proven effects: _____   Risks: _____

Proven effects

a. Has little effect on strength, power, and local muscular endurance.
b. Reduces plasma volume, which reduces maximal cardiac output, which in turn reduces aerobic capacity.
c. Causes apparent improvement in speed, power, endurance, concentration, and fine motor coordination.

d. Impairs performance of skills requiring hand-eye coordination, fast reaction time, motor coordination, tracking ability, and perceptual accuracy.

e. Impairs performance by negatively affecting psychomotor skills, such as reaction time, movement time, speed, sensorimotor coordination, and information processing.

f. Is detrimental or of little value to athletic performance. Can result in lower $\dot{V}O_2$max than nonusers; increased heart rate, blood pressure, and autonomic reactivity; vasoconstriction; decreased peripheral circulation; increased secretion of antidiuretic hormone and catecholamines; and increased blood lipid levels, plasma glucose, glucagon, insulin, and cortisol.

g. Can cause a "motivational syndrome," characterized by apathy, impaired judgment, loss of ambition, and an inability to carry out long-term plans.

h. Has no ergogenic effects on strength, power, speed, local muscular endurance, or cardiorespiratory endurance.

i. Leads to significant weight loss.

j. Improves endurance performance, perhaps through increased FFA mobilization, and lowers the perception of effort at a given rate of work.

k. Reduces maximal oxygen uptake, maximal ventilatory capacity, submaximal and maximal heart rate, maximal cardiac output, and blood pressure.

l. Stimulates the CNS: Increases mental alertness, increases concentration, elevates mood, decreases fatigue and delays its onset, decreases reaction time, enhances catecholamine release, increases FFA mobilization, and increases the use of muscle triglycerides.

m. No evidence of ergogenic properties.

n. Stimulates the CNS: Increases mental alertness, elevates mood, decreases the sense of fatigue, and produces euphoria.

o. Is ergogenic for shooting sports, due to the slowing of heart rate; but ergolytic for activities requiring aerobic capacity.

Risks

aa. Increased risk of injury due to its depressant effects on the CNS, which dull the sensation of pain.

bb. Fatigue, bronchospasm, and cardiovascular complications.

cc. Negative behavioral effects such as extreme nervousness, acute anxiety, aggressive behavior, and insomnia.

dd. Increased risk of dehydration and heat-related illnesses when performing in hot environments.

ee. Hypotension (lowered blood pressure).

ff. Psychological and physical addiction.

gg. Physically addictive: Abrupt disruption can result in severe headache, fatigue, irritability, and gastrointestinal distress.

hh. Dehydration: It suppresses the release of ADH, which causes the body to excrete more water in the urine.

ii. Negative behavioral effects such as nervousness, restlessness, insomnia, and tremors.

jj. Increased risk of hypothermia in cold environments, due to peripheral vasodilation.

kk. Increased risk of cardiac arrhythmia or death: This agent elevates heart rate and blood pressure, which places great stress on the cardiovascular system; this agent might also delay the *sensation* of fatigue, enabling athletes to push themselves beyond normal limits to the point of circulatory failure.

ll. Depending on method of ingestion, increased risk of lung cancer; cancers of the mouth, pharynx, and larynx; and emphysema.

mm. Physiological problems such as inflammation and destruction of nasal tissues, and cardiac arrhythmias because of the agent's increasing norepinephrine's effects on the heart.

nn. Impaired short-term memory.

oo. Impaired thermoregulation due to reduced plasma volume.

pp. Psychological problems such as agitation, irritability, restlessness, anxiety, insomnia, hallucinations, and paranoia.

qq. Electrolyte imbalances, which can cause fatigue, muscle cramping, exhaustion, cardiac arrhythmias, and cardiac arrest.

rr. Decreased circulating testosterone levels.

ss. Increased susceptibility to respiratory infections.

tt. Hallucinations and psychotic-like behavior with heavy use.

uu. Very high risk of physical addiction.

vv. Cardiovascular changes: Raises blood cholesterol levels, promotes atherosclerosis, impairs circulation to the extremities (increased risk of frostbite when performing in cold environments), and can cause peripheral vascular disease.

For an extra challenge . . . Keep track of your alcohol, caffeine, and nicotine use for one week. See table 13.4 on page 422 of *Physiology of Sport and Exercise* to help you track your caffeine intake. Write the amount of each item you consumed here:

Alcohol: _____ oz

Nicotine: _____ mg of tar (Include cigarettes as well as smokeless tobacco in the form of chewing tobacco, snuff, or compressed tobacco.)

Caffeine: _____ mg

1. If you were an athlete competing during the week you recorded your intake, how might these pharmacological agents have affected your performance?

2. Based on information provided in *Physiology of Sport and Exercise,* what health risks are you subjecting yourself to by ingesting these substances?

Activity 13.3

Hormonal Agents

Do this activity after reading pages 427-432 of *Physiology of Sport and Exercise*.

Hormonal agents are a group of hormones believed by some athletes to have ergogenic properties. The three most commonly used or abused hormones are anabolic steroids, human growth hormone, and, to some extent, oral contraceptives. Although numerous scientific studies have been conducted on anabolic steroids and sport, little is known about the effects of human growth hormone and birth control pills on sport performance. Read the following case studies about athletes attempting to use these hormones; then answer, on a separate sheet of paper, the questions regarding the hormones' proven effects and risks.

Darren is 13 years old and just beginning the eighth grade. American football is a huge sport in his small town, and Darren's dream for next year is to make the high school football team, which has won the state championship three times in the last 5 years. But Darren is small for his age; he has not even begun his growth spurt. The guys he hangs around with start talking about steroids and showing Darren some of the pills they are taking. They say these pills are making them grow faster and making their muscles stronger. Soon, Darren decides to buy some anabolic steroids from his friends. What can it hurt? Maybe it will help him grow tall enough and gain enough strength over the next year to make the junior varsity high school football team.

1. Darren is not all wrong about the ways in which anabolic steroids might affect his performance. What are the proven effects of anabolic steroids?

2. Darren does not realize it, but there are some serious health risks to taking anabolic steroids. What are they? Given Darren's stage of maturation, what might be the most serious health risk for him?

3. We often think of males taking steroids to increase strength, but some females also take anabolic steroids without realizing the medical consequences. In addition to the risks that are similar to those of men, what are the health risks specific to women who take anabolic steroids?

Peter plays on his university's rugby team. Peter's coach is pleased with the team's endurance, but has been pressuring Peter and his teammates to increase their muscle strength so they can tackle with greater force. Peter has heard stories of how anabolic steroids and human growth hormone can help athletes gain strength. He has also wondered about the claims that human growth hormone assists in the healing of injuries. He makes a couple of contacts and soon has some human growth hormone in his possession.

4. As in Darren's situation, there is some truth to what Peter has heard. What are the proven effects of human growth hormone?

5. There are some very serious health risks to taking human growth hormone. What medical consequences might Peter experience if he uses human growth hormone?

Lauren is an elite cyclist. Her coach has noticed that Lauren's performances vary quite a bit and has started plotting the performances. When she shows the records to Lauren, Lauren sees a pattern—her performances typically dip several days before menstruation. She tells her coach how awful she feels on those days, with bloating, cramps, and irritability distracting her from the competition. Lauren's times are only split seconds lower on those days, but at her level of competition, every hundredth of a second counts. The World Championships are several months away. Lauren's coach suggests that she take oral contraceptives continuously (not cyclically) until 10 days before the Worlds. Lauren will have some withdrawal bleeding about 3 days after she discontinues the contraceptives, and then she will be left with low levels of estrogen and progesterone and will be in the follicular phase of her menstrual cycle at the time of the event.

6. While many women take oral contraceptives for birth control or to assist with medical conditions (e.g., irregular periods and other conditions), for what performance reasons might an elite athlete desire to take oral contraceptives?

7. If Lauren were a recreational cyclist or even an amateur competitor instead of an elite cyclist, would you recommend she use oral contraceptives as an ergogenic aid? Why or why not?

8. If you did not already answer this in question 7, list the risks of oral contraceptive use.

Activity 13.4	# Physiological Agents

Do this activity after reading pages 433-441 of *Physiology of Sport and Exercise*.

The goal of using physiological agents is to improve the body's physiological response during exercise. With these agents, the athlete typically adds more of something that already occurs naturally in the body to try to improve performance. The reasoning is that if natural levels of a substance are beneficial to performance, higher levels should be even better. However, not every physiological agent improves performance, nor is every agent safe at any level.

Read pages 433-441 in *Physiology of Sport and Exercise* to learn the proven effects of each physiological agent as well as the risks of using it. Then, without looking in your textbook, try to match the physiological agents with their proven effects and risks. You will use more than one answer in some blanks, *and you may use an answer more than once.*

Physiological agent

1. Alcohol   Proven effects: _____   Risks: _____

2. Erythropoietin   Proven effects: _____   Risks: _____

3. Oxygen supplementation   Proven effects: _____   Risks: _____

4. Aspartic acid   Proven effects: _____   Risks: _____

5. Bicarbonate loading   Proven effects: _____   Risks: _____

6. Phosphate loading   Proven effects: _____   Risks: _____

Proven effects

a. Inconclusive research evidence, with some possibility of improvements in $\dot{V}O_2$max and time to exhaustion.
b. Inconclusive research evidence, with some possibility of improved endurance.
c. Improved blood buffering capacity.
d. Limited improvements in the amount of work and rate of work when administered immediately before a short bout of exercise; definite improvements in the amount of work and rate of work when administered during exercise; no effect when administered postexercise.
e. Improved performance of all-out, maximal anaerobic activities of 1- to 7-min duration.
f. Enhanced lactate removal from muscle.
g. Improved $\dot{V}O_2$max and improved endurance performance.

Risks

aa. Gastrointestinal discomfort, including diarrhea, cramps, and bloating.
bb. Cardiovascular complications caused by excessive blood viscosity.
cc. No known risks.
dd. Unpredictable amount of red blood cell production, which could lead to cardiovascular complications caused by excessive blood viscosity.
ee. Allergic reactions or infections resulting from blood infusions.

Activity 13.5

Nutritional Agents

Do this activity after reading pages 442-444 of *Physiology of Sport and Exercise.*

Many nutritional agents have been proposed to have specific ergogenic properties, but most of them have not been studied adequately. The mechanisms through which these nutritional agents work lead researchers to believe they might have ergogenic properties, yet for the most part, the evidence is inconclusive. Using the information in your textbook, fill in the table below to learn the proposed mechanisms and whether or not the nutritional agent has been found to be ergogenic. One row is filled in for you as an example.

Nutritional agent	Proposed mechanism	Ergogenic?
L-tryptophan	L-tryptophan is the first precursor of serotonin, a potent CNS neurotransmitter that acts as an analgesic, delaying fatigue.	No evidence of ergogenic effects.
Branched-chain amino acids		
L-carnitine		
Creatine		
Chromium		

Putting It All Together: Ergogenic Aids and Performance

Activity 13.6

Do this activity after reading chapter 13 of *Physiology of Sport and Exercise.*

In this chapter, we have looked at the proposed benefits of ergogenic aids, their proven effects, and the risks of using them. We have also discussed the mechanisms through which these agents might work. All athletes must recognize the legal, ethical, moral, and medical consequences of using any ergogenic agent. Athletes who use banned substances risk disqualification from a particular competition, being banned from competition in their sport for a year or more, and serious health risks.

Without looking in your textbook, and recognizing that not all of these effects have been fully proven, place a black dot in the appropriate columns in the table on the next page to indicate the mechanisms through which each ergogenic aid is proposed to work. You might have more than one black dot in each row.

Sample Test Questions for Chapter 13

Test yourself on your knowledge of this chapter by taking this self-test. Write the correct answers on a separate sheet of paper.

Multiple Choice

1. This pharmacological agent acts primarily as a central nervous system depressant:

    a. Amphetamines;   b. Caffeine;   c. Alcohol;   d. Cocaine

2. Which statement best describes the mechanism exerted by beta blockers?

    a. Beta blockers stimulate the beta-adrenergic receptors, which in turn stimulate the central nervous system.
    b. Beta blockers prevent binding of the neurotransmitter epinephrine, and this greatly reduces the effects of stimulation by the sympathetic nervous system.
    c. Beta blockers improve the binding of the neurotransmitter epinephrine, and this greatly increases the effects of stimulation by the sympathetic nervous system.
    d. None of the above.

3. An athlete who takes diuretics can expect

    a. to gain weight.
    b. an increase in maximal cardiac output.
    c. an increase in aerobic capacity.
    d. performance to be impaired.

4. At present, this is the proven effect of anabolic steroids:

    a. Increased fat-free muscle mass and strength
    b. Increased aerobic power
    c. Improved recovery from high-intensity training
    d. Increased capacity for muscular exercise

5. This person's performance is most likely to improve due to oxygen supplementation:

    a. The football player who breathes oxygen on the sidelines during a game
    b. The miler who breathes oxygen for several minutes prior to running the mile
    c. The rower who breathes oxygen upon completing a rowing match
    d. The research subject who breathes oxygen during a treadmill test

Proposed Ergogenic Aids and Mechanisms Through Which They Might Work

	Act on heart, blood, circulation, and aerobic endurance	Increase oxygen delivery	Supply fuel for muscle and general muscle function	Act on muscle mass and strength	Result in weight loss or weight gain	Counteract or delay onset or sensation of fatigue	Counteract CNS inhibition	Aid in relaxation and stress reduction
Pharmacological agents								
Alcohol								
Amphetamines								
Beta blockers								
Caffeine								
Cocaine and marijuana								
Diuretics								
Nicotine								
Hormones								
Anabolic steroids								
Human growth hormone								
Oral contraceptives								
Physiological agents								
Aspartic acid salts								
Bicarbonate loading								
Blood doping								
Erythropoietin								
Oxygen								
Phosphate loading								
Nutritional agents								
Amino acids								
Chromium								
Creatine								
L-carnitine								

Adapted from E.L. Fox, R.W. Bowers, and M.L. Foss, 1988, *The physiological basis of physical education and athletics* (Philadelphia: Saunders College Publishing), 632. Copyright 1988 The McGraw-Hill Companies. Adapted by permission of The McGraw-Hill Companies.

True-False

6. The observation of performance improvements after use of a particular substance automatically means that the substance possesses ergogenic properties.

7. Alcohol is an excellent source of carbohydrates.

8. Amphetamines increase one's state of arousal, which leads to a sense of increased energy, self-confidence, and faster decision making.

9. The use of oral contraceptives is entirely safe, and it is quite advisable for female athletes to use oral contraceptives to manipulate their menstrual cycles in order to improve performance.

10. Because physiological agents occur naturally in the body, they are safe to use at any level.

11. Performance improvements from blood doping result from increased cardiac output due to an expanded plasma volume.

12. Bicarbonate loading is proposed to work by increasing plasma bicarbonate levels, thereby providing additional buffer capacity, which would allow higher concentrations of lactate in the blood.

Fill in the Blank

13. The phenomenon by which your expectations of a substance determine your body's response to it is known as the _____.

14. The lower $\dot{V}O_2$max values smokers experience are associated with increased _____ binding to hemoglobin, which reduces _____ capacity.

15. With _____ use, no one can predict how much red blood cell production will occur.

Short Answer

16. Explain how the decreased sense of fatigue brought on by amphetamine use poses a health risk.

17. Through what mechanism does cocaine stimulate the central nervous system?

18. Although growth hormone is thought to stimulate bone growth and increase blood glucose levels, how can these same properties become dangerous when athletes use growth hormone after their bones have fused?

19. Explain the physiological mechanisms whereby creatine supplementation could increase performance of high-intensity, intermittent exercise but not of endurance exercise.

Essay

20. Describe the research difficulties of evaluating the efficacy of a potential ergogenic aid.

21. Discuss the risks of anabolic steroid use. For each risk, explain the physiological mechanism that leads to the health risk.

Answers to Selected Chapter 13 Activities

13.1 The Placebo Effect and Limitations of Research

In a laboratory testing, the environment can be carefully controlled, yet the findings will not always accurately reflect natural results. The opposite is true of field tests: Although the results will be reflective of the natural situation, the environment cannot be carefully controlled.

13.2 Pharmacological Agents

1. Alcohol *Proven effects:* e, h;   *Risks:* aa, ee, hh, jj
2. Amphetamines *Proven effects:* c, n;   *Risks:* cc, ff, kk
3. Beta blockers *Proven effects:* a, k, o;   *Risks:* bb
4. Caffeine *Proven effects:* j, l;   *Risks:* dd, gg, ii
5. Cocaine *Proven effects:* m;   *Risks:* mm, pp, uu
6. Diuretics *Proven effects:* b, i;   *Risks:* oo, qq
7. Marijuana *Proven effects:* d, g;   *Risks:* nn, rr, tt
8. Nicotine *Proven effects:* f;   *Risks:* ll, ss, vv

13.3 Hormonal Agents

1. Anabolic steroids can lead to increased fat-free body mass and increased muscle size and strength. They do not increase endurance capacity, and their ability to facilitate recovery from exhaustive exercise has not been proven.

2. The health risks of anabolic steroids include testicular atrophy, reduced sperm counts, and breast enlargement in males; liver damage; cardiomyopathy; personality changes; and of most serious concern for Darren, interruption of normal bone growth in adolescents, which would be counterproductive to Darren's desire to grow tall.

3. In addition to the risks shared by men and women, women who take anabolic steroids are at increased risk for breast regression, masculinization, and menstrual cycle disruption.

4. Taking human growth hormone seems to increase fat-free mass and decrease body fat.

5. Peter could experience acromegaly, which results in bone thickening, skin thickening, and soft tissue growth. With acromegaly, internal organs enlarge and ultimately the victim suffers muscle and joint weakness and often heart disease. Peter is also putting himself at increased risk for cardiomyopathy, glucose intolerance, diabetes, and hypertension.

6. Most female athletes find that their performance is unaffected by their menstrual cycle, but for those who have cyclic fluctuations in their performance due to premenstrual syndrome, their menstrual cycle can be manipulated with oral contraceptives.

7. It is rarely advisable or necessary to manipulate an athlete's menstrual cycle to improve her performance.

8. Women who take oral contraceptives are at increased risk for nausea, weight gain, fatigue, hypertension, liver tumors, blood clots, stroke, and heart attack.

13.4   Physiological Agents

1. Blood doping *Proven effects:* i;   *Risks:* bb, ee
2. Erythropoietin *Proven effects:* g;   *Risks:* dd
3. Oxygen supplementation *Proven effects:* d;   *Risks:* cc
4. Aspartic acid *Proven effects:* b;   *Risks:* cc
5. Bicarbonate loading *Proven effects:* c, e, f;   *Risks:* aa
6. Phosphate loading *Proven effects:* a;   *Risks:* cc

13.5   Nutritional Agents

Nutritional agent	Proposed mechanism	Ergogenic?
L-tryptophan	L-tryptophan is the first precursor of serotonin, a potent CNS neurotransmitter that acts as an analgesic, delaying fatigue.	No evidence of ergogenic effects.
Branched-chain amino acids	Exercise-induced increases in the plasma-free tryptophan: BCAA ratios are associated with increased brain serotonin and the onset of fatigue during prolonged exercise. Theoretically, increasing the BCAA would reduce the ratio and delay the onset of fatigue.	No evidence of ergogenic effects.
L-carnitine	Assists in the transfer of fatty acids from the cytosol across the inner mitochondrial membrane for β oxidation. Increasing L-carnitine might facilitate the oxidation of lipids. By relying more on fat as an energy source, you could spare glycogen and increase aerobic endurance capacity.	Inconclusive. Most studies show no ergogenic effect.
Creatine	Increases muscle PCr levels, thus enhancing the ATP-PCr energy system by better maintaining muscle ATP levels.	Yes. Increases performance of high-intensity, intermittent exercise, except for sprint running and sprint swimming. Does not improve endurance exercise. Might improve strength.
Chromium	Not clear. Appears to potentiate the action of insulin. Chromium picolinate supplementation might increase glycogen synthesis, improve glucose tolerance and lipid profiles, and increase amino acid incorporation in muscle.	Inconclusive. May increase fat-free mass and decreased fat mass.

13.6 Putting It All Together: Ergogenic Aids and Performance

	Act on heart, blood, circulation, and aerobic endurance	Increase oxygen delivery	Supply fuel for muscle and general muscle function	Act on muscle mass and strength	Result in weight loss or weight gain	Counteract or delay onset or sensation of fatigue	Counteract CNS inhibition	Aid in relaxation and stress reduction
Pharmacological agents								
Alcohol	•		•					•
Amphetamines	•					•	•	
Beta blockers	•							•
Caffeine	•		•			•		
Cocaine and marijuana	•							•
Diuretics	•				•			
Nicotine	•							•
Hormones								
Anabolic steroids				•	•			
Human growth hormone				•	•			
Oral Contraceptives								•
Physiological agents								
Aspartic acid salts						•		
Bicarbonate loading						•		
Blood doping	•	•				•		
Erythropoietin	•	•				•		
Oxygen	•	•				•		
Phosphate loading	•	•				•		
Nutritional agents								
Amino acids	•		•	•	•	•		
Chromium			•	•	•			
Creatine			•	•	•	•		
L-carnitine			•			•		

Adapted from E.L. Fox, R.W. Bowers, and M.L. Foss, 1988, *The physiological basis of physical education and athletics* (Philadelphia: Saunders College Publishing), 632. Copyright 1988 The McGraw-Hill Companies. Adapted by permission of The McGraw-Hill Companies.

Answers to Selected Chapter 13 Test Questions

Multiple Choice

1. c   2. b;   3. d;   4. a;   5. d

True-False

6. False;   7. False;   8. True;   9. False;   10. False;   11. False;   12. True

Fill in the Blank

13. placebo effect

14. carbon monoxide; oxygen transport

15. erythropoietin

Short Answer and Essay

For questions 16 to 21, check your answers against the explanations given in the textbook.

14

Nutrition and Nutritional Ergogenics

concepts

- Food can be categorized into six nutrient classes: carbohydrate, fat (lipid), protein, vitamins, minerals, and water.

- While carbohydrate is the primary fuel source for most athletes, the use of fat for energy production can delay exhaustion.

- Water balance depends on electrolyte balance, and vice versa. At rest, water intake equals water output. During exercise, water loss increases at a faster rate than does water production.

- The greater the amount of glycogen stored, the better the potential endurance performance, because fatigue will be delayed. Thus, an athlete's goal is to begin an exercise bout or competition with as much stored glycogen as possible, and an athlete recovering from an exhaustive endurance event should ingest sufficient carbohydrate as soon after exercise as is practical.

- The faster the rate of gastric emptying—that is, the emptying of food from the stomach into the small intestine—the faster the nutrients are absorbed into the blood. The volume of stomach contents, the type and concentration of the ingestate, and even exercise intensity affect the rate of gastric emptying.

- No ideal sports drink has been identified. In terms of absorption from the gastrointestinal tract, plain water is good, and adding carbohydrate is probably better.

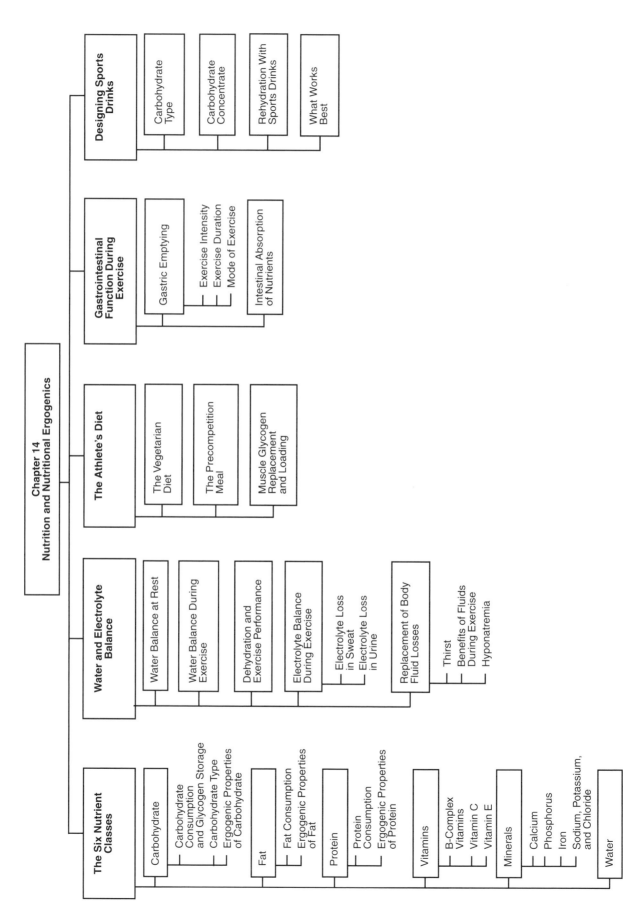

Chapter 14
Nutrition and Nutritional Ergogenics

The Six Nutrient Classes

- Carbohydrate
  - Carbohydrate Consumption and Glycogen Storage
  - Carbohydrate Type
  - Ergogenic Properties of Carbohydrate
- Fat
  - Fat Consumption
  - Ergogenic Properties of Fat
- Protein
  - Protein Consumption
  - Ergogenic Properties of Protein
- Vitamins
  - B-Complex Vitamins
  - Vitamin C
  - Vitamin E
- Minerals
  - Calcium
  - Phosphorus
  - Iron
  - Sodium, Potassium, and Chloride
- Water

Water and Electrolyte Balance

- Water Balance at Rest
- Water Balance During Exercise
- Dehydration and Exercise Performance
- Electrolyte Balance During Exercise
  - Electrolyte Loss in Sweat
  - Electrolyte Loss in Urine
- Replacement of Body Fluid Losses
  - Thirst
  - Benefits of Fluids During Exercise
  - Hyponatremia

The Athlete's Diet

- The Vegetarian Diet
- The Precompetition Meal
- Muscle Glycogen Replacement and Loading

Gastrointestinal Function During Exercise

- Gastric Emptying
  - Exercise Intensity
  - Exercise Duration
  - Mode of Exercise
- Intestinal Absorption of Nutrients

Designing Sports Drinks

- Carbohydrate Type
- Carbohydrate Concentrate
- Rehydration With Sports Drinks
- What Works Best

Activity 14.1

Functions of Nutrients

Do this activity after reading pages 452-469 of *Physiology of Sport and Exercise.*

All foods can ultimately be broken down to carbohydrate, fat, or protein; and a person's diet should contain a relative balance of each of these. It is recommended that of the total calories consumed, 55% to 60% should come from carbohydrate; no more than 30% should come from fat; and 10% to 15% should come from protein. Why are these nutrients so important? Obviously, they play key roles in the normal functioning of the body and in helping us to accomplish physical feats.

In the list of functions below, fill in the blank with a "C" if the function describes carbohydrate, an "F" if it describes fat, and a "P" if it describes protein. Try to do this without referring to *Physiology of Sport and Exercise.*

_____ 1. Serves as a major energy source, especially during high-intensity exercise.

_____ 2. Serves as a primary energy source, providing up to 70% of our total energy when we are at rest.

_____ 3. Not a primary source of energy production, but can be used for energy production as an auxiliary fuel during endurance exercise.

_____ 4. Regulates fat and protein metabolism.

_____ 5. Is the sole provider of energy for the nervous system.

_____ 6. Supports and cushions vital organs.

_____ 7. Is an essential component of cell membranes and nerve fibers.

_____ 8. Is the major structural component of the cell.

_____ 9. All steroid hormones in the body are produced from a form of it.

_____ 10. Is used for growth, repair, and maintenance of body tissues.

_____ 11. Produces hemoglobin, enzymes, and many hormones.

_____ 12. Serves as an insulating layer to preserve body heat.

_____ 13. Normal blood osmotic pressure is maintained by this nutrient in the plasma.

_____ 14. Muscle and liver glycogen are synthesized from it.

_____ 15. Antibodies are formed from it.

_____ 16. Some vitamins gain entry into, are stored in, and are transported throughout the body via this nutrient.

We need vitamins in relatively small quantities, but without them we could not use the other nutrients we ingest. We need some minerals in larger quantities, but many trace elements in very small amounts; yet all these minerals are important for normal cellular functions. Water is seldom thought of as a nutrient, yet its importance in maintaining life is second only to the importance of oxygen. What do these nutrients do that makes them so important?

In the list of functions on the next page, fill in the blank with the specific name of the vitamin (e.g., "Vitamin A") if it describes a vitamin, the name of the mineral (e.g., "Calcium") if it describes a mineral, and "Water" if it describes water. Try to do this without referring to *Physiology of Sport and Exercise.* You may have more than one answer in a blank.

_____ 17. Is essential for normal growth and development, because it plays an integral role in bone development.

_____ 18. Is essential for intestinal absorption of calcium and phosphorus, and thus for bone development and strength. By regulating calcium absorption, also plays a key role in neuromuscular function.

_____ 19. Is an intermediate in the electron transport chain, making it important for oxidative phosphorylation.

_____ 20. Play an essential role in cellular metabolism. For example, they serve as cofactors in various enzyme systems involved in the oxidation of food and the production of energy.

_____ 21. Is important in the formation and maintenance of collagen, a crucial protein found in connective tissue; therefore, it is essential for healthy bones, ligaments, and blood vessels.

_____ 22. Functions in the metabolism of amino acids.

_____ 23. Functions in the synthesis of some hormones and the anti-inflammatory corticoids.

_____ 24. Promotes iron absorption from the intestine.

_____ 25. Enhances the activity of vitamins A and C by preventing their oxidation.

_____ 26. Acts as an antioxidant, disarming free radicals that could otherwise damage cells and disrupt metabolic processes.

_____ 27. Is essential for building and maintaining healthy bones.

_____ 28. Is essential for nerve impulse transmission.

_____ 29. Plays a major role in enzyme activation and regulation of cell membrane permeability.

_____ 30. Is essential for normal muscle function.

_____ 31. Provides strength and rigidity to bones.

_____ 32. Is essential in metabolism, cell membrane structure, and the buffering system; is an essential component of ATP.

_____ 33. Crucial for oxygen transportation, and required for the formation of hemoglobin and myoglobin.

_____ 34. Enable neural impulses to control muscle activity.

_____ 35. Are responsible for maintaining water balance and distribution, normal osmotic equilibrium, acid-base balance, and normal cardiac rhythm.

_____ 36. Regulates body temperature.

_____ 37. Maintains blood pressure.

_____ 38. Is the primary ingredient of blood plasma, which, among other things, carries oxygen to active muscles; transports nutrients such as glucose, fatty acids, and amino acids to muscles; clears carbon dioxide and other metabolic wastes; transports hormones that regulate metabolism and muscular activity during exercise.

_____ 39. Is the primary ingredient of body fluids, which, among other things, contain buffering agents to maintain proper pH when lactate is being formed.

Ergogenic Properties of Carbohydrate, Fat, and Protein

Activity 14.2

Do this activity after reading pages 452-461 of *Physiology of Sport and Exercise*.

Carbohydrate, fat, and protein play particularly important roles for athletes. Though the RDA for these nutrients is sufficient for the average person, the athlete may need to make adjustments in order to improve performance. To test your knowledge of the ergogenic properties of these nutrients, read the case studies and answer the questions that follow (on a separate piece of paper, if necessary).

Tom is a long-distance runner. His usual diet consists of 40% carbohydrate, 40% fat, and 20% protein.

1. What effects could this diet have on Tom's competitive running performance?

2. How would you adjust Tom's diet to help him improve his running performance?

3. What could Tom do during competition to help delay fatigue?

Tom, the long-distance runner, overcorrects and decides to eat a daily diet of 75% carbohydrate, 5% fat, and 20% protein.

4. What will be the likely effects of this diet on Tom's running performance?

5. Why could Tom's low fat intake actually adversely affect his performance?

Beth is a 25-year-old female elite competitive weightlifter. Beth weighs 59 kg (130 lb); she ingests 47.2 g of protein per day, which is about 0.8 g of protein per kg of body weight.

6. How could Beth improve her diet to facilitate muscle development?

7. How would this change in diet facilitate muscle development?

► Activity 14.3

Water and Electrolyte Balance ◄

Do this activity after reading pages 469-475 of *Physiology of Sport and Exercise*.

For optimal performance, the body's water and electrolyte contents should remain relatively constant. However, this does not always happen during exercise. How do we lose water and electrolytes, how does exercise affect the rate of loss, and how can we replace them?

Using pages 469-475 in *Physiology of Sport and Exercise* as a guide, fill in the blanks below to learn (1) how we lose water and electrolytes, (2) how we replace fluid, and (3) how our body responds to fluid and electrolyte needs during exercise.

Fluid Loss and Replacement

How do we replace fluid?

1. _____

2. _____

3. _____

How do we lose water and electrolytes?
(See p. 469 in textbook for help)

Water loss

4. _____

5. _____   Electrolyte loss

6. _____   8. _____

7. _____   9. _____

During exercise

10. Factors that increase water loss

_____

11. Factors that try to minimize water loss

_____

_____

12. Factors that increase electrolyte loss

_____

13. Factors that try to minimize electrolyte loss

_____

10a. What three factors affect the amount of sweat lost during exercise?

_____

_____

12a. What three factors affect sweat's electrolyte concentration?

_____

_____

Dehydration, Fluid Intake During Exercise, and Hyponatremia

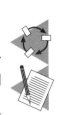

Activity 14.4

Do this activity after reading pages 469-475 of *Physiology of Sport and Exercise.*

Because water loss accelerates during exercise, we need to replace lost fluids. But how much should we replace? How might inadequate fluid replacement affect our performance and health? And is it actually possible to take in too much fluid? In this activity, we will first look at what causes dehydration; we will then examine the mechanisms and benefits of fluid replacement; and, finally, we will review the causes of hyponatremia.

Dehydration and Exercise Performance

1. Draw a flowchart (on a separate sheet of paper) to show the cycle of dehydration. Start with the body temperature rising during exercise (see the bottom of page 469 in the textbook), include the steps that cause rapid water losses, and end with the impact of dehydration on the cardiovascular and thermoregulatory systems (see the bottom of page 470 in the textbook). Assume inadequate fluid replacement.

2. Circle the three athletes whose performances would be most affected by dehydration:

Marathon runner   Discus thrower

Weight lifter   Cross-country skier

Wrestler who dehydrates before   Mountain biker on a 2-h ride
weigh-in and rehydrates before
the competition

Fluid Intake During Exercise

For questions 3 to 5, fill in the blanks with the correct answers.

3. Dehydration triggers the release of the hormone _____, which stimulates renal reabsorption of _____. This elevates the body's sodium content and increases the plasma's _____ pressure. In turn, this increased pressure causes the _____ to trigger thirst.

4. You do not sense thirst until well after _____ begins.

5. During exercise, water intake will minimize _____, _____, and _____.

If you get a chance in the next few days, compare two exercise bouts:

- *Exercise bout 1:* Do not drink any water immediately beforehand; during the exercise bout drink only when you become thirsty. (Do not do this for an exercise session longer than 30 min.)

- *Exercise bout 2:* Drink a good amount of water before you exercise, even if you are not thirsty; during the exercise bout, keep yourself fully hydrated, drinking even when you are not thirsty.

Did you notice a difference in your fatigue level between these exercise bouts? What probably accounted for this difference?

Hyponatremia

6. Define hyponatremia.

7. What type of athlete is most likely to suffer from hyponatremia?

8. What are the possible causes of hyponatremia?

9. What are the possible ways to prevent hyponatremia?

Designing Precompetition and Postcompetition Diets

Do this activity after reading pages 475-479 of *Physiology of Sport and Exercise*.

The athlete's diet can mean the difference between exceptional performance and merely sufficient performance, between completing the competition in top form and slowing or dropping out of it because of fatigue. Proper physical training obviously contributes to successful physical performance; proper nutrition can also significantly impact an athlete's health and level of performance. In this activity, we will look at three aspects of the athlete's diet: glycogen loading, the precompetition meal, and the postcompetition diet (glycogen replenishment).

Glycogen Loading

Zack is competing in his first mini-triathlon a week from today. This is his plan for the coming week:

Day 7	Complete an exhaustive training bout
Days 6-4	Markedly reduce training intensity and volume
	Eat fat and protein almost exclusively
Days 3-1	Continue with reduced training intensity and volume
	Eat a carbohydrate-rich diet

1. What are the positive physiological benefits of this regimen? What are the mechanisms underlying these benefits?

2. What are the possible negative consequences of this regimen?

3. How would you redesign this plan to eliminate some of the possible negative consequences?

4. What is the theory behind muscle glycogen loading?

The Precompetition Meal

Today is the day Zack is competing in his first mini-triathlon. Thirty minutes before competing, Zack eats the following meal:

Two eggs

A side of steak

Two slices of bacon

A glass of water

5. What is wrong about *when* Zack ate his meal?

6. In general, what are the problems with Zack's menu selections?

7. Design an appropriate precompetition meal for Zack.

8. What are the physiological goals of the precompetition meal?

The Postcompetition Diet

For the first few hours after completing the mini-triathlon, Zack drinks a lot of water but does not eat anything. About 5 hours after competing, Zack eats a slice of ham, a side serving of corn, and a glass of decaffeinated iced tea.

9. What is wrong about *when* Zack started eating after competing?

10. In general, what else is wrong with Zack's postcompetition diet?

11. Design an appropriate postcompetition diet for Zack.

12. What are the physiological goals of the postcompetition diet?

Activity 14.6

Gastrointestinal Function

Do this activity after reading pages 479-481 of *Physiology of Sport and Exercise*.

Athletes are particularly interested in gastrointestinal function, because the quicker digestion occurs and nutrients are absorbed into the blood, the sooner their bodies can take advantage of the ingested nutrients. Complete this activity to ensure your understanding of gastrointestinal function.

Gastric Emptying at Rest

1. List the 10 factors that affect the rate at which a solution passes through the stomach when a person is at rest. (If you get stuck, compare your answers to page 479 of *Physiology of Sport and Exercise*.)

a. _____ f. _____

b. _____ g. _____

c. _____ h. _____

d. _____ i. _____

e. _____ j. _____

Gastric Emptying During Exercise

2. In each pair of activities listed, circle the athlete who would likely exhibit a faster rate of gastric emptying. If there would be no difference in the rate of gastric emptying, circle both activities.

   a. Person running at 80% $\dot{V}O_2$max

   Person running at 35% $\dot{V}O_2$max

   b. Person walking

   Person walking and talking with a friend

   c. Person exercising at 55% $\dot{V}O_2$max

   Same person sitting in front of a television

   d. A highly trained athlete swimming at a pace of 3.0 km/h (1.86 mi/h)

   An untrained person swimming at a pace of 3.0 km/h (1.86 mi/h)

   e. Person cycling for 15 min at 65% $\dot{V}O_2$max

   Person cycling for 2 h at 65% $\dot{V}O_2$max

   f. Person running for 20 min

   Person cycling for 20 min

Intestinal Absorption of Nutrients

3. Define intestinal absorption.

4. During what type of exercise is intestinal absorption most likely to be delayed?

Activity 14.7

Sports Drinks

Do this activity after reading pages 481-484 of *Physiology of Sport and Exercise.*

The sports drink industry is very interested in the type of research that is discussed in this chapter, especially regarding the athlete's need for carbohydrate and the factors that affect gastrointestinal function. In this activity, you will analyze various nutrition labels to see how the sports drink industry has responded to this research.

Use the four nutrition labels on the next page to answer the questions in this activity. Write your answers to the questions on a separate sheet of paper.

Gatorade

NO FRUIT JUICE

Nutrition Facts

Serving Size 8 fl oz (240 mL)
Servings Per Container 4

Amount Per Serving

Calories 50

	% Daily Value*
Total Fat 0g	**0**%
Sodium 110mg	**5**%
Potassium 30mg	**1**%
Total Carbohydrate 14g	**5**%
Sugars 14g	
Protein 0g	

Not a significant source of Calories from Fat, Saturated Fat, Cholesterol, Dietary Fiber, Vitamin A, Vitamin C, Calcium, Iron

*Percent Daily Values are based on 2,000 calorie diet.

INGREDIENTS: WATER, SUCROSE SYRUP, GLUCOSE-FRUCTOSE SYRUP, CITRIC ACID, NATURAL ORANGE FLAVOR WITH OTHER NATURAL FLAVORS, SALT, SODIUM CITRATE, MONOPOTASSIUM PHOSPATE, YELLOW 6, ESTER GUM, BROMINATED VEGETABLE OIL.

Hansen's Energy Smoothie

Fat Free Non-Dairy Beverage
35% Fruit Juice

Nutrition Facts

Serving Size 8 fl oz (240 mL)
Servings Per Container About 2

Amount per Serving

Calories 120

	% Daily Value*
Total Fat 0g	0%
Cholest 0mg	0%
Sodium 25mg	1%
Potassium 110mg	3%
Total Carb 29g	10%
Sugars 29g	
Protein 0g	0%

Vitamin C 100%•Calcium 2%•Iron 5%

Vitamin B-2, B-6, B-12 5%•Niacin 5%

*Percent Daily Values are based on a 2,000 calorie diet.

CONTAINS: FILTERED WATER, GLUCOSE, HIGH FRUCTOSE CORN SYRUP, PINEAPPLE, PEAR, WHITE GRAPE, APPLE AND ORANGE CONCENTRATES, NATURAL FRUIT FLAVORS, PASSION FRUIT JUICE, MANGO AND BANANA PUREES, NATURAL GUMS, BETA CAROTENE, TAURINE, VITAMIN C, GINSENG, VITAMINS B-2, B-6, B-12 AND NIACIN.

POWERaDE

NO LEMON/LIME JUICE
LOW SODIUM

Nutrition Facts

Serving Size 8 fl oz (240 mL)
Servings Per Container 4

Amount per Serving

Calories (Energy) 70

	% Daily Value*
Total Fat 0g	0%
Sodium 55mg	2%
Potassium 30mg	1%
Total Carbohydrate 15g	6%
Sugars 15g	
Protein 0g	

Not a significant source of calories from fat, saturated fat, cholesterol, dietary fiber, vitamin A, vitamin C, calcium or iron.

*Percent Daily Values are based on a 2,000 calorie diet.

WATER, HIGH FRUCTOSE CORN SYRUP, MALTODEXTRIN (GLUCOSE POLYMERS), CITRIC ACID, ACACIA, POTASSIUM CITRATE, SALT, POTASSIUM PHOSPATE, NATURAL FLAVORS, GLYCEROL ESTER OF WOOD ROSIN, BROMINATED VEGETABLE OIL, YELLOW 5.

All Sport

Nutrition Facts

Serv. Size 8 fl oz (240 mL)
Serv. Per Container 4
Calories 70

Not a significant source of fat, saturated fat, cholesterol, dietary fiber, vitamin A, vitamin C, calcium, iron, riboflavin and folate.

Amount serving		Amount serving	
Total Fat 0g	0%	Total Carb. 20g	7%
Sodium 55mg	2%	Sugars 19g	
Potassium 50mg	1%	Protein 0g	

Thiamine 10% •	Niacin 10% • Vitamin B6 10%
Vitamin B12 10%	Pantothenic acid 10%

*Percent Daily Values are based on a 2,000 calorie diet.

CONTAINS: WATER, HIGH FRUCTOSE CORN SYRUP, CARBON DIOXIDE, CITRIC ACID, NATURAL FLAVORS, SODIUM POLYPHOSPHATES, POTASSIUM BENZOATE (PRESERVES FRESHNESS), MONO-POTASSIUM PHOSPHATE, SODIUM CHLORIDE, PHOSPHORIC ACID, GUM ARABIC, RED 40, CALCIUM CHLORIDE, ESTER GUM, CALCIUM DISODIUM EDTA (TO PROTECT FLAVOR), BLUE 1, B VITAMINS: NIACINAMIDE, CALCIUM PANTOTHENATE, THIAMINE MONONITRATE, PYRIDOXINE HYDRO-CHLORIDE, AND VITAMIN B12.   PLEASE RECYCLE • STORE IN A COOL PLACE

1. What types of carbohydrate are used in each of these beverages?

2. Why do all of these use some form of fructose?

3. What are the advantages and disadvantages of a high carbohydrate concentration?

4. According to *Physiology of Sport and Exercise,* how much carbohydrate does an athlete need to consume to improve performance? What are the problems in consuming this amount of carbohydrate?

5. Which product has the highest carbohydrate concentration? Which one has the lowest carbohydrate concentration? How many g of carbohydrate per 100 mL does each of these two drinks have?

6. What might be the disadvantages of using the beverage with the highest carbohydrate concentration as a sports drink?

7. Compare and contrast the amount of sodium in each of the four products shown.

8. What rationale is used to justify including sodium in sports drinks?

9. If you can, conduct a taste test on as many of these products as possible. Which product tastes the best to you? Do you think your answer would be different if you were in the middle of exercising intensely? Explain.

10. Based on your observations in this activity and what you have learned in this chapter, which of the products listed (or any others you examined) would receive your highest recommendation as a sports drink?

11. Based on your observations in this activity and what you have learned in this chapter, which of the products listed seems to be more of an energy beverage than a sports drink?

Putting It All Together: Nutrition and Nutritional Ergogenics

| Activity 14.8 |

Do this activity after reading chapter 14 of *Physiology of Sport and Exercise.*

This chapter examined nutritional needs, especially those of athletes. We learned that a balanced diet is important not only for general health but also for performance. So, how are *you* doing nutritionally? Apply what you have learned to your own diet. Write your answers to the following questions on a separate piece of paper.

1. Track your own diet for 1 day. Write down everything you eat, including breakfast, lunch, supper, and any snacks. Beside each food item, write down the amount of carbohydrate, fat, protein, vitamins, and minerals that it supplied you. Do the best you can with this: To be most accurate, find nutrition labels of the products you ate and compile information from them. You might need to go to a grocery store and look at the labels of comparable items, or, if you ate fast food, ask whether the restaurant offers a nutritional guide. If you do not have access to nutrition labels, simply analyze the foods yourself (for instance, you know that meats supply mostly protein, breads supply mostly carbohydrates, etc.).

2. Compare your actual intake with your dietary needs, as shown in the Recommended Dietary Allowances (RDA) in the tables on pages 460, 462, and 465 of *Physiology of Sport and Exercise*. For each nutrient, explain how and by how much you need to modify your diet to match the RDA (e.g., "reduce protein intake by 8 g"). Leave blank any nutrients you were unable to track.

Nutrient	RDA for my gender and age	My intake	Modifications I need to make to match the RDA
Protein			
Vitamin A			
Vitamin D			
Vitamin E			
Vitamin K			
Vitamin C			
Thiamine (B$_1$)			
Riboflavin (B$_2$)			
Niacin (B$_3$)			
Vitamin B$_6$			
Folate (folic acid)			
Vitamin B$_{12}$			
Calcium			
Phosphorus			
Magnesium			
Iron			
Zinc			
Iodine			
Selenium			
Chromium			
Copper			
Fluoride			

3. Evaluate what percentage of your total calories is from carbohydrate, and what percentage is from fat. (See page 458 of *Physiology of Sport and Exercise* for help.) To do this, you will need to know the total number of calories you ingested. You can get this information from nutrition labels. Carbohydrate and protein provide 4 calories per g; fat provides 9 calories per g. So if you ate 200 g of carbohydrate, you would multiply 200 × 4 to see that you received 800 of your calories from carbohydrate. Once you know your total number of calories ingested (say it was 2,000), you would divide the amount of calories from carbohydrate (800) by the total calories (2,000) to see the percentage of calories you ingested from carbohydrate (40%).

Nutrient	Recommended percentage	My intake	Modifications I need to make
Carbohydrate	*Nonathletes:* 45% to 50% of total calories *Nonendurance athletes:* At least 50% of total calories *Endurance athletes:* 55% to 65% of total calories		
Fat	Below 30% of total calories		

4. Plan a new daily menu (breakfast, lunch, and supper) for yourself, making the modifications you have listed in order to ensure a complete RDA and the right percentages of calories from carbohydrate and fat. If you are a competitive athlete, take the recommendations for athletes provided in this chapter into account as you adjust these menus.

Sample Test Questions for Chapter 14

Test yourself on your knowledge of this chapter by taking this self-test. Write the correct answers on a separate sheet of paper.

Multiple Choice

1. This is the primary reason athletes should eat a high percentage of carbohydrates.

   a. Fat-soluble vitamins gain entry into, are stored in, and are transported through the body via carbohydrate.
   b. Normal blood osmotic pressure is maintained by carbohydrate in the plasma.
   c. Excess carbohydrate is stored as glycogen in the muscles and liver, and serves as the primary fuel source for most exercise.
   d. Carbohydrate can promote the use of fat and improve prolonged exhaustive exercise.

2. Which of the following foods are the best sources of carbohydrate?

   a. Shrimp and lobster
   b. Grains, fruits, and vegetables
   c. Beef and poultry
   d. Cheese and eggs

3. Given the ergogenic properties of protein, which athlete would benefit the least from a slightly increased protein intake?

   a. Marathon runner
   b. Competitive rock climber
   c. Recreational walker
   d. Weightlifter

4. An athlete who is suffering from fatigue, little aerobic capacity, and headaches might have a deficiency of

   a. calcium.
   b. manganese.
   c. vitamin A.
   d. iron.

True-False

5. The precompetition meal should ensure that the stomach is full at the start of the competition.

6. Simple carbohydrates are absorbed from the digestive system more quickly than complex carbohydrates.

7. Eating fat stimulates muscles to burn fat.

8. Protein is a primary source of energy in our bodies.

9. When no deficiency exists, supplementation of B-complex vitamins, vitamin C, and vitamin E does not improve athletic performance.

10. A water loss of only 9% to 12% of a person's total body weight can be fatal.

11. When exercising, it is better to drink fluids that are near one's body temperature to prevent shock.

12. There is no reason for an athlete to ingest fluids until he or she feels thirsty.

13. A vegetarian diet is very unsafe for athletes.

14. Gastric emptying slows significantly during intense exercise.

Fill in the Blank

15. Carbohydrate should constitute at least _____ percent of an athlete's total caloric intake. For endurance athletes, carbohydrate intake should constitute _____ percent of the total caloric intake.

16. When carbohydrate intake is higher than can be used or stored within the cells, the excess carbohydrate is converted to _____.

17. Excessive _____ [unsaturated, saturated] fat consumption is a risk factor for numerous diseases. Fats derived from _____ sources generally contain more saturated fatty acids than fats derived from _____.

18. Mineral compounds that can dissociate into ions in the body are called
_____.

19. _____ vitamins are stored in the body, so excessive intake can
cause toxic accumulations.

20. The two major routes for electrolyte loss are _____ and
_____.

Short Answer

21. List the four ways in which your body loses water at rest.

22. Explain the role of aldosterone in triggering thirst.

23. What are the benefits of fluid intake during exercise?

24. Explain how and why the volume and the fat content of food ingested can affect
gastric emptying.

Essay

25. Explain what events lead to dehydration, and how dehydration impacts the cardiovascular and thermoregulatory systems.

26. Muscle glycogen loading has been of great interest to athletes for many years.
Explain the main goals of glycogen loading, the two leading glycogen loading
regimens, and the advantages and disadvantages of each.

27. No ideal sports drink solution has been identified to date. Discuss the current
rationales for including carbohydrate, for using a strong carbohydrate concentration, and for including sodium in sports drinks.

Answers to Selected Chapter 14 Activities

14.1   Functions of Nutrients

1. C; 2. F; 3. P; 4. C; 5. C; 6. F; 7. F; 8. P; 9. F; 10. P; 11. P; 12. F; 13. P;
14. C; 15. P; 16. F

17. Vitamin A; 18. Vitamin D; 19. Vitamin K; 20. B-complex vitamins; 21. Vitamin C;
22. Vitamin C; 23. Vitamin C; 24. Vitamin C; 25. Vitamin E; 26. Vitamin E; 27. Calcium; 28. Calcium; 29. Calcium; 30. Calcium; 31. Phosphorus; 32. Phosphorus;
33. Iron; 34. Sodium, potassium, and chloride; 35. Sodium, potassium, and chloride;
36. Water; 37. Water; 38. Water; 39. Water

14.2   Ergogenic Properties of Carbohydrate, Fat, and Protein

1. Muscle glycogen is a major energy source during exercise. A diet low in carbohydrates could lead to muscle glycogen depletion and early fatigue.

2. Tom should increase his carbohydrate intake to 55% to 65%, lessen his fat intake
to under 30%, and lessen his protein intake.

3. Carbohydrate feedings during exercise might help preserve liver glycogen, helping the exercising muscles to rely more on blood glucose for energy late in the
exercise.

4. Tom will likely fatigue earlier than he used to.

5. Muscle and liver glycogen stores in the body are limited, so the use of fat for energy production can delay exhaustion. Without an adequate intake of fat, Tom's body will have to rely on glycogen as its primary energy source. Once that source is depleted, Tom will become fatigued.

6. Beth could ingest 1.2 to 1.8 g of protein per kg of body weight daily—up to about 106.2 g of protein.

7. Protein is essential for growth and development of body tissues. Strength training requires additional amino acids as the building blocks for muscle development, so a diet a little more rich in protein could be beneficial to Beth's strength-training goals.

14.3   Water and Electrolyte Balance

1. Fluids we drink (60% at rest)

2. Fluids in the food we consume (30% at rest)

3. Fluid produced in cells during metabolism (10% at rest)

4. Evaporation from the skin

5. Evaporation from the respiratory tract

6. Excretion from the kidneys

7. Excretion from the large intestine

8. Sweating

9. Urine production

10. Mainly increased sweating and increased insensible water loss (from skin and respiration)

10a. Environmental temperature, body size, and metabolic rate

11. Increased oxidative metabolism naturally produces more water; decreased urine production rate

12. Heavy sweating

12a. Rate of sweating, state of training, and state of heat acclimatization

13. Decreased urine production rate

14.4   Dehydration, Fluid Intake During Exercise, and Hyponatremia

1. Flowchart might include these steps: Body temperature rises; sweating increases to avoid overheating; metabolic rate increases, producing some water, but also increasing body temperature; sweating increases to avoid overheating; rapid losses of water occur; fluid loss decreases plasma volume; decreased plasma volume decreases blood pressure; decreased blood pressure reduces blood flow to the muscles and the skin; in an effort to overcome this, heart rate increases; less blood reaches the skin, hindering heat dissipation; body retains more heat (bringing the cycle full circle, and without fluid replacement, the cycle repeats, becoming more serious).

2. Marathon runner, cross-country skier, mountain biker on a 2-h ride

3. aldosterone, sodium, osmotic, hypothalamus

4. dehydration

5. dehydration, body temperature increases, and cardiovascular stress

6 Hyponatremia is a blood sodium concentration below the normal range of 136 to 143 mmol/L.

7. It seems that ultra-endurance athletes—for example, ultramarathoners who run 160 km (100 mi)—are most likely to succumb to hyponatremia.

8. Hyponatremia seems to be caused by consuming a large amount of fluid that contains too little sodium, and this dilutes the blood sodium content.

9. Ideally, one would replace water at the exact rate that it is being lost, or one would add sodium to the ingested fluid. But even the amount of sodium in sports drinks is too weak to prevent sodium dilution, and stronger concentrations cannot be tolerated.

14.5 Designing Precompetition and Postcompetition Diets

1. This regimen can elevate the muscle glycogen stores to twice the normal level. The 3-day fat and protein diet increases the activity of glycogen synthase, an enzyme responsible for glycogen synthesis. Then when the athlete switches to the 3-day carbohydrate-rich diet, the increased glycogen synthase activity helps the carbohydrate diet result in greater muscle glycogen storage.

2. During the 3 days of low-carbohydrate intake, athletes find training difficult. They can also be irritable and show signs of low blood sugar, such as muscle weakness and disorientation. The exhaustive depletion bout of exercise 7 days before the competition can impair glycogen storage and expose athletes to possible injury or overtraining.

3. Answers may vary, but in general the athlete should reduce training intensity a week before competition, while eating a normal mixed diet of 55% carbohydrate, until 3 days before the competition. In the last 3 days before competition, training should be reduced to a daily warm-up of 10 to 15 minutes of activity, and the diet should be rich in carbohydrates.

4. The greater the amount of glycogen that is stored, the better the endurance performance.

5. The precompetition meal should be eaten at least 2 h before the competition to ensure that the meal is digested and the nutrients are absorbed prior to competing.

6. In general, Zack's meal is too high in calories; it is also very high in protein and low in carbohydrates. Instead, Zack should eat a lighter precompetition meal— one that consists of 200 to 500 kcal and is high in easily digested carbohydrates.

7. Answers will vary, but a bowl of carbohydrate-rich cereal, a slice of whole grain toast, and a glass of orange juice would be sufficient. Some athletes prefer liquid meals to avoid nervous indigestion, nausea, vomiting, and abdominal cramps.

8. This meal will contribute little to muscle glycogen stores, but it can ensure a normal blood glucose level and prevent hunger.

9. Zack should have started ingesting carbohydrates as soon after the mini-triathlon as possible. By waiting 5 h, Zack deprived his body of carbohydrates during a period in which the rate of muscle glycogen resynthesis is somewhat faster than the normal rate.

10. Zack's postcompetition diet consisted of one meal, whereas high-carbohydrate feedings every 2 h after the competition would have helped promote faster replacement of muscle glycogen. Zack's one meal was not very high in carbohydrates. The corn would have supplied some, but not enough, carbohydrate.

11. Answers will vary, but should include high-carbohydrate feedings every 2 h after competition. Carbohydrate-rich foods include grains, fruits, vegetables, milk, and concentrated sweets.

12. The goal of the postcompetition diet is to replace muscle and liver glycogen stores as rapidly as possible. Liver glycogen stores are replenished within a few h of eating a carbohydrate-rich meal. Muscle glycogen resynthesis takes several days to accomplish after an exhaustive exercise bout such as a marathon.

14.6   Gastrointestinal Function

1. Volume of the solution, caloric content, osmolarity, temperature, pH, caffeine, emotional distress, diurnal variations, environmental conditions, and phase of the menstrual cycle

2a. Person running at 35% $\dot{V}O_2$max;   b. Person walking and talking with a friend; c. These would have the same rate of gastric emptying;   d. A highly trained athlete swimming at a pace of 3.0 km/h (1.86 mi/h);   e. These would have the same rate of gastric emptying;   f. Person running for 20 minutes

3. Intestinal absorption is the movement of nutrients through the intestinal wall into the blood.

4. Intestinal absorption is most likely to be delayed during highly intense endurance exercise, such as long-distance running and triathlon competitions.

14.7   Sports Drinks

1. Gatorade and Hansen's both use sucrose and glucose. All Sport uses just fructose. POWERaDE uses fructose and maltodextrin.

2. Fructose has been shown to leave the stomach faster than other carbohydrates and, when given at low enough concentrations, does not inhibit gastric emptying, whereas some other forms of sugar might.

3. Increasing the glucose concentration drastically reduces the gastric emptying rate, but when even a small amount of a strong glucose drink leaves the stomach, it can contain more sugar than a larger amount of a weaker solution.

4. To improve performance, athletes should consume at least 50 g of sugar per h. Only drinks containing at least 11 g of carbohydrate per 100 mL would be of any energy value, but such a rich mixture might be delayed in the stomach, draw water from the stomach's lining, and cause an uncomfortable feeling of fullness.

5. Hansen's has the highest carbohydrate concentration, with 12.08 g per 100 mL; Gatorade has the lowest carbohydrate concentration, with 5.8 g per 100 mL.

6. Although Hansen's could meet the carbohydrate needs of the athlete, it might also be delayed in the stomach, draw water from the stomach's lining, and cause an uncomfortable feeling of fullness.

7. Gatorade has the highest amount of sodium, with 110 mg; All Sport and POWERaDE each have 55 mg of sodium; Hansen's has the lowest amount, with 25 mg of sodium.

8. Although the interactions of sodium and glucose are unconfirmed, there is some thought that sodium is required for glucose transportation. Also, when sodium is retained, water is retained.

9. Answers will vary.

10. Answers will vary; not enough research in the area to know which is truly best.

11. Hansen's

Answers to Selected Chapter 14 Test Questions

Multiple Choice

1. c;   2. b;   3. c;   4. d

True-False

5. False;   6. True;   7. False;   8. False;   9. True;   10. True;   11. False;   12. False;   13. False;   14. True

Fill in the Blank

15. 50%, 55% to 65%

16. fat

17. saturated, animal, plants

18. electrolytes

19. fat-soluble

20. sweating, urine production

Short Answer and Essay

For questions 21 to 27, check your answers against the explanations given in the textbook.

Optimal Body Weight for Performance

concepts

- Body composition refers to the body's chemical composition and can be expressed in terms of fat mass and fat-free mass. Fat mass is often discussed in terms of relative body fat, which is the percentage of the total body mass that is composed of fat. Fat-free mass is composed of all of the body's nonfat tissue including bone, muscle, organs, and connective tissue.

- Although total body size and weight are important for most athletes, an athlete's body composition is generally more valuable for predicting performance potential. Body weight standards should be based on body composition and should emphasize relative body fat rather than total body mass.

- Densitometry is the method of choice for assessing body composition, although it does carry certain risks of error. Multiple skinfold fat thickness measurements and other field techniques also provide a good estimate of body composition and are less costly and more accessible than are laboratory techniques.

- The ideal body composition varies with different sports, but in general, the less fat mass, the better the performance.

- Severe weight loss in athletes can cause health problems such as dehydration, chronic fatigue, disordered eating, menstrual dysfunction, and bone mineral disorders.

- The preferred approach to weight loss is to combine moderate dietary restriction and increased exercise to result in gradual weight loss.

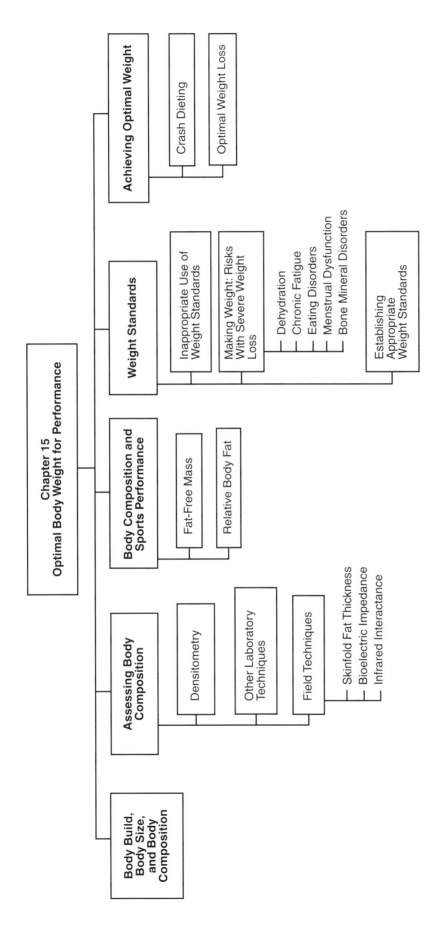

Chapter 15
Optimal Body Weight for Performance

Body Build,
Body Size,
and Body
Composition

Assessing Body
Composition
- Densitometry
- Other Laboratory
  Techniques
- Field Techniques
  - Skinfold Fat Thickness
  - Bioelectric Impedance
  - Infrared Interactance

Body Composition and
Sports Performance
- Fat-Free Mass
- Relative Body Fat

Weight Standards
- Inappropriate Use of
  Weight Standards
- Making Weight: Risks
  With Severe Weight
  Loss
  - Dehydration
  - Chronic Fatigue
  - Eating Disorders
  - Menstrual Dysfunction
  - Bone Mineral Disorders
- Establishing
  Appropriate
  Weight Standards

Achieving Optimal Weight
- Crash Dieting
- Optimal Weight Loss

What Is My Body Build, Body Size, and Body Composition?

> **Activity 15.1**

Do this activity after reading pages 492-494 of *Physiology of Sport and Exercise.*

Have you ever noticed that Olympic figure skaters seem thin, small, and light; and heavyweight weightlifters seem large and muscular, sometimes even fat? By noticing these characteristics, you are paying attention to body build, body size, and body composition. Appropriate size, build, and composition are critical to success in almost all athletic endeavors. Imagine trying to do a triple axel in figure skating if you weighed 109 kg (240 lb), or blocking a tackle in American football if you were slight in build and not very muscular. The results would not be pleasant! In this activity, you will reflect on your own characteristics and how they could impact your performance.

1. The three major components of body build (morphology) are muscularity, linearity, and fatness. Describe your own body build in general terms using these categories. You might, for example, say that you are "not very muscular," "quite linear," and "thin."

   Muscularity:

   Linearity:

   Fatness:

2. Describe your body size in specific terms of height and mass, for example, "173 cm (5 ft 8 in), 65 kg (143 lb)."

   Height:

   Mass (weight):

3. Body composition refers to the body's chemical composition. The model used in *Physiology of Sport and Exercise* considers two components: fat mass and fat-free mass. The next time you see a piece of meat with some fat on it—perhaps a steak, some pork, or a slice of ham with some fat around the edges—notice how the fat is truly a separate entity from the rest of the meat, and yet it makes up part of the total composition. In the same way, our fat mass is a separate entity from our fat-free mass, and yet it makes up part of our total body composition.

   See the far right bar in figure 15.1 on page 493 of *Physiology of Sport and Exercise*. Divide the bar on the next page into fat mass and fat-free mass portions to represent what you believe your body composition to be. Label each section with the percentage you think is true of your body composition. (So, if you think your body composition is 40% fat mass and 60% fat-free mass, you would divide the bar slightly above the middle and label the top portion "Fat mass 40%" and the bottom portion "Fat-free mass 60%.")

   Your instructor will likely lead you in lab activities to calculate your body composition in several ways. See how close your estimate here comes to your actual body composition.

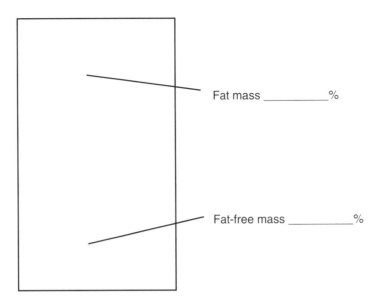

Fat mass _____%

Fat-free mass _____%

4. What is the body's fat-free mass composed of?

5. Even though you may not yet have read the rest of the chapter, for which physical activities do you think you are best suited, given your body build, size, and composition?

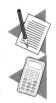

| Activity 15.2 | **Assessing Body Composition** |

Do this activity after reading pages 494-499 of *Physiology of Sport and Exercise.*

Standard height-weight tables are not accurate because they do not take into account the composition of the weight. Various laboratory and field tests can be conducted to determine an athlete's body composition. In this activity, we will focus on the laboratory method of densitometry and three field techniques for measuring body composition. After reading pages 494-499 in *Physiology of Sport and Exercise,* match the characteristics listed below with the method. Try to do this without looking in your textbook. You will have more than one letter in each blank, but you will use each letter only once.

Methods of Assessing Body Composition

Method

_____ 1. Densitometry

_____ 2. Skinfold fat thickness

_____ 3. Bioelectric impedance

_____ 4. Infrared interactance

Characteristic

a. Using this method, the relative body fat in lean athletic populations tends to be overestimated because of the nature of the equations used.

b. This is the most widely applied field technique for measuring body composition.

c. This technique measures the density of the athlete's body.

d. This procedure is based on the principles of light absorption and reflection. A probe placed on the skin emits electromagnetic radiation, and optic fibers on the same probe absorb the energy reflected back from the tissues. The amount of energy that is reflected indicates the composition of the tissue directly under the probe.

e. An undetectable current is passed through two distal electrodes (hand and foot) to two proximal electrodes (wrist and ankle). The amount of current flow through the tissues reflects the relative amount of fat contained in that tissue.

f. To use this method, one must know the athlete's body volume, which is often obtained via hydrostatic weighing.

g. Inaccuracies in this method largely reflect the variation in density of the fat-free mass from one individual to another, which can be affected by age, sex, and race.

h. This method relies on the fact that conductivity is much greater in the fat-free mass than in the fat mass, since the fat-free mass contains almost all the body water and the conducting electrolytes.

i. Studies conducted to date are insufficient to determine this method's validity for athletic populations.

j. Measurements are taken at one or more sites and then summed and used in a quadratic, curvilinear equation to estimate body density.

Calculating Relative Body Fat Using Densitometry

Your instructor will likely lead you in lab activities calculating your body composition in several ways. However, due to time considerations and equipment costs, you will probably not be able to see densitometry with hydrostatic weighing in action. To compensate for this, complete the following calculations.

Debra is 173 cm (68 in.) tall. She weighs 55 kg (121 lb). She is weighed hydrostatically, and her underwater weight is 3.0 kg.

5. What is Debra's body volume?

Scale weight – Underwater weight = Volume (L)

6. What is Debra's body density?

$D_{body} = M_{body} \div V_{body}$

7. What is Debra's relative body fat?

% body fat = $(495 \div D_{body}) - 450$

8. What is Debra's fat weight?

Fat weight = Scale weight × Percent relative fat

9. What is Debra's fat-free weight?

Fat-free weight = Scale weight − Fat weight

Activity 15.3

Body Composition and Sport Performance

Do this activity after reading pages 499-502 of *Physiology of Sport and Exercise*.

Performance can actually be affected by body composition. In general, the less fat mass, the better the performance, and yet this is not always true. Read pages 499 to 502 in *Physiology of Sport and Exercise*. Then circle the athlete in each pair who would perform better than the other if performance success were based solely on body composition. In the space after each pair, explain why you chose the athlete you did as the one who would perform better.

1. a. A 50-kg (110-lb) female marathon runner with 90% fat-free mass

   b. A marathon runner who has worked to increase her fat-free mass so that she weighs 55 kg (121 lb) and has 90% fat-free mass

   Explanation:

2. a. The 100-kg (220.5-lb) defensive lineman in American football with 80% fat-free mass

   b. The defensive lineman in American football who has worked to increase his fat-free mass so that he weighs 105 kg (231.5 lb) and has 85% fat-free mass

   Explanation:

3. a. A 42-kg (93-lb) gymnast with 10% relative body fat

   b. A 42-kg (93-lb) gymnast with 6% relative body fat

   Explanation:

4. a. A heavyweight weightlifter who weighs 109 kg (240 lb) and has 40% relative body fat

   b. A heavyweight weightlifter who weighs 114 kg (251 lb) and has 45% relative body fat

   Explanation:

5. a. A 72.5-kg (160-lb) long jumper with 8% relative body fat

b. A 72.5-kg (160-lb) long jumper with 11% relative body fat

Explanation:

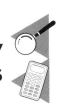

Activity 15.4

Using Weight Standards Appropriately and the Risks of Severe Weight Loss

Do this activity after reading pages 502-507 of *Physiology of Sport and Exercise*.

Although well intended, using standard height-weight charts to guide athletes' weight loss is fraught with dangers. Not only can inappropriate weight loss lead to poor performance, but it can also affect the health of the athlete. In this activity, we will review the risks of using weight guidelines inappropriately, and we will see how they can be used appropriately in tandem with body composition information.

1. Circle the examples below that illustrate an appropriate use of weight standards. Cross out the examples that illustrate an inappropriate use of weight standards. For those you cross out, be ready to explain on a test why that use is not appropriate.

   a. A swimming coach decides that all of the swimmers on the women's team need to attain 10% relative body fat, the low end of the recommended range for that sport.

   b. A gymnastics coach notices that one of his gymnasts has lost a drastic amount of weight and her performance is suffering. The coach meets with the athlete and uses weight standards along with body composition measurements to show the gymnast that if she loses more fat-free mass, she will be unable to compete because of fatigue and the potential for injury.

   c. The manager of a baseball team dictates that all players must report to training camp at a weight within the range recommended on standard height-weight tables in order to avoid a financial penalty.

   d. A wrestling coach uses standard height-weight tables to organize the team so that every athlete is wrestling in the division just below his optimal weight.

   e. A coach works with a rugby player to figure out a weight-loss goal based on the percentage of fat-free mass that is desired.

   f. A basketball coach tells both his men's and women's teams that he wants their relative body fat to be 10% or less.

2. This section of *Physiology of Sport and Exercise* discusses risks of severe weight loss. The female athlete triad is mentioned and will be discussed in more depth in chapter 18. Three disorders seem to be linked together and seem to result from each other; that is, one leads to the next, which can lead to the next. Fill in the blanks below in the order these symptoms often occur.

   a. _____ → b. _____ → c. _____

3. Dehydration and chronic fatigue are two other symptoms of inappropriate weight loss. Dehydration was discussed in depth in chapter 14. But what causes chronic fatigue? There are several possibilities. Explain them on a separate piece of paper in your own words.

Neural and hormonal causes:

Substrate depletion:

4. A 63.5-kg (140-lb) female skier with 23% body fat wants to lose weight in order to have only 17% body fat. Compute her weight goal, following the guidelines on page 506 of *Physiology of Sport and Exercise.*

For an extra challenge . . . Choose the activity of most interest to you:

1. Find a grouping of women's magazines—for example, you might look at the checkout lanes at a grocery store or the magazine section of a retail store or library—and figure out the percentage of magazine covers that list a story about weight loss or eating right. What about this percentage surprises you? How might this phenomenon contribute to the development of disordered eating in women? If your instructor asks you to do so, write a one-page paper summarizing your findings.

2. Search the Internet for information about the health risks of severe weight loss. Especially look for information on athletes and weight loss, and how severe weight loss can impair performance. If your instructor asks you to do so, write a one-page paper summarizing your findings.

| Activity 15.5 |

Risks of Crash Dieting: Losing Weight Safely

Do this activity after reading pages 507-510 of *Physiology of Sport and Exercise.*

Now that we have seen the benefits of having an optimal body composition for sport and exercise performance, how does one achieve it? Many athletes try to make weight or to lose weight in unhealthy ways—ways that give the outward appearance of weight loss but wreak havoc on the internal workings of the body and therefore performance. Answer the questions below on a separate piece of paper to ensure your understanding of optimal weight-loss strategies.

1. Rapid weight loss is associated with water loss and other health concerns. Using pages 507-509 in *Physiology of Sport and Exercise* as your guide, draw a flowchart that shows the effects of severe dieting. The first step in your flowchart should be something like "Food intake is reduced." Once you have drawn the flowchart, highlight or circle all the times water loss appears.

2. *Physiology of Sport and Exercise* gives the example of a football player returning to training camp in 4 weeks. The football player embarks on a crash diet in order to avoid the financial penalty of coming to camp weighing more than his agreed-upon playing weight. Due to his crash diet, the events depicted in your flowchart occur. When the football player reports to training camp, how will his diet affect his performance? Given what you see in your flowchart, what consequence would be of particular importance to the athlete's well-being? Why?

3. If this football player puts his performance success above financial gain, what are the general guidelines he should follow in order to lose weight safely? Fill in the blanks below to answer this question.

   a. A person trying to lose weight should combine increased _____ with reduced _____ in order to prevent any significant loss of fat-free mass.

   b. If the player exceeds the upper end of the weight range for his position, he should lose no more than _____ to _____ kg (less than _____ lb) per week.

   c. Once he reaches the upper limit of the range, he should lose no more than _____ kg (_____ lb) per week. If combined with a sound exercise program, decreasing caloric intake by _____ to _____ kcal per day will be sufficient to accomplish this goal. Total daily calories should be consumed over at least _____ meals a day.

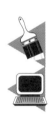

Putting It All Together: Optimal Body Weight for Performance

Activity 15.6

Do this activity after reading chapter 15 of *Physiology of Sport and Exercise*.

After studying this chapter, you probably have new appreciation for the role body composition plays in performance. But as with many things in life, reaching a particular body composition is easier said than done, and, as we learned, if a person attempts to reach a certain weight improperly, without considering body composition, both performance and general health can be compromised.

Go to the Shape Up America! Cyberkitchen at **http://www.shapeup.org/kitchen/index.htm**, and go through the process outlined at that site to estimate a daily calorie goal and eating plans for yourself. Be sure to use the "fat calculator" to estimate the maximum amount of dietary fat you should consume each day. The goal of this site is to show you how to balance the food you eat with physical activity so that you can achieve and maintain a healthy weight. Write your answers to the questions below on a separate piece of paper.

1. From what you have learned in this chapter, what is good about the approach this site takes to weight control, whether it be weight loss, weight maintenance, or weight gain?

2. From what you have learned in this chapter, what is missing from the approach this Web site takes to weight control?

3. How might you need to adjust your weight goal and body composition goal if you were going to compete in the following activities? (If you measured your percent body fat in lab activities, use your actual body composition as a starting point for your answers.)

gymnastics, weight lifting, endurance running, archery, swimming:

Sample Test Questions for Chapter 15

Test yourself on your knowledge of this chapter by taking this self-test. Write the correct answers on a separate sheet of paper.

Multiple Choice

1. Which of the following items is a key component of body composition?

   a. Height
   b. Muscularity
   c. Fat mass
   d. Linearity

2. Which method of body composition assessment would the coach of an elite athlete use to obtain the most accurate results?

   a. Infrared interactance
   b. Bioelectric impedance
   c. Skinfold fat thickness
   d. Densitometry

3. Which best describes the female athlete triad?

   a. Disordered eating leads to menstrual dysfunction, which leads to osteoporosis.
   b. Anorexia nervosa or bulimia nervosa leads to menstrual dysfunction, which leads to bone mineral disorders.
   c. Disordered eating leads to early menarche, which leads to enhanced bone growth.
   d. Anorexia nervosa leads to low bone density, which leads to amenorrhea.

4. Which of the following examples represents the best use of weight standards?

   a. A cycling coach requires both male and female cyclists to attain 6% relative body fat.
   b. A tennis coach tells all his male tennis players that they must weigh the minimum for their range on standard height-weight charts.
   c. A coach works with an athlete to set a weight-loss goal based on the percentage of fat-free mass that is desired.
   d. None of the above.

True-False

5. Standard height-weight tables provide accurate estimates of what an athlete should weigh.

6. Inaccuracies in densitometry result from variation in the density of fat-free mass among individuals of different ages, sexes, and races.

7. Increased fat-free mass is undesirable for the endurance runner, high jumper, and long jumper.

8. Realistic weight standards for athletes are best set by using a range of relative fat values that are considered acceptable for the sport and the athlete's age and sex.

9. Over 70% of the weight lost during crash diets comes from stored fat.

10. A person can safely lose 2.3 kg (5 lb) per week without losing any fat-free mass.

Fill in the Blank

11. A person's body build, or the form and structure of the body, is also called one's _____.

12. Fat-free mass is composed of all of the body's nonfat tissue, including _____, _____, _____, and _____.

Short Answer

13. Explain the method of measuring body composition by using skinfold fat thickness. Why is this method the most widely used field technique for measuring body composition?

14. Explain how percentage of relative body fat contributes to gender differences in running performance.

Essay

15. Do standard height-weight tables provide accurate estimates of what an athlete should weigh? Why or why not? Give an example that supports your answer.

16. Describe in detail how crash diets can lead to dehydration and declines in performance.

Answers to Selected Chapter 15 Activities

15.1 What Is My Body Build, Body Size, and Body Composition?

4. All nonfat tissue, including bone, muscle, organs, and connective tissue

15.2 Assessing Body Composition

1. c, f, g;   2. b, j;   3. e, h;   4. d, i

5. $55 - 3 = 52$ L

6. $D_{body} = 55$ kg $\div$ 52 L = 1.058 g/mL

7. % body fat = $(495 \div 1.058) - 450 = 467.86 - 450 = 17.86$

8. Fat weight = $55 \times 0.1786 = 9.823$ kg (21.66 lb)

9. Fat-free weight = $55 - 9.823 = 45.18$ kg (99.62 lb)

15.3 Body Composition and Sports Performance

1. a; Even though the marathoner in "b" has more fat-free mass, this additional weight could decrease performance, because the distance runner must move the additional load horizontally for an extended period of time.

2. b; Maximizing fat-free mass is desirable for athletes involved in activities that require strength, power, and muscular endurance, all of which might be important to the defensive lineman. In this case, Subject b has about 9 more kg (20 more lb) of fat-free mass and about 4.25 fewer kg (9.37 fewer lb) of relative body fat than Subject a.

3. b; In general, leaner athletes perform better. Higher percentages of body fat have been associated with poorer performance on tests of balance, agility, and jumping, all important skills to the gymnast.

4. b; Heavyweight weightlifters might be an exception to the rule that less fat is better. These athletes add large amounts of fat weight just before competition, on the premise that the additional weight will lower their centers of gravity and give them a greater mechanical advantage in lifting.

5. a; The long jumper with less body fat will generally perform better, because there is less extra (and inactive) body fat to move through space.

15.4 Using Weight Standards Appropriately and the Risks of Severe Weight Loss

1. b and e should be circled; a, c, d, and f should be crossed out.

2. a. anorexia nervosa or bulimia nervosa; b. menstrual dysfunction; c. bone mineral disorders

3. Neural and hormonal causes: When an athlete is underweight, the sympathetic nervous system is inhibited, and the parasympathetic system dominates. The hypothalamus does not function normally, and immune function seems impaired. All of these changes lead to a number of symptoms that include chronic fatigue.

   Substrate depletion: If an athlete trains hard, but eats an inadequate diet—one that is deficient either in total calories or in total carbohydrate calories—carbohydrate stores become depleted. Liver and muscle glycogen levels decrease, which in turn reduce blood glucose levels. Muscle protein can also become depleted as the body looks for new energy sources. All of this can lead to chronic fatigue and declines in performance.

4. Weight: 63.5 kg (140 lb)

   Relative fat: 23%

   Fat weight: Weight × 23% = 63.5 kg (140 lb) × 0.23 = 14.6 kg (32.2 lb)

   Fat-free weight: Weight – fat weight = 63.5 kg (140 lb) – 14.6 kg (32.2 lb) = 48.9 kg (107.8 lb)

   Relative fat goal: 17% (= 83% fat-free)

   Weight goal: Fat-free weight ÷ 83% = 48.9 kg (107.8 lb) ÷ 0.83 = 58.9 kg (130 lb)

   Weight-loss goal: Current weight – weight goal = 63.5 kg (140 lb) – 58.9 kg (130 lb) = 4.6 kg (10 lb)

15.5 Risks of Crash Dieting: Losing Weight Safely

1. Presentation will vary, but, in general, the flowchart would include these steps: food intake is reduced, *water (not fat) is lost rapidly,* protein is lost, reduced carbohydrate intake results in depleted carbohydrate stores, reduced carbohydrate storage leads to *reduced water storage,* the body relies more on free fatty acids for energy, ketone bodies accumulate in the blood resulting in ketosis, *ketosis increases water loss.*

2. The football player will likely not perform nearly as well as desired. He will find it difficult to train very hard with reduced glycogen stores and dehydration. Of particular concern, the dehydration resulting from the diet could lead to undesired effects, especially relating to kidney and cardiovascular function; these effects include decreased blood volume and blood pressure, decreased maximal cardiac output, decreased blood flow to and from the kidneys, and impaired thermoregulation (of great concern to these athletes who attend training camps at the warmest time of the year).

3. a. exercise or activity, dietary intake or caloric intake

   b. 0.5 to 1 kg (less than 2 lb)

   c. 0.5 kg (1 lb), 200 to 500 kcal, three

Answers to Selected Chapter 15 Test Questions

Multiple Choice

1. c ;   2. d;   3. b;   4. c

True-False

5. False;   6. True;   7. True;   8. True;   9. False;   10. False

Fill in the Blank

11. morphology

12. bone, muscle, organs, connective tissue

Short Answer and Essay

For questions 13 to 16, check your answers against the explanations given in the textbook.

Growth, Development, and the Young Athlete

concepts

- Girls mature physiologically about 2 to 2.5 years earlier than boys do.

- Prior to adulthood, marked development occurs in height, weight, bone, muscle, fat, and the nervous system.

- The function of almost all physiological systems, and therefore the ability to perform physical feats, improves until full maturity is reached or shortly before. After that, physiological function plateaus for a period of time before starting to decline with advancing age.

- Prepubescent children can improve their strength with resistance training. These strength gains are due largely to neurological factors, with little or no change in the size of the muscle.

- Aerobic training in preadolescents does not alter $\dot{V}O_2$max as much as would be expected, but endurance performance does improve with aerobic training; in addition, a child's anaerobic capacity increases with anaerobic training.

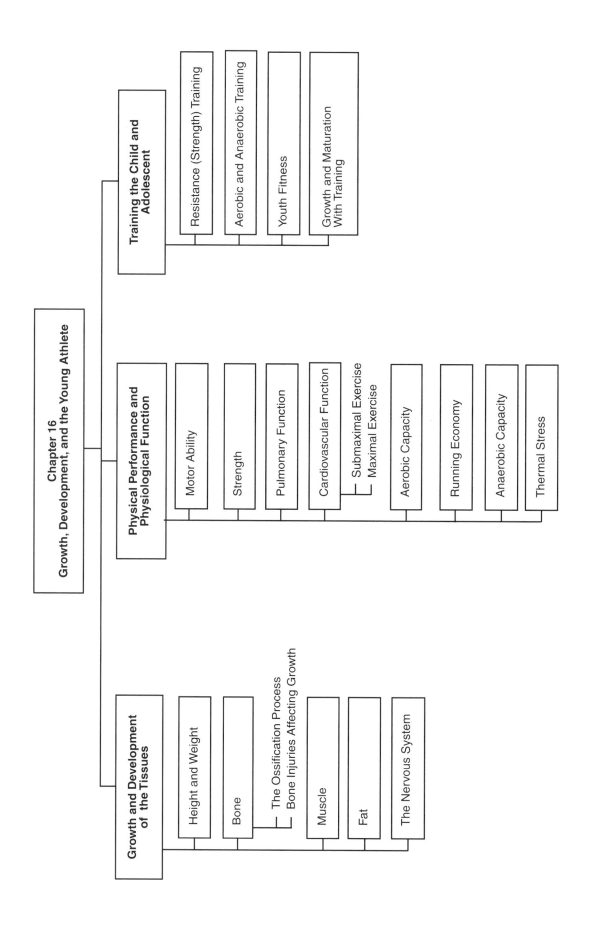

Chapter 16
Growth, Development, and the Young Athlete

Growth and Development of the Tissues

Height and Weight

Bone
- The Ossification Process
- Bone Injuries Affecting Growth

Muscle

Fat

The Nervous System

Physical Performance and Physiological Function

Motor Ability

Strength

Pulmonary Function

Cardiovascular Function
- Submaximal Exercise
- Maximal Exercise

Aerobic Capacity

Running Economy

Anaerobic Capacity

Thermal Stress

Training the Child and Adolescent

Resistance (Strength) Training

Aerobic and Anaerobic Training

Youth Fitness

Growth and Maturation With Training

Activity 16.1

Definitions of Terms

Do this activity after reading page 518 of *Physiology of Sport and Exercise.*

This chapter uses a variety of terms to describe periods of life and changes that occur in the body. To get off to a good start with this chapter, read page 518 of *Physiology of Sport and Exercise*, and then without looking in your textbook, match each term with both its correct definition and the example that best illustrates that term. You will use each letter only once, but you will have two letters in each blank (one definition and one example).

Term

_____ 1. Growth

_____ 2. Development

_____ 3. Maturation

_____ 4. Infancy

_____ 5. Childhood

_____ 6. Adolescence

_____ 7. Puberty

Definition

a. The first year of life.
b. The point at which a person becomes physiologically capable of reproduction.
c. An increase in the size of the body or any of its parts.
d. The period of life between childhood and adulthood; the onset of puberty marks its beginning.
e. The process by which the body takes on adult form and becomes fully functional; often defined by the system or function being considered.
f. Changes that occur in the body starting at conception and continuing through adulthood; the differentiation of cells along specialized lines of function, reflecting functional changes that occur with growth.
g. The period of life between the first birthday and the onset of puberty.

Example

h. Sharese's membranes and cartilage are being transformed into bone through ossification, or bone formation. What type of change does this describe?
i. Florence has developed secondary sex characteristics and has just started menstruating. She has just experienced the onset of what event?
j. John is 16 years old. He is capable of sexual reproduction, but has not yet attained his adult height. What phase is he in?
k. All of Tony's bones have completed normal growth and ossification. What type of change does this describe?
l. Mary has not yet reached her first birthday. What phase is she in?
m. Steve celebrated his first birthday long ago, but has not yet reached adolescence. What phase is he in?
n. Tanya's height has increased by 4 in. this year. What type of change does this describe?

Activity 16.2

Growth and Development of the Tissues

Do this activity after reading pages 518-525 of *Physiology of Sport and Exercise.*

Before we can understand the physical capabilities of children, we must first understand the physical state of their bodies. In this activity, we will take a look at when and how certain tissues grow and develop prior to adulthood.

What: Height

When: Height increases rapidly during the first _____ years of life. After this, height increases at a progressively slower rate throughout childhood. Just before _____, the rate of change in height increases markedly, with the peak rate of growth in height at about age _____ in girls and age _____ in boys. This is followed by an exponential decrease in rate until full height is attained at about _____ years in girls and _____ years in boys.

What: Weight

When: Weight increases in a similar fashion to height, but the peak rate of growth in body weight occurs at about age _____ in girls and age _____ in boys.

What: Bone

When: Bones begin to develop during the _____ stage of development. Bones continue to develop for the first _____ to _____ years of life.

How: Bones develop from these two types of tissues: _____ and _____. Ossification, which means _____, begins at this area: _____. Ossification is initiated when the perichondrium is penetrated by _____. Once the perichondrium is vascularized, it is called the _____, and the chondrocytes in it become bone-forming cells called _____. Osteoblasts secrete substances that form a _____ around the diaphysis. The cartilage cells in the diaphysis undergo a series of changes that eventually result in calcification of the bone. This area of bone formation is then known as the _____ _____. Shortly after birth, secondary ossification centers arise in the _____ and the epiphyses begin to ossify. The plate of cartilage between the diaphysis and each epiphysis is known as the _____ or _____. Ossification, and therefore bone growth, is completed when the _____ cease to grow and the epiphyseal plates are replaced by _____.

Exercise primarily affects bone _____, _____, and _____.

The figure below illustrates the anatomy of a long bone once bone formation has begun in the diaphysis and epiphyses after birth. Fill in the correct labels without looking in *Physiology of Sport and Exercise*.

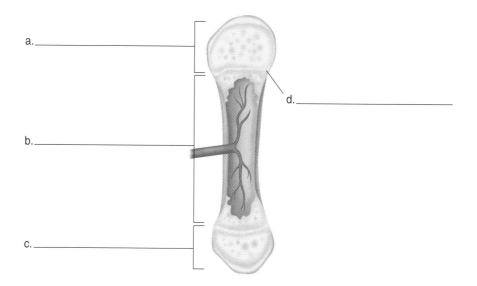

What: Muscle

When: The body's muscle mass steadily increases, along with weight gain, from birth to this stage: _____. Muscle mass peaks in females at ages _____ to _____ and in males at ages _____ to _____.

How: Increases in muscle mass with age result primarily from increased _____ _____ (hyperplasia or hypertrophy?) of existing fibers, with little or no increase in fiber _____ (hyperplasia or hypertrophy?). Increases in muscle length as young bones elongate result from increases in the number and length of _____.

What: Fat

When: Fat cells form and fat deposition begins early during the _____ stage of development. Each fat cell can increase in size at any age from _____ to _____.

How: At birth, _____% to _____% of total body weight is fat. At physical maturity, fat content reaches about _____% of total body weight in males and about _____% of total body weight in females. This sex difference is primarily due to _____ differences. Once existing fat cells are filled to a certain critical volume, _____ _____ _____ are formed. The amount of fat that accumulates with growth and aging depends on _____, _____, and _____.

What: The Nervous System

When: Myelination of the cerebral cortex occurs most rapidly during the stage of _____, but continues well beyond puberty.

How: _____ of nerve fibers must be completed before fast reactions and skilled movements can occur. Conduction of an impulse along a nerve fiber is considerably _____ (slower or faster?) if myelination is absent or incomplete. Although practicing an activity or skill can improve performance, the full development of that activity or skill depends on full maturation of the _____.

Observing Children's Physiological Development

Activity 16.3

Do this activity after reading pages 525-535 of *Physiology of Sport and Exercise.*

The amount of development that takes place during childhood is truly amazing. The functioning of almost all physiological systems improves until full maturity is reached or shortly before. In this activity, you will get a sense of the amount of development that needs to take place before all systems are fully functional.

Observe children age 10 or younger—perhaps a younger sibling, a child you babysit, a group of schoolchildren playing at recess, or children participating in a sport during physical education class or at a YMCA. Find evidence of their lack of maturity in these areas, and write your answers on a separate sheet of paper:

Motor ability

1. What evidence did you observe of lack of maturity in the children's motor ability?

2. What do the improvements in motor ability with age result from?

3. What three factors help explain the plateau of motor ability in girls around the age of puberty?

Strength

4. What evidence did you observe of lack of maturity in the children's strength?

5. What three factors contribute to increasing strength with age?

Pulmonary function, cardiovascular function, and aerobic capacity

6. What evidence did you observe of lack of maturity in the children's pulmonary function, cardiovascular function, and aerobic capacity?

7. For what reasons are submaximal and maximal heart rates higher in children than in adults?

8. How do the results of measuring $\dot{V}O_2$max in L/min versus measuring $\dot{V}O_2$max relative to body weight (in ml $\cdot$ kg^{-1} $\cdot$ min^{-1}) differ?

Running economy

9. What evidence did you observe of lack of maturity in children's running economy?

10. Which of the factors that Rowland has hypothesized as affecting running economy in children do your observations support? (See page 531 in *Physiology of Sport and Exercise* for a list of these factors.)

Anaerobic capacity

11. What evidence did you observe of lack of maturity in the children's anaerobic capacity (look for children giving all-out effort in short bouts of 60 s or less)?

12. What are the possible reasons for lower anaerobic capacity in children when compared with adults?

Thermal stress

13. What evidence did you observe of lack of maturity in the children's ability to tolerate heat or cold stress?

14. What factors may cause children to be more susceptible than adults to hypothermia in cold environments?

15. What factors may cause children to be more susceptible than adults to hyperthermia in hot environments?

For an extra challenge... In addition to generally observing children in this activity, look for differences in development in younger children versus older children and in boys versus girls. What evidence do you see of differing physiological maturity levels based on age or gender?

Activity 16.4   Physical Training for the Child and Adolescent

Do this activity after reading pages 535-540 of *Physiology of Sport and Exercise.*

Children are physiologically distinct from adults and must be considered differently. How should these differences affect training, and how do they affect children's adaptations to training? After reading pages 535 to 540 in *Physiology of Sport and Exercise,* fill in the table below, assessing the risks and benefits of training as well as what factors result in changes in strength, aerobic capacity, and anaerobic capacity in children.

Type of training	Risks for children and adolescents	Benefits for children and adolescents	How capacity is increased
Resistance training			*Prepubescent:*
			Adolescent:
Aerobic training			*What limits improvements in aerobic capacity in children?*
Anaerobic training			

Putting It All Together: Growth, Development, and the Young Athlete

Activity 16.5

Do this activity after reading chapter 16 of *Physiology of Sport and Exercise.*

Having learned about the growth and development of children through studying this chapter, you should now be able to discern what types of activities and training are appropriate for children and what effects the training will have on children's development.

Read the scenarios below and decide how you would respond in each situation. You do not need to write your answers here (unless your instructor asks you to), but you should know how you would respond in each situation and you should be ready to defend your position.

Craig is 10 years old and a pitcher on his youth baseball team. His dad is really proud of him, because he can pitch the ball at speeds up to 113 km/h (70 mph).

1. What type of injury is Craig at risk for, and what are the possible consequences of such an injury?

2. If you were the coach of Craig's team, what modifications would you make to prevent such an injury?

3. If you were Craig's parent, what alternate sports or positions would you guide Craig to participate in?

Tori, age 8, recently suffered a fracture to an epiphyseal plate in her tibia during an auto accident.

4. In what ways can such an injury cause disruption of growth?

5. What are the possible lifelong consequences of such an injury?

Todd is 9 years old and wants to train with weights in order to be stronger and more muscular by the time of his park district's summer youth football camp.

6. Can Todd gain strength through resistance training at such an early age?

7. If so, what mechanisms may lead to his strength gains?

8. Is Todd likely to reach his goal of gaining muscle size through his resistance-training program?

9. If you were Todd's parent, what would you look for in a strength-training instructor and program?

Kristina's mom is running a 5K in 3 months, and Kristina, who is 10 years old, wants to run the 5K with her mom. She has begun running long distances after school in order to prepare for the event.

10. How will Kristina's training affect her $\dot{V}O_2$max? What are the possible reasons for these changes or lack thereof?

11. Will Kristina's running performance likely increase because of her aerobic training? Why?

12. If you were Kristina's mother, and wanted your daughter to continue enjoying physical activities of all types, what nonphysiological responses would you monitor as your young daughter trains for this event?

Jake is 11 years old and loves swimming for his YMCA's swim team. He is especially gifted at short sprints. In fact, his swim coach has suggested to Jake that he sprint train in order to improve his times in his favorite events—the 50 m and 100 m freestyle events.

13. Can Jake's anaerobic capacity be improved through anaerobic training at such a young age?

14. What physiological improvements can Jake expect after training?

15. If you were Jake's coach, desiring that Jake stick with swimming for a long time to come, what nonphysiological responses would you monitor as your young student trains under your supervision?

Sample Test Questions for Chapter 16

Test yourself on your knowledge of this chapter by taking this self-test. Write the correct answers on a separate sheet of paper.

Multiple Choice

1. Exercise does *not* affect bone's

   a. width;   b. strength;   c. length;   d. density

2. Regular physical training in children can result in all of these *except*

   a. lower total body fat;   b. higher total body mass;   c. increased height;
       d. higher fat-free mass

3. From what you have read in this chapter, which sport seems least likely to cause epiphyseal injuries in children?

   a. competitive baseball;   b. slow-pitch softball;   c. swimming;   d. tennis

4. Which of these factors is least likely to cause strength gains from resistance training in prepubescent boys?

   a. improved motor skill coordination;   b. increased motor unit activation;
       c. neurological adaptations;   d. increased muscle size

True-False

5. Because bone is not a living tissue, it does not receive a blood supply.

6. Girls mature physiologically about 2 to 2.5 years earlier than boys do.

7. When injury occurs, more calcium is deposited in the affected bone.

8. When extra stress is placed on a bone, such as during exercise, more calcium is deposited in the bone matrix.

9. Epiphyseal injuries always result in crippling or permanent trauma.

10. The number of fat cells cannot increase throughout life; instead, only the size of existing fat cells can increase.

11. As body size increases with growth and development, so does lung size and function.

Fill in the Blank

12. Fractures at the _____ can disturb the bone's nutrient supply and disrupt the growth process.

13. A child's lower capacity for evaporative heat loss is largely the result of a lower _____.

Short Answer

14. Explain how high and low calcium levels affect bone health.

15. Explain the role that myelination plays in children's reaction time, skill development, and strength development.

16. What factors limit children's anaerobic capacity?

Essay

17. Discuss the changes that occur in cardiovascular function as children grow and age. Focus on submaximal and maximal exercise and include discussion of blood pressure, cardiac output, heart size, heart rate, stroke volume, total blood volume, and arterial-venous difference.

18. Explain this apparent contradiction: When children's $\dot{V}O_2$max is expressed relative to body weight, their $\dot{V}O_2$max is at or near adult values; yet in an activity where body weight is the major resistance to movement, such as running, children cannot maintain a running pace as fast as adults.

Answers to Selected Chapter 16 Activities

16.1   Definitions of Terms

1. c, n;   2. f, h;   3. e, k;   4. a, l;   5. g, m;   6. d, j;   7. b, i

16.2   Growth and Development of the Tissues

Height *When:* 2, puberty, 12, 14, 16.5, 18.0

Weight *When:* 12, 14.5

Bone *When:* fetal, 14, 22 *How:* cartilage and fibrous membranes, bone formation, diaphysis, blood vessels, periosteum, osteoblasts, collar of bone, primary ossification center, epiphyses, epiphyseal plate, growth plate, cartilage cells, bone, width, density, strength (last three are interchangeable) *Figure labels: a.* epiphysis, *b.* diaphysis, *c.* epiphysis, *d.* epiphyseal growth plate

Muscle *When:* adolescence, 16, 20, 18, 25 *How:* hypertrophy (size), hyperplasia (number), sarcomeres

Fat *When:* fetal, birth, death *How:* 10, 12, 15, 25, hormonal, new fat cells, diet, exercise, heredity (last three are interchangeable)

The Nervous System *When:* childhood *How:* Myelination, slower, nervous system

16.3 Observing Children's Physiological Development

1. Answers will vary.

2. Development of the neuromuscular and endocrine systems, and secondarily from the children's increased activity.

3. Increase in estrogen levels at puberty leads to increased fat deposition, and performance tends to decrease as fat increases; girls have less muscle mass; around puberty, many girls assume a more sedentary lifestyle than boys.

4. Answers will vary.

5. Increased muscle mass, increased testosterone levels in males at puberty, and maturation of the nervous system.

6. Answers will vary.

7. The heart rate response in children is a compensatory mechanism in response to the child's smaller heart size, smaller total blood volume, and lower stroke volume.

8. When measured in L/min, aerobic capacity increases from age 6 to between ages 17 and 21 and is lower in children than in adults. When expressed relative to body weight, there is little or no difference in aerobic capacity between children and adults; values in boys change little from age 6 to young adulthood; values in girls change little from age 6 to 13, but gradually decrease after age 13.

9. Answers will vary.

10. Answers will vary.

11. Answers will vary.

12. Children have a lower glycolytic capacity, possibly because of a limited amount of phosphofructokinase. Children cannot attain high respiratory exchange ratios during maximal or exhaustive exercise, suggesting less lactate production.

13. Answers will vary.

14. Children appear to have greater conductive heat loss than adults, due to larger surface area–to–mass ratios.

15. Children sweat at a lower rate—individual sweat glands in children form sweat more slowly and are less sensitive to increases in the body's core temperature than those in adults—so their capacity to lose heat through evaporation is lower than it is in adults.

16.4   Physical Training for the Child and Adolescent

Type of training	Risks for children and adolescents	Benefits for children and adolescents	How capacity is increased
Resistance training	Some risk of injury, though very low. If program is designed and supervised appropriately, there is generally no more risk of injury than for other physical activities or as compared with adult participation.	Increased strength. Might offer some protection against injury by strengthening muscles.	*Prepubescent:* Improved motor skill coordination, increased motor unit activation, other neurological adaptations. *Adolescent:* Neural adaptations and increases in both muscle size and specific tension.
Aerobic training	None.	Improved general fitness, although no significant increases in $\dot{V}O_2$max until child reaches puberty.	*What limits improvements in aerobic capacity in children?* Stroke volume, and therefore smaller heart size.
Anaerobic training	None.	Improved anaerobic capacity.	Increased resting levels of PC, ATP, and glycogen; increased PFK activity; increased maximal blood lactate.

Answers to Selected Chapter 16 Test Questions

Multiple Choice

1. c ;   2. c   3. b;   4. d

True-False

5. False;   6. True;   7. True;   8. True;   9. False;   10. False;   11. True

Fill in the Blank

12. epiphyseal plate

13. sweating rate

Short Answer and Essay

For questions 14 to 18, check your answers against the explanations given in the textbook.

Aging and the Older Athlete

concepts

- Most athletic performance declines steadily during middle and older age, primarily due to decrements in endurance and strength.

- Cardiorespiratory endurance declines with age, although continued physical training significantly reduces this decline. It is unclear how much these decreases are due to physical aging alone and how much are due to deconditioning because of decreased activity.

- Muscle strength is reduced with age, primarily due to a loss of muscle mass. Training cannot preclude age-related changes in muscle, but it can lessen the rate of muscle strength loss.

- Aging does not reduce our capacity to perform normal activity at high altitude; however, aging does reduce our ability to adapt to exercise in the heat.

- With age, body-fat content increases, while at the same time fat-free mass decreases. Training can help delay these changes.

- Older people have considerable ability to increase their endurance capacity and strength with aerobic training and strength training.

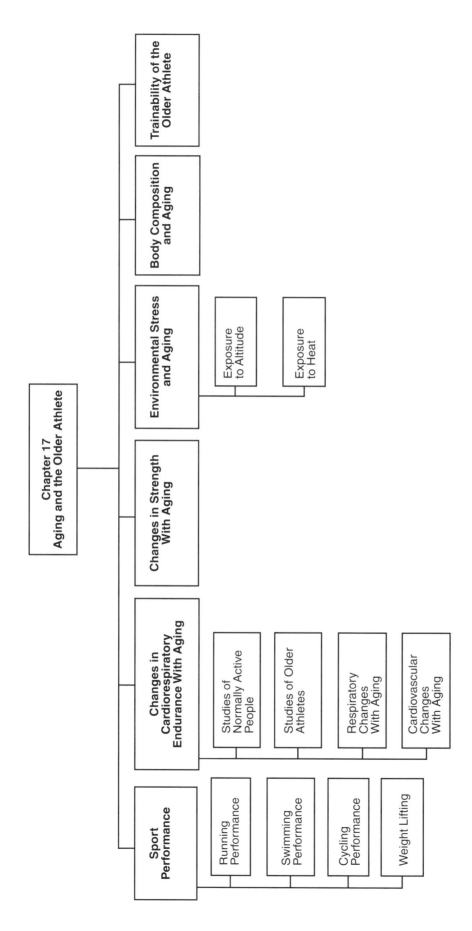

How Does Sport Performance Change With Age?

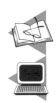

Activity 17.1

Do this activity after reading pages 545-549 of *Physiology of Sport and Exercise*.

In many sports, performance begins to decline once we reach the physical prime of our 20s and early 30s. Conduct a study to see if your results match those of the textbook. Search the Internet or other sources for performance times of elite athletes of several age groups for two or three sports. For example, if you choose swimming, you might search for national or world records of the women's 100-m freestyle for ages 25, 45, and 65 (these are only examples; use whatever ages are available between the 20s and 80s). Record your findings below. Then calculate the percent decline per decade and year, and describe how these compare to the findings presented on pages 545 to 549 of *Physiology of Sport and Exercise*.

In order to find performance times of older athletes, search the Internet for "masters running," "masters swimming," and so forth. Some Web sites you might find useful include

http://www.nationalmastersnews.com/ (presenting U.S. track and field, long-distance running, and race-walking news)

http://www.nationalseniorgames.net/ (presenting information on this U.S. organization)

http://www.masters.cwfhc.ca/ (home site of Canadian Masters Weightlifting)

http://www.modernmedia.demon.co.uk/swim/masters.htm (home site for English Masters Swimming; European results available here)

http://www.fina.org/masterswldrecords.html (masters swimming world records)

Event/gender (e.g., women's 100-m freestyle):

Age and time (e.g., 25 yr; 57.09 s):

Age and time:

Age and time:

% decline per decade:

% decline per year:

How compares with findings in *Physiology of Sport and Exercise:*

Event/gender:

Age and time:

Age and time:

Age and time:

% decline per decade:

% decline per year:

How compares with findings in *Physiology of Sport and Exercise:*

Event/gender:

Age and time:

Age and time:

Age and time:

% decline per decade:

% decline per year:

How compares with findings in *Physiology of Sport and Exercise:*

| Activity 17.2 | Physiological Changes With Age |

Do this activity after reading pages 549-562 of *Physiology of Sport and Exercise.*

Performance declines in sport and exercise are likely related to the natural physiological changes that come with aging as well as to decreased activity, which leads to deconditioning. Your text describes many of the physiological changes that take place as we age. List them below, along with the underlying reasons for the change. Use this listing as a study tool for the exam for this chapter. The first row is filled in as an example for you.

Parameter	Change	Mechanisms that cause change (if noted in textbook)
Cardiorespiratory endurance $\dot{V}O_2$max	Declines on average 1% per year beginning around age 25 for men and late teens for women.	Reduction in maximum heart rate and stroke volume.
Vital capacity (VC)		
Forced expiratory volume (FEV)		
Residual volume (RV)		
Total lung capacity (TLC)		
RV: TLC ratio		
Maximal expiratory ventilation ($\dot{V}$Emax)		

Parameter	Change	Mechanisms that cause change (if noted in textbook)
Cardiorespiratory endurance *(continued)*		
Maximum heart rate (HRmax)		
Maximal stroke volume (SVmax)		
Maximal cardiac output		
Strength		
Maximal strength		
Muscle fibers (number, size, type)		
Speed of movement		
Environmental stress		
Ability to exercise at high altitude		
Ability to exercise in the heat		
Body composition		
Relative body fat		
Fat-free mass		

The Effect of Training on Physiological Changes

Activity 17.3

Do this activity after reading pages 549-564 of *Physiology of Sport and Exercise.*

For many parameters it is unclear how much the declines in performance and function depend on physical aging alone and how much are because of decreased activity; however, it is quite clear that physical training can lessen the rate of decline. In fact, older people have considerable ability to increase their endurance capacity and strength with training and are capable of exceptional performances.

Review pages 549 to 564 in *Physiology of Sport and Exercise,* and jot notes (on a separate piece of paper) explaining how training impacts each parameter as we get older. Use this listing as a study tool for the exam for this chapter. The first row is filled in as an example for you. For instance, for $\dot{V}O_2$max you might write, "Highly intense training substantially slows rate of decrease from about age 30 to 50; it has less effect after 50 years of age."

- Maximum heart rate (HRmax)
- Elasticity of lungs and chest wall
- Maximal stroke volume (SVmax)
- Maximal cardiac output
- Peripheral blood flow
- a-$\bar{v}O_2$ diff
- Muscle strength
- Ratio of muscle to fat
- Composition of muscle fiber type
- Muscle mass (number and size of muscle fibers)
- Speed of movement
- Body weight (see pp. 561 and 562)
- Body-fat content (see pp. 561 and 562)
- Longevity (the length of one's life)

Cardiorespiratory Changes: What About You?

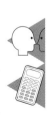

Activity 17.4

Do this activity after reading pages 549-564 of *Physiology of Sport and Exercise.*

As we age, our bodies will change in many ways. We will be able to prevent or minimize some of these changes, but not others. This activity challenges you to reflect on two cardiorespiratory changes that take place as we age. The first, maximum heart rate, seems to decrease as we age regardless of activity level. But the second, maximal oxygen uptake, can be maintained quite well through regular endurance exercise.

Maximum Heart Rate

To see how your maximum heart rate (HRmax) will change over the years, calculate your current HRmax as well as the HRmax for each subsequent decade. Remember that this equation is only an average. Your actual HRmax might be up to 20 beats/min higher or lower than what you calculate here.

HRmax = 220 – age

Current HRmax (age _____):

HRmax 10 years from now (age _____):

HRmax 20 years from now (age _____):

HRmax 30 years from now (age _____):

HRmax 40 years from now (age _____):

HRmax 50 years from now (age _____):

Maximal Oxygen Uptake (Aerobic Capacity)

To see how your aerobic capacity will change over the years *if you lead a sedentary lifestyle,* let us look at your $\dot{V}O_2$max levels. If you know your current $\dot{V}O_2$max from previous testing in this course, fill it in below. If you do not know your $\dot{V}O_2$max and have no way of measuring it, use these guidelines to select an estimate:

- If you are relatively sedentary, use 47 mL · kg^{-1} · min^{-1} if you are male and 38 mL · kg^{-1} · min^{-1} if you are female.

- If you are relatively active, use 60 mL · kg^{-1} · min^{-1} if you are male and 55 mL · kg^{-1} · min^{-1} if you are female.

Current $\dot{V}O_2$max (age _____):

$\dot{V}O_2$max 10 years from now (age _____):

[Without intense exercise, $\dot{V}O_2$max decreases by about 10% each decade.]

$\dot{V}O_2$max 20 years from now (age _____):

$\dot{V}O_2$max 30 years from now (age _____):

$\dot{V}O_2$max 40 years from now (age _____):

$\dot{V}O_2$max 50 years from now (age _____):

What Can You Do?

Although maximum heart rate decreases with age regardless of exercise levels, your aerobic capacity or $\dot{V}O_2$max can be maintained quite well through regular intense exercise. What plans do you have to maintain your aerobic capacity throughout your lifetime?

> **Activity 17.5**

Putting It All Together: Aging and the Older Athlete

Do this activity after reading chapter 17 of *Physiology of Sport and Exercise.*

Now that you have learned from the textbook what changes take place as we get older and how training can affect those changes, take some time to observe these changes in people around you. Choose one of the two options in this activity to broaden your understanding of aging and the older athlete.

Option 1: Observation

Observe older people to find evidence of changes in the following physiological parameters. You might arrange to volunteer at a nursing home or retirement village for a few hours; observe older people at a YMCA or JCC; or go to a shopping mall and watch how older people navigate the task of shopping or exercising, as many health-conscious seniors walk for fitness in indoor malls. Record evidence you witness of age-related declines in physical performance *and* any evidence you see of how regular exercise slows these declines.

- Cardiorespiratory endurance
- Strength
- Environmental stress
- Body composition

Option 2: Interview

Interview an older person in your life to find out how that person perceives physical performance to have changed with age. You might interview an older coach, an instructor or professor, a parent or grandparent, or even your boss. You do not need to interview someone extremely old—even adults in their late 30s and 40s have likely noticed physical changes as they have gotten older.

You can use the following questions or create ones more specific or appropriate to the situation. Summarize the person's responses on a separate sheet of paper. Your instructor may or may not require you to bring your summary to class for discussion.

1. How has your activity level changed from the time you were in your 20s?

2. What are the general changes you have noticed in your fitness level as you have gotten older? (Lead the individual to describe these as specifically as possible.)

3. What is your favorite physical activity? How has your performance in this activity changed over the years? Do you think this is caused more by getting older or by a change in how often or how intensely you train?

4. How would you compare your current endurance levels with those of your early 20s?

   Strength levels?

   Your ability to exercise in the heat?

5. What activities do you find more difficult to do now than when you were in your 20s and 30s? Are there any activities that you simply cannot do anymore? (Answers here may vary considerably by age—people in their 70s and 80s might remark about activities of daily living; younger people might have more difficulty answering this question.)

6. If you were to change anything about your exercise habits, what would you change?

Sample Test Questions for Chapter 17

Test yourself on your knowledge of this chapter by taking this self-test. Write the correct answers on a separate sheet of paper.

Multiple Choice

1. Which of the following does *not* apparently contribute to the reduction in $\dot{V}O_2$max with age?

   a. reduced maximal heart rate
   b. reduced stroke volume
   c. decreased cardiorespiratory endurance activity
   d. reduced total lung capacity

2. Which activity is the best choice for increasing muscle mass and decreasing fat?

   a. long-distance running;   b. playing soccer;   c. lifting weights;   d. walking

3. Due to physiological changes that accompany aging, in which of the following situations might a 55-year-old person actually have an advantage over a 20-year-old?

   a. competing at altitude;   b. competing in the heat   c. running a marathon;
      d. performing a 1RM lift

4. Limited data supports the contention that if you exercise regularly as you age you will

   a. be more prone to injuries.
   b. achieve the performance standards established by younger athletes.
   c. increase your lifespan by about 2 years.
   d. increase your body-fat content through training.

True-False

5. It is not possible to improve our physical performances as we age.

6. Maximum heart rate (HRmax) generally decreases with age despite physical training.

7. Maximal cardiac output generally decreases with age, although the rate of decrease can be reduced with endurance training.

8. With age, body-fat content increases despite physical conditioning.

9. Aging impairs a person's ability to increase muscle strength and muscle hypertrophy.

10. Endurance training produces similar gains in healthy people, regardless of their ages.

Fill in the Blank

11. Aging accompanied by decreased activity results in (increased or decreased) _____ muscle mass, _____ proportion of ST fibers to FT fibers, and _____ number and size of muscle fibers.

12. Aging reduces thermal tolerance partly because aging reduces _____, which means that less heat can be lost via _____.

Short Answer

13. Describe the possible reasons for the reductions in maximum heart rate regardless of physical training.

14. Explain how changes in the nervous system affect cardiorespiratory endurance and strength as we grow older.

Essay

15. Explain the changes in lung function that might contribute to age-related decreases in cardiorespiratory endurance. Comment on VC, FEV, RV, TLC, $\dot{V}Emax$, and elasticity.

16. A previously sedentary 60-year-old man asks you to design a program for him that will improve his strength and endurance. What elements would you include in this program to allow him to best reach his goals (include comments about type of activity, intensity, frequency, volume)?

17. The 60-year-old man embarks on the fitness program you have designed for him. What physiological changes can be expected? You should be able to describe at least five specific physiological changes (although there are many more).

Answers to Selected Chapter 17 Test Questions

Multiple Choice

1. d;   2. c;   3. a;   4. c

True-False

5. False;   6. True;   7. True;   8. True;   9. False;   10. True

Fill in the Blank

11. decreased, increased, decreased

12. sweat production, evaporation

Short Answer and Essay

For questions 13 to 17, check your answers against the explanations given in the textbook.

Sex Differences and the Female Athlete

concepts

- Until puberty, girls and boys do not differ significantly in body size and composition. At puberty, body composition changes markedly, so that at maturity, women in general are shorter, weigh less, have more body fat, and have less fat-free mass than men.

- Women and men respond differently to acute bouts of exercise, but women respond to physical training in the same manner as men do, experiencing up to 40% increases in strength and $\dot{V}O_2$max.

- For almost every physiological measure, there is overlap between the sexes. For instance, some average-sized women have remarkable strength, exceeding that of some average-sized men.

- Female athletes can experience menstrual dysfunction, most often secondary amenorrhea and oligomenorrhea, which are likely caused by inadequate nutrition and training-induced hormonal changes.

- Disordered eating, part of the female athlete triad, has become a major concern in female athletes.

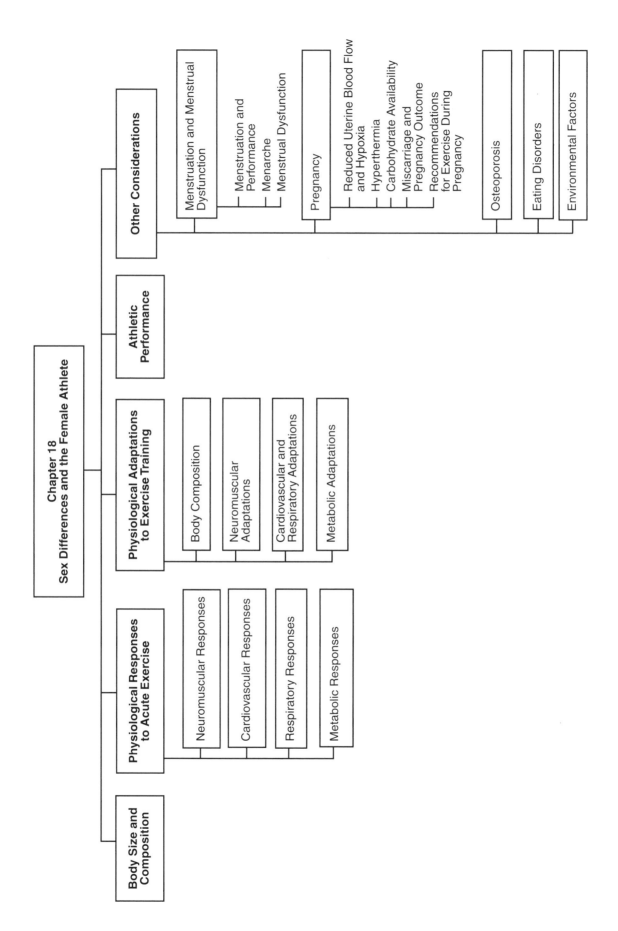

Chapter 18
Sex Differences and the Female Athlete

- Body Size and Composition
- Physiological Responses to Acute Exercise
  - Neuromuscular Responses
  - Cardiovascular Responses
  - Respiratory Responses
  - Metabolic Responses
- Physiological Adaptations to Exercise Training
  - Body Composition
  - Neuromuscular Adaptations
  - Cardiovascular and Respiratory Adaptations
  - Metabolic Adaptations
- Athletic Performance
- Other Considerations
  - Menstruation and Menstrual Dysfunction
    - Menstruation and Performance
    - Menarche
    - Menstrual Dysfunction
  - Pregnancy
    - Reduced Uterine Blood Flow and Hypoxia
    - Hyperthermia
    - Carbohydrate Availability
    - Miscarriage and Pregnancy Outcome
    - Recommendations for Exercise During Pregnancy
  - Osteoporosis
  - Eating Disorders
  - Environmental Factors

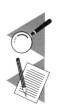

| **Activity 18.1** | **Body Size and Composition** |

Do this activity after reading pages 572-576 of *Physiology of Sport and Exercise*.

Prior to puberty, girls and boys have similar body composition. (1) Observe children of both sexes under age 12 at some public area—a playground; a YMCA, YWCA, or JCC; or a recess area at a local school. Pay attention to the *similarities* in height, weight, and girth of children of similar ages but different sexes. (2) Now spend some time observing men and women on your college campus. Pay attention to the *differences* in height, weight, and girth of men and women of similar ages. Briefly compare and contrast the findings of your two observations—children versus college-age adults—here:

At puberty, estrogen and testosterone begin to cause drastic changes in body composition in women and men, respectively. List these changes in the correct column below.

Changes caused by estrogen secretion in women	Changes caused by testosterone secretion in men

The effects of estrogen in women and testosterone in men lead to differences in body composition in women and men at maturity. Circle the correct choices in each phrase below:

When compared with men, women are generally

1. shorter/taller?

2. lighter in total weight/heavier in total weight?

3. lighter in fat-free mass/heavier in fat-free mass?

4. heavier in fat mass/lighter in fat mass?

5. higher in relative body fat/lower in relative body fat?

Sex-Related Responses to Acute Exercise and Exercise Training

> **Activity 18.2**

Do this activity after reading pages 576-586 of *Physiology of Sport and Exercise.*

When men and women are exposed to an acute bout of exercise, characteristic responses differ between the sexes. But when men and women engage in long-term physical training, their responses are very similar.

Complete the following table, placing an **X** in the second column if men's and women's responses are similar and an **X** in the third column if they are different. If the responses are different, use the fourth column to note what those differences are and why they occur.

Use your completed table as a study tool for your chapter exam.

Parameter	Women and men *similar* or *same*	Women and men *different*	If different . . . What are differences? What causes differences?
Responses to acute exercise Innate quality of muscle and its mechanisms of motor control			
Lower-body strength relative to FFM			
Lower-body strength relative to body weight			
Upper-body strength relative to FFM or body weight			
Muscle fiber type distribution in same sport or event			
Muscle fiber cross-sectional areas and amount of muscle mass			
HR response for any absolute level of sub-maximal exercise			
Stroke volume			

Parameter	Women and men *similar* or *same*	Women and men *different*	If different . . . What are differences? What causes differences?
Responses to acute exercise *(continued)*			
Cardiac output for same same absolute submaximal power output			
Potential to increase a-$\bar{v}O_2$ diff			
Breathing frequency at same relative power output			
Breathing frequency at same absolute power output			
Tidal volume and ventilatory volume			
$\dot{V}O_2$max			
Oxygen consumption ($\dot{V}O_2$) for same absolute power output			
Peak blood lactate values in active but untrained individuals			
Lactate threshold for equally trained individuals when expressed in relative (% $\dot{V}O_2$max) terms			
In summary, responses to acute exercise			

(continued)

(continued)

Parameter	Women and men *similar* or *same*	Women and men *different*	If different . . . What are differences? What causes differences?
Responses to exercise training			
Losses in total body mass with training			
Losses of fat mass with training			
Losses of relative fat with training			
Gains in fat-free mass with training			
Bone and connective tissue adaptations with training			
Magnitude of changes in strength with training			
Muscle girth (hypertrophy) with training			
Increases in maximal cardiac output with training			
Decreases in HR for any given rate of work with training			
Increases in maximal muscle blood flow and muscle capillary density			
Relative increases in $\dot{V}O_2$max with cardio-respiratory endurance training			
In summary, responses to exercise training			
Performance in athletic activities that can be objectively measured by distance and time			

Activity 18.3

Menstrual Dysfunction

Do this activity after reading pages 586-592 of *Physiology of Sport and Exercise.*

Although it is not entirely clear how menstruation affects physical performance and how sports competition affects menstruation, researchers are beginning to understand the causes of menstrual dysfunction. Recent studies have called into question the idea that intense competition on its own causes menstrual dysfunction. Instead, many factors seem to be at play.

In the blank after each scenario, write the disorder or dysfunction the athlete is experiencing.

1. Lavon competes on her high school gymnastics team. Even though she is 16 years old, she still has not started menstruating. _____

2. Julie is a long-distance runner. She is 22 years old and has never menstruated. _____ .

3. Corrin is a bodybuilder who has been training since she was 18. She started menstruating when she was 13, but several months after she began serious training for bodybuilding competitions, she stopped menstruating. _____ _____ .

4. Jan competes on her university's swimming team, swimming several hours each day and working out intensely in the off-season. Although she does menstruate, she does so infrequently, only a few times a year. _____

5. List the six possible causes of oligomenorrhea and secondary amenorrhea given in *Physiology of Sport and Exercise.*

   _____   _____

   _____   _____

   _____   _____

6. According to *Physiology of Sport and Exercise,* which of these seems the most plausible cause of menstrual dysfunction? _____

Activity 18.4

Pregnancy and Exercise

Do this activity after reading pages 592-595 of *Physiology of Sport and Exercise.*

Many women wonder whether they should exercise during pregnancy, and how much exercise is safe. What are the risks to the baby? Are there any risks for the mother? Not all of the research is conclusive, but it is clear that exercise provides many benefits during pregnancy. Read pages 592 to 595 of *Physiology of Sport and Exercise,* and then, without looking in your textbook, answer the following questions.

1. Summarize the four main physiological concerns associated with exercise during pregnancy:

   _____   _____

   _____   _____

2.   Following are several exercise choices a woman could make during pregnancy. Put a slash through the circle next to the choices that would be contraindicated (not recommended) or not preferable.

a. Start an intense running program.   O

b. Exercise in cool, not humid environments.   O

c. Avoid liquids before and after exercise.   O

d. Avoid strenuous exercise during the first trimester.   O

e. Exercise when tired.   O

f. Exercise in the supine (flat-on-back) position
   when at all possible.   O

g. Avoid exercise as much as possible while pregnant.   O

h. Obtain medical clearance.   O

i. Try not to take rest breaks while exercising.   O

Activity 18.5   # Osteoporosis

Do this activity after reading pages 595-597 of *Physiology of Sport and Exercise.*

Osteoporosis is characterized by decreased bone mineral content, which causes increased bone porosity. Do a search online to find illustrations and further information about osteoporosis. You might find some of the Web sites listed here interesting. Then answer the questions that follow.

http://www.courses.washington.edu/bonephys/opgallery.html (Click on the photo of "Osteoporosis" and the movie of "Estrogen Deficiency.")

http://www.osteoporosis_centre.org/oc_thin.htm (Illustrations of normal bone and loss of spinal trabecular bone)

http://www.nof.org/ (The National Osteoporosis Foundation)

http://www.effo.org/real_index.html (The International Osteoporosis Foundation)

http://www.osteo.org/osteo.html

http://www.endocrineweb.com/osteoporsis/

1. Define osteoporosis.

2. What is the major health risk of someone with osteoporosis?

3. At what point in a woman's life does the occurrence of osteoporosis become more likely?

4. What are the three major contributing factors common to postmenopausal women?

5. In addition to postmenopausal women, what other women are at great risk for osteoporosis?

6. Although there is not sufficient data to draw firm conclusions about the effects of exercise and amenorrhea on osteoporosis, what three actions can women take to preserve healthy bones?

Activity 18.6

Eating Disorders and Disordered Eating

Do this activity after reading pages 597-600 of *Physiology of Sport and Exercise.*

Although both men and women suffer from eating disorders, these disorders are much more prevalent in women. Read pages 597 to 600 of *Physiology of Sport and Exercise,* and then test your knowledge of eating disorders and disordered eating by completing this activity.

After each description, fill in the blank with the disorder the description best describes. Your choices include anorexia nervosa, bulimia nervosa, and disordered eating.

1. Refusal to maintain body weight over a minimally normal weight for age and height, with body weight maintained 15% below that expected. _____

2. Binge eating combined with compensatory behaviors (use of laxatives, self-induced vomiting, or excessive exercise in order to prevent weight gain) twice a week for 3 months. _____

3. Binge eating and compensating for it with laxatives or vomiting once every 3 or 4 weeks. _____

4. Distorted body image. _____

5. Intense fear of gaining weight or becoming fat, even though 15% underweight.

   _____

6. Eating an amount of food that is definitely larger than most people would eat in a similar period of time in similar circumstances, and a sense of a lack of control over eating during the episode. _____

7. In postmenarchal women, having amenorrhea. _____

8. Failure to make expected weight gain during period of growth, leading to body weight below 5% of that expected. _____

9. Read about the female athlete triad on page 600 of *Physiology of Sport and Exercise,* and then draw a brief flowchart showing the sequence of events in the triad.

Putting It All Together: Sex Differences and the Female Athlete

Activity 18.7

Do this activity after reading chapter 18 of *Physiology of Sport and Exercise*.

You should have learned through studying this chapter that there is no "weaker" sex. Instead, men's and women's bodies were simply designed differently, to perform different and unique functions. Some women are stronger than some men, and some men are stronger than some women. For the most part, the physiological differences that occur are easily explained by the innate and unique design of the male and female bodies. Take a moment to jot down the reasons for these physiological and performance differences and similarities, and note how all of these have rational physiological explanations.

What are the primary reasons for the *differences* between women and men in

1. body composition?
2. strength?
3. cardiovascular responses?
4. respiratory responses?
5. metabolic responses (e.g., $\dot{V}O_2max$)?
6. cold exposure?
7. disposition to osteoporosis?
8. disposition to eating disorders?

What are the primary reasons for the *similarities* between women and men in

9. body composition adaptations to training?
10. neuromuscular adaptations to training?
11. cardiovascular and respiratory adaptations to training?
12. metabolic adaptations to training?
13. responses to exercise in the heat?
14. responses to exercise at altitude?

Sample Test Questions for Chapter 18

Test yourself on your knowledge of this chapter by taking this self-test. Write the correct answers on a separate sheet of paper.

Multiple Choice

1. Which of the following does not contribute to osteoporosis?

   a. estrogen deficiency
   b. inadequate calcium intake
   c. inadequate sodium intake
   d. inadequate physical activity

2. Of the following choices, which is the safest form of exercise during pregnancy?

a. sit-ups
b. jogging
c. jump-roping
d. swimming

3. Inadequate nutrition can lead to menstrual dysfunction because

a. the resulting low body weight triggers changes in the menstrual cycle.
b. the reduced calcium intake disrupts the normal menstrual cycle.
c. the resulting energy deficit leads to reductions in luteinizing hormone pulse frequency.
d. the reduced fiber intake disrupts the normal menstrual cycle.

4. During which phase of the menstrual cycle is women's sports performance the best?

a. the flow phase
b. the proliferative phase
c. the secretory phase
d. There is no evidence that performance is best in any one phase

True-False

5. For the same amount of muscle, there are no differences in strength between the sexes.

6. Some average-sized women have remarkable strength, exceeding that of some average-sized men.

7. The only reason women have less muscle mass than men is because they are more sedentary than men.

8. Women respond to physical training in the same manner as men do.

9. It has been conclusively proven that intense sports training delays menarche.

10. Eating disorders can lead to death from failure of the cardiovascular system.

11. Women are at a distinct disadvantage to men when exercising at altitude.

12. Because women have a lower sweat rate than men, they do not tolerate heat as well.

Fill in the Blank

13. The group of disorders including disordered eating, secondary amenorrhea, and bone mineral disorders has been collectively termed the _____.

14. Refusal to maintain body weight over a minimally normal weight for age and height is characteristic of individuals suffering from _____.

Short Answer

15. Explain how women achieve similar cardiac outputs as comparably trained men for the same rate of work.

16. Explain why women have a slight advantage over men during cold exposure, but are at a disadvantage to men in extreme cold.

Essay

17. Compare and contrast the roles of testosterone and estrogen in leading to sex-related differences in body composition of adult men and women.

18. Explain the role of lipoprotein lipase activity and lypolytic activity in the hips and thighs of women and why these roles make it difficult for women to lose fat from these areas.

Answers to Selected Chapter 18 Activities

18.1 Body Size and Composition

Changes caused by estrogen secretion in women	Changes caused by testosterone secretion in men
Broadening of pelvis	Increased bone formation
Breast development	Larger bones
Increased fat deposition, especially in thighs and hips	Increased muscle mass
Increased growth rate of bone, so that bones in females reach their final length earlier than in males	

1. shorter
2. lighter in total weight
3. lighter in fat-free mass
4. heavier in fat mass
5. higher in relative body fat

18.2 Sex-Related Responses to Acute Exercise and Exercise Training

(See table on pages 311 through top of page 313.)

18.3 Menstrual Dysfunction

1. delayed or later menarche; 2. primary amenorrhea; 3. secondary amenorrhea; 4. oligomenorrhea; 5. prior history of menstrual dysfunction, acute effects of stress, high quantity or intensity of training, low body weight or body fat, inadequate nutrition (energy deficit) and disordered eating, hormonal alterations; 6. energy deficit resulting from inadequate nutrition

Parameter	Women and men *similar* or *same*	Women and men *different*	If different . . . What are differences? What causes differences?
Responses to acute exercise			
Innate quality of muscle and its mechanisms of motor control	X		
Lower-body strength relative to FFM	X		
Lower-body strength relative to body weight		X	The reasons for this are not clear.
Upper-body strength relative to FFM or body weight		X	Women generally have less upper-body strength than men. Women have a higher percentage of their FFM below the waist than men; this implies there is also more muscle there than in the upper body. Women use lower-body muscle mass more than they use their upper-body muscle mass.
Muscle fiber type distribution in same sport or event	X		
Muscle fiber cross-sectional areas and amount of muscle mass		X	Increased testosterone secretion in males causes increased muscle mass in males as compared with females.
HR response for any absolute level of sub-maximal exercise		X	In women, a higher HR compensates for a lower stroke volume.
Stroke volume		X	This is usually lower in women because of smaller hearts and smaller blood volume, both the result of women's smaller body size.
Cardiac output for same absolute submaximal power output	X		
Potential to increase a-$\bar{v}O_2$ diff		X	Potential is lower in women due to lower hemoglobin content, which results in lower arterial oxygen content and reduced muscle oxidative potential.
Breathing frequency at same relative power output	X		
Breathing frequency at same absolute power output		X	Women's smaller body size causes them to work at a higher percentage of $\dot{V}O_2$max than men at the same absolute power output.

(continued)

(continued)

Parameter	Women and men *similar* or *same*	Women and men *different*	If different . . . What are differences? What causes differences?
Responses to acute exercise (continued)			
Tidal volume and ventilatory volume		X	Generally lower in women due to smaller body size than men.
$\dot{V}O_2$max		X	Women's greater sex-specific essential body-fat stores, lower hemoglobin levels, and lower maximal cardiac output reduces the ability to achieve $\dot{V}O_2$max levels as high as men, although considerable overlap between the sexes occurs.
Oxygen consumption ($\dot{V}O_2$) for same absolute power output	X		
Peak blood lactate values in active but untrained individuals		X	Generally lower in women, but the reasons for this are not clear.
Lactate threshold for equally trained individuals when expressed in relative (% $\dot{V}O_2$max) terms	X		
In summary, responses to acute exercise		X	
Responses to exercise training			
Losses in total body mass with training	X		
Losses of fat mass with training	X		
Losses of relative fat with training	X		
Gains in fat-free mass with training		X	Women generally gain much less FFM than men, because of hormonal differences.
Bone and connective tissue adaptations with training	X		
Magnitude of changes in strength with training	X		
Muscle girth (hypertrophy) with training		X	Women generally exhibit less hypertrophy to a given training stimulus than men do, although overlap between the sexes occurs. The differences are likely the result of hormonal differences.
Increases in maximal cardiac output with training	X		

Parameter	Women and men *similar* or *same*	Women and men *different*	If different . . . What are differences? What causes differences?
Responses to exercise training *(continued)* Decreases in HR for any given rate of work with training	X		
Increases in maximal muscle blood flow and muscle capillary density	X		
Relative increases in $\dot{V}O_2$max with cardio-respiratory endurance training	X		
In summary, responses to exercise training	X		
Performance in athletic activities that can be objectively measured by distance and time		X	The gap between the sexes is narrowing, but women are still outperformed by men, especially where high levels of upper body strength are crucial. Despite similarities in responses to training, innate sex-specific differences preclude elite women from performing as well as elite men in the same sport.

18.4   Pregnancy and Exercise

1. fetal hypoxia, fetal hyperthermia, reduced carbohydrate availability, miscarriage
2. a. Ø   f. Ø
   b. O   g. Ø
   c. Ø   h. O
   d. O   i. Ø
   e. Ø

18.5   Osteoporosis

1. Osteoporosis is decreased bone mineral content, which causes increased bone porosity.
2. A person with osteoporosis has a greater risk of suffering from bone fractures.
3. After the onset of menopause.
4. Estrogen deficiency, inadequate calcium intake, and inadequate physical activity.

5. Women with anorexia nervosa and women with amenorrhea.

6. Increase physical activity, ensure adequate calcium intake, and ensure adequate caloric intake.

18.6   Eating Disorders and Disordered Eating

1. anorexia nervosa;   2. bulimia nervosa   3. disordered eating;   4. anorexia nervosa;
5. anorexia nervosa;   6. bulimia nervosa;   7. anorexia nervosa   8. disordered eating
9. disordered eating → secondary amenorrhea → bone mineral disorders

18.7   Putting It All Together: Sex Differences and the Female Athlete

1. Differences between men's and women's body compositions is primarily due to hormonal differences—that is, the different effects of testosterone in men and estrogen in women.

2. Women possess smaller muscle fiber cross-sectional areas and typically less muscle mass than men.

3. Women typically have smaller hearts and less blood volume.

4. Respiratory responses are different because of women's smaller body size.

5. Differences in metabolic responses are generally related to women's greater essential body-fat stores, and to a lesser extent, their lower hemoglobin levels, which result in a lower oxygen content of the arterial blood.

6. Women have more subcutaneous fat and are therefore at a slight advantage over men during cold exposure; however, their smaller muscle mass is a disadvantage in extreme cold, because shivering is the major adaptation for generating body heat.

7. After menopause, many women experience estrogen deficiency, inadequate calcium intake, and inadequate physical activity. Men experience osteoporosis less than women as a result of a slower rate of bone mineral loss.

8. Females are more likely to experience an eating disorder, probably from social/cultural/media pressures; and female athletes are even more prone to experience an eating disorder, perhaps because the female athlete often matches the profile of the female at high risk for eating disorders and because of pressures on athletes to keep weight down for certain sports.

9. The magnitude of the change in body composition is related more to the total energy expenditure than to the participant's sex.

10. Gains in muscle strength usually occur because of neural factors rather than because of hypertrophy.

11. Women experience the same relative increases in $\dot{V}O_2$max that men experience with endurance training.

12. Increases in $\dot{V}O_2$max that accompany training are primarily due to increased maximal muscle blood flow and muscle capillary density, and these adaptations are not sex specific.

13. Women and men acclimatize to the heat in similar ways—the internal temperature at which sweating and vasodilation begin is similarly lowered in women and men, and the sensitivity of the sweating response increases by a similar amount in both sexes following both physical training and heat acclimatization.

14. Studies report no difference between men's and women's responses to maximal exercise at altitude.

Answers to Selected Chapter 18 Test Questions

Multiple Choice

1. c;   2. d;   3. c;   4. d

True-False

5. True   6. True;   7. False;   8. True;   9. False;   10. True;   11. False;   12. False

Fill in the Blank

13. female athlete triad

14. anorexia nervosa

Short Answer and Essay

For questions 15 to 18, check your answers against the explanations given in the textbook.

Prescription of Exercise for Health and Fitness

concepts

- Physical activity is vital to your body's health.

- Before beginning any exercise program, men over age 40, women over age 50, and anyone who is considered to be at high risk for coronary artery disease or cardiopulmonary disease should have a complete medical evaluation.

- The four basic factors in an exercise prescription are exercise mode, frequency, duration, and intensity. A minimum threshold for the last three factors must be met to attain any aerobic benefits.

- Exercise intensity can be monitored on the basis of training heart rate, metabolic equivalent, or rating of perceived exertion.

- The exercise prescription is integrated into a total exercise program, which includes a warm-up, endurance training, a cool-down, flexibility training, resistance training, and recreational activities.

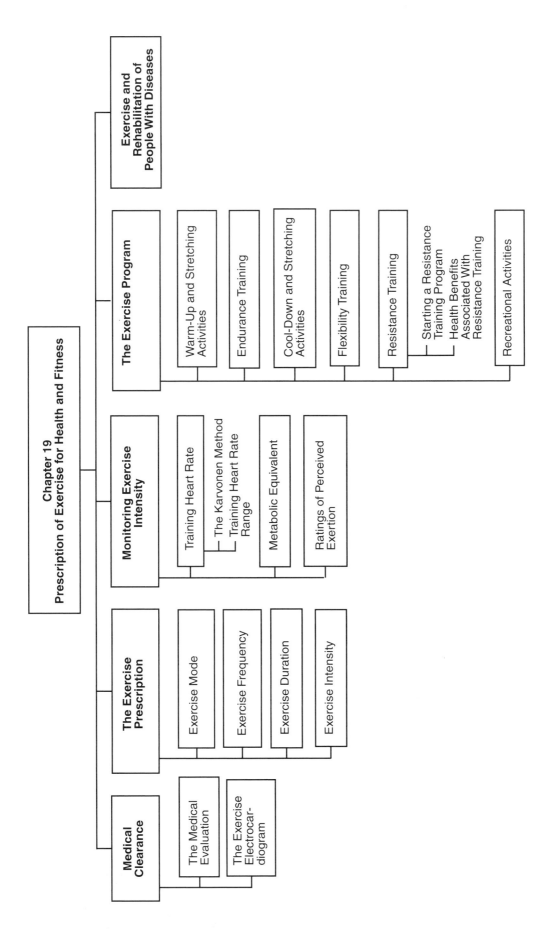

Identifying Individuals Who Need Medical Clearance

Activity 19.1

Do this activity after reading pages 610-613 of *Physiology of Sport and Exercise*.

Although a medical evaluation is useful and desirable before prescribing exercise, it is not practical or necessary to require this for all people who want to start an exercise program. However, some people are at a higher risk than others for medical complications and should meet with a physician to assess their general health and to discuss any medical contraindications to the proposed activity. Pages 612 to 613 of your text provide guidelines for assessing who should have a complete medical examination prior to embarking on an exercise program.

Read each of the situations below and write "yes" in the blank if the person should undergo a medical evaluation prior to starting an exercise program and "no" if a medical evaluation is not necessary.

Yes/No

_____ 1. Cheryl, 34 years old, is an avid runner and softball player who wants to take up roller-blading. She has no risk factors for coronary artery disease and no symptoms or signs of cardiopulmonary disease.

_____ 2. Rhonda is 29 years old and fairly active. Although her mother died suddenly of a heart attack at 64, Rhonda has no other risk factors for coronary artery disease. She has no symptoms or signs suggestive of cardiopulmonary disease.

_____ 3. Harry is 46 years old and in very good health. He has no risk factors for coronary artery disease and no symptoms or signs of cardiopulmonary disease.

_____ 4. Dan is 55 years old and would like to start bicycling on a regular basis with his wife. He has smoked since he was in high school. When he was 40, Dan was diagnosed with hypertension and is on medication to control his blood pressure. Lately, he has noticed that climbing a short set of steps or even walking his dog at a casual pace makes him out of breath.

_____ 5. Martha is 63 years old and wants to start fitness walking in the mall every morning with her friends. She really has not exercised much since her college years, when she enjoyed intramural sports. Martha spends her days reading and visiting on the phone with her friends. She thinks the daily exercise will do her some good.

The Exercise Electrocardiogram

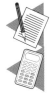

Activity 19.2

Do this activity after reading pages 613-616 of *Physiology of Sport and Exercise*.

The exercise electrocardiogram is an extremely important part of the medical evaluation; a small, but significant, percentage of the adult population have abnormalities in ECGs taken during or following exercise, even though they have normal resting ECGs. These abnormalities often indicate the presence of coronary artery disease.

Definitions

Match the definitions with the terms that are important in understanding exercise ECGs:

_____ 1. Exercise electrocardiogram (ECG)

_____ 2. Graded exercise test (GXT)

_____ 3. Sensitivity

_____ 4. Specificity

_____ 5. Predictive value of an abnormal exercise test

a. A test's ability to correctly identify subjects who fit the criteria being tested (in this case, subjects who have coronary artery disease).

b. The accuracy with which abnormal test results reflect presence of a disease.

c. A test in which the rate of work is increased progressively until the maximal rate of work is achieved.

d. A recording of the heart's electrical activity during exercise; this test can detect undiagnosed coronary artery disease and other cardiac abnormalities.

e. A test's ability to correctly identify subjects who do not fit the criteria being tested (in this case, subjects who do not have coronary artery disease).

Test Accuracy

Without looking in your textbook, fill in the blanks with the correct percentages:

6. Past studies show that exercise ECG sensitivity averages from ____% to _____%, indicating that between _____% and _____% of those with coronary artery disease are correctly identified by exercise ECGs as having the disease.

7. This means that _____% to _____% of those with the disease are incorrectly diagnosed as disease free based on exercise ECGs.

8. Average specificity values range from _____% to _____%, indicating that _____% to _____% of those without disease are correctly identified as disease free.

9. This means that _____% to _____% of the population is incorrectly identified as having the disease.

10. The predictive value of an abnormal exercise test is generally _____ (low or high?) in a population with a low prevalence of coronary artery disease, but it is quite _____ (low or high?) in a population with a high prevalence of coronary artery disease.

Calculating Sensitivity, Specificity, and Predictive Value

Given the following data, calculate the sensitivity, specificity, and predictive value of exercise stress testing for this group:

Total positive tests = 12   Total negative tests = 58

True positive = 9   True negative = 50

False positive = 3   False negative = 8

Write your answers here:

11. Sensitivity: _____

12. Specificity: _____

13. Predictive value: _____

Activity 19.3

Exercise Prescription

Do this activity after reading pages 617-620 of *Physiology of Sport and Exercise.*

An exercise prescription involves individualizing exercise mode, frequency, duration, and intensity in order to reach a specific goal. Answer the following questions without looking in the textbook.

Jared runs for 30 min 3 days a week at 60% $\dot{V}O_2$max. What is Jared's

1. mode of exercise? _____

2. frequency of participation? _____

3. duration of each exercise bout? _____

4. intensity of each exercise bout? _____

Assuming the goal is to improve aerobic capacity and an individual has reached the minimum threshold, what is the optimal

5. frequency of exercise participation? _____

6. duration of exercise? _____

7. intensity of the exercise bout? _____

Activity 19.4

Monitoring Exercise Intensity

Do this activity after reading pages 620-624 of *Physiology of Sport and Exercise.*

The intensity of the exercise bout appears to be the most important factor in attaining aerobic fitness. After a person has decided what type of exercise to do (mode), how often to exercise (frequency), how long each exercise bout should be (duration), and how intensely he or she should exercise, the key is monitoring exercise intensity. Several methods have been proposed for doing this. Let us take a look at each of them.

Training Heart Rate

1. Use the formulas on page 621 of *Physiology of Sport and Exercise,* illustrating the Karvonen method, to calculate your own training heart rate (THR) range of 50% to 74% of your maximal heart rate reserve.

    a. Estimate your maximum heart rate (HRmax). Recall that this is 220 – your age: _____

    b. Take your resting heart rate (HRrest). Recall from chapter 7 that your HRrest should be taken under conditions of total relaxation, such as early in the morning before rising from a restful night's sleep. _____

    c. Now fill in these two formulas to find your training heart rate range:

    $THR_{50\%}$ = HRrest + 0.50 (HRmax – HRrest)

$$THR_{74\%} = HRrest + 0.74 (HRmax - HRrest)$$

d. My training heart rate range for 50% to 74% of my maximal heart rate reserve (HRmax reserve) is _____.

Metabolic Equivalent

2. Define *metabolic equivalent (MET)*, including the metabolic rate that one MET equals:

3. Using table 19.5 on page 622 of *Physiology of Sport and Exercise*, calculate how much oxygen your body has used in the last hour.

   a. Total METs expended in last hour: _____

   b. Amount of oxygen used (multiply total number of METs by 3.5): _____ mL O_2 · kg^{-1} · min^{-1}

Ratings of Perceived Exertion

4. Look over Borg's ratings of perceived exertion in table 19.6 on page 623 of *Physiology of Sport and Exercise*.

   a. Take a break from studying and do an aerobic endurance exercise of some sort (e.g., walking, running, cycling, hiking, swimming). Increase your exertion until you believe you are working "somewhat hard"—at the 12 to 13 range of Borg's rating of perceived exertion.

   b. While you are working at the 12 to 13 level of perceived exertion, take your heart rate. Is your heart rate within your training heart rate (THR) range as calculated earlier in this activity? If your heart rate is above your estimated THR range, decrease your exercise intensity; you might be working too hard. But if your heart rate has not quite reached your estimated THR range, increase your intensity a bit to see if you can exercise within your THR.

> **Activity 19.5**

Benefits of the Total Exercise Program

Do this activity after reading pages 624-629 of *Physiology of Sport and Exercise*.

Once the exercise prescription has been determined, it is integrated into a total exercise program, which consists of a warm-up and stretching activities, endurance training, a cool-down and stretching activities, flexibility training, resistance training, and recreational activities. Each of these portions of the program benefits the participant in unique and specific ways.

On a separate sheet of paper, list the benefits of each portion of the total exercise program:

- Warm-up and stretching activities
- Endurance training
- Cool-down and stretching activities
- Flexibility training
- Resistance training
- Recreational activities

Putting It All Together: Prescription of Exercise for Health and Fitness
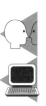

> **Activity 19.6**

Do this activity after reading chapter 19 of *Physiology of Sport and Exercise*.

Throughout this chapter, we have emphasized how important physical activity is to your general health. This closing activity will give you the opportunity to apply what you have learned to your own situation. Write your plans and responses on a separate sheet of paper.

1. Having read pages 612 to 616 of *Physiology of Sport and Exercise*, should you seek medical clearance, perhaps including an exercise ECG, prior to participating in an exercise program? You can also go to **http://www.phys.com/f_fitness/ 01self_analysis/05assess/assess.html** and take this risk assessment test to find out if it is safe for you to exercise without a doctor's approval.

2. Create an exercise prescription for yourself. Choose your desired mode of exercise (see page 617), and a frequency, duration, and intensity that match the recommendations in the text as well as ensure that you are exceeding your minimum threshold. Write down your plans.

3. How will you monitor your exercise intensity? At what intensity will you try to exercise? See your responses in activity 19.4 for guidance.

4. Now map out an entire exercise program for yourself, incorporating your exercise prescription from number 2 into the "endurance training" portion of the program.

See pages 624 to 629 of *Physiology of Sport and Exercise* for guidelines. Write down both the types of activities and the frequency with which you will do them for each portion of the program:

Warm-up and stretching activities

Frequency

Activities

Endurance training

Incorporate your exercise prescription here.

Cool-down and stretching activities

Frequency

Activities

Flexibility training

Frequency

Activities

Resistance training

Frequency

Activities

Recreational activities

Frequency

Activities

Now all that is left to do is to carry out the program! If you do so, you will be well on your way to a lifetime of physical fitness and good health.

Sample Test Questions for Chapter 19

Test yourself on your knowledge of this chapter by taking this self-test. Write the correct answers on a separate sheet of paper.

Multiple Choice

1. People with hypertension should be cautioned to avoid

   a. bicycling;   b. running;   c. activities that use isometric actions;   d. all resistance-training activities

2. Which of the following best describes test sensitivity?

   a. The test's ability to correctly identify people who do not have the disease
   b. The test's ability to correctly identify people with a given disease
   c. The accuracy with which abnormal test results reflect presence of the disease
   d. The accuracy with which normal test results reflect lack of presence of the disease

3. Which of the following is *not* one of the basic factors of exercise prescription?

   a. duration;   b. intensity;   c. mode;   d. gender

4. Which of the following would *not* be a recommended guideline for starting a resistance training program?

   a. Start with a weight that is exactly one half of your maximal strength.
   b. When a given weight brings you to fatigue by the 8th or 10th repetition in your first set, this is your appropriate starting weight.
   c. Perform three to four sets of each lift per day, 5 to 7 days per week.
   d. When you reach 15 repetitions on the first set, you are ready to progress to the next higher weight.

True-False

5. During the "fitness boom" of the 1970s and 1980s, the majority of American adults exercised at levels that would increase or maintain their aerobic fitness.

6. A medical evaluation before prescribing exercise for a population presumed healthy has been proven to reduce the medical risks associated with exercise.

7. A negative exercise test implies that no disease was detected, but a positive exercise test implies that disease was detected.

8. Exercise ECGs are 100% accurate.

9. Recommendations for minimum thresholds of frequency, duration, and intensity are the same for all exercisers.

10. A man over age 45 with non-insulin-dependent diabetes mellitus should have a complete medical examination prior to embarking on an exercise program.

Fill in the Blank

11. A test in which the rate of work is increased progressively until the maximal rate of work is achieved is called a _____.

12. The _____ of the exercise bout appears to be the most important factor in improving aerobic conditioning.

Short Answer

13. Who is at high risk and in need of medical clearance prior to starting an exercise program?

14. Why is an exercise ECG an important part of the medical evaluation?

15. Why is the metabolic equivalent (MET) system not as useful for a guideline for training as are ratings of perceived exertion and the Karvonen method?

Essay

16. Why is a medical evaluation prior to starting an exercise program useful and important? Provide at least four reasons.

17. Why is exercise testing of limited value in screening young, apparently healthy individuals before prescribing exercise to them? Provide at least three reasons.

Answers to Selected Chapter 19 Activities

19.1   Identifying Individuals Who Need Medical Clearance

1. No. Cheryl is in no high-risk categories.

2. No. Rhonda is below the age cutoff and has only one positive risk factor for coronary artery disease.

3. Yes. Harry is over age 40.

4. Yes. Dan is above the age cutoff, and even though he has only one risk factor (smoking) for coronary artery disease, he has one major symptom (shortness of breath) suggestive of cardiopulmonary disease. Dan should definitely see a doctor, even if he does not plan to start an exercise program.

5. Yes. Martha has two risk factors for coronary artery disease: She is over age 55 and she is likely part of the least active 25% of the population. Her desire for exercise is commendable, but she should have a thorough physical examination before embarking on such a program.

19.2   The Exercise Electrocardiogram

1. d;   2. c;   3. a;   4. e;   5. b

6. 50, 80, 50, 80;   **7.** 20, 50;   **8.** 80, 90, 80, 90;   **9.** 10, 20;   **10.** low, high

11. Sensitivity [SN] = [TP/(TP + FN)] $\times$ 100% = [9/(9 + 8)] $\times$ 100% = 0.5294 $\times$ 100% = 52.9%

12. Specificity [SP] = [TN/(FP + TN)] $\times$ 100% = [50/(3 + 50)] $\times$ 100% = 0.9433 $\times$ 100% = 94.3%

13. Predictive Value [PV] = [TP/(TP + FP)] $\times$ 100% = [9/(9 + 3)] $\times$ 100% = 0.75 $\times$ 100% = 75.0%

19.3   Exercise Prescription

1. running;   **2.** 3 days a week;   **3.** 30 min;   **4.** 60% $\dot{V}O_2$max;   **5.** 3 to 5 days a week;   **6.** 20 to 30 min per day;   **7.** at least 60% $\dot{V}O_2$max

19.4   Monitoring Exercise Intensity

1. Answers will vary.

2. A metabolic equivalent is a unit used to estimate the metabolic cost (oxygen consumption) of physical activity. One MET equals the resting metabolic rate of approximately 3.5 mL $O_2 \cdot kg^{-1} \cdot min^{-1}$.

3. Answers will vary.

4. Answers will vary.

19.5   Benefits of the Total Exercise Program

See pages 624 to 629 of *Physiology of Sport and Exercise* for answers to this activity.

Answers to Selected Chapter 19 Test Questions

Multiple Choice

1. c   2. b;   3. d;   4. c

True-False

5. False;   6. False;   7. True;   8. False;   9. False;   10. True

Fill in the Blank

11. graded exercise test; 12. intensity

Short Answer and Essay

For questions 13 to 17, check your answers against the explanations given in the textbook.

Cardiovascular Disease and Physical Activity

concepts

- Cardiovascular diseases—including coronary artery disease, hypertension, stroke, and congestive heart failure—are the number one cause of death in the United States, accounting for more than two out of every five deaths.

- Atherosclerosis begins in childhood and progresses at different rates, depending primarily on heredity and lifestyle choices.

- More than 90% of people with hypertension have idiopathic hypertension, meaning its cause is unknown.

- There are both alterable and unalterable risk factors for coronary artery disease and hypertension. Physical inactivity is a risk factor for both, and one that individuals can easily alter.

- Physical inactivity doubles the risk of having a fatal heart attack.

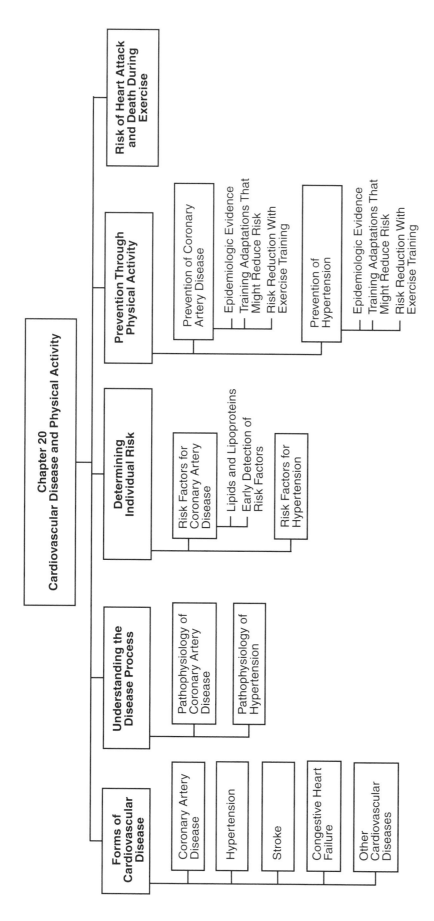

Chapter 20
Cardiovascular Disease and Physical Activity

Forms of Cardiovascular Disease
- Coronary Artery Disease
- Hypertension
- Stroke
- Congestive Heart Failure
- Other Cardiovascular Diseases

Understanding the Disease Process
- Pathophysiology of Coronary Artery Disease
- Pathophysiology of Hypertension

Determining Individual Risk
- Risk Factors for Coronary Artery Disease
  - Lipids and Lipoproteins
  - Early Detection of Risk Factors
- Risk Factors for Hypertension

Prevention Through Physical Activity
- Prevention of Coronary Artery Disease
  - Epidemiologic Evidence
  - Training Adaptations That Might Reduce Risk
  - Risk Reduction With Exercise Training
- Prevention of Hypertension
  - Epidemiologic Evidence
  - Training Adaptations That Might Reduce Risk
  - Risk Reduction With Exercise Training

Risk of Heart Attack and Death During Exercise

Activity 20.1

Extent of Cardiovascular Disease

Do this activity after reading pages 635-637 of *Physiology of Sport and Exercise.*

Cardiovascular diseases are the major cause of serious illness and death in the United States. You probably know someone who has suffered a heart attack or a stroke, has had heart surgery of some sort, or has high blood pressure. To see how pervasive these illnesses are in our society, add bars to the graph below to illustrate the correct data for each category.

Note that United States data is provided in *Physiology of Sport and Exercise* and can be filled in on the graph below. If you live in a country other than the United States, see if you can find data for your nation. If this is not possible, simply use the United States data from the textbook.

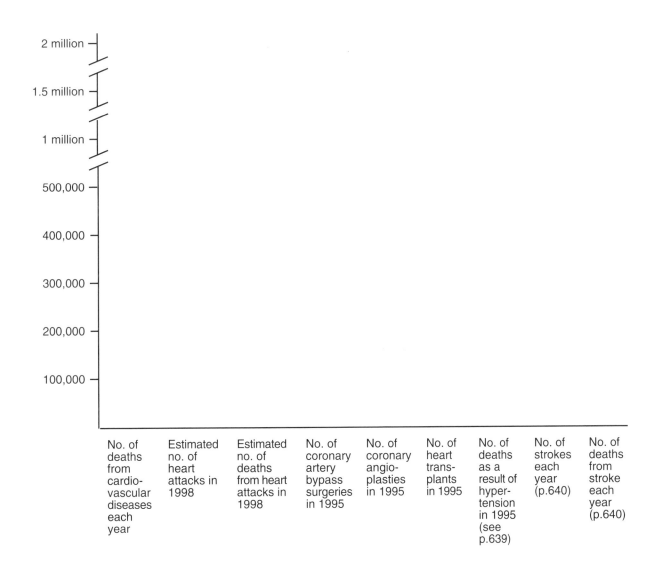

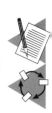

Activity 20.2

Forms of Cardiovascular Disease

Do this activity after reading pages 638-642 of _Physiology of Sport and Exercise._

In this activity, we focus on learning basic terminology surrounding the major cardiovascular diseases and on seeing how these diseases lead to illness and death.

Match each term in the left column below with its correct definition by writing the letter of the corresponding definition in the blank.

Term

_____ 1. Coronary artery disease

_____ 2. Plaque

_____ 3. Atherosclerosis

_____ 4. Ischemia

_____ 5. Myocardial infarction

_____ 6. Fatty streaks

_____ 7. Hypertension

_____ 8. Diastolic blood pressure

_____ 9. Systolic blood pressure

_____ 10. Stroke

_____ 11. Cerebral infarction

_____ 12. Congestive heart failure

_____ 13. Peripheral vascular diseases

_____ 14. Arteriosclerosis

_____ 15. Valvular heart diseases

_____ 16. Rheumatic heart disease

_____ 17. Congenital heart disease

Definition

a. Death of heart tissue that results from insufficient blood supply to part of the myocardium, commonly called a heart attack.

b. A condition that involves loss of elasticity, thickening, and hardening of the arteries.

c. A clinical condition in which the myocardium becomes too weak to maintain adequate cardiac output to meet the body's oxygen demands.

d. Progressive narrowing of the coronary arteries.

e. The lowest arterial pressure, resulting from ventricular diastole (the resting phase).

f. A form of valvular heart disease involving a streptococcal infection that has caused acute rheumatic fever, typically in children between ages 5 and 15.

g. A form of arteriosclerosis that involves changes in the lining of the arteries and plaque accumulation, leading to progressive narrowing of the arteries.

h. The greatest arterial blood pressure, resulting from systole (the contracting phase of the heart).

i. A heart defect present at birth that occurs from abnormal prenatal development of the heart and associated blood vessels.

j. A buildup of lipids, smooth muscle cells, connective tissue, and debris that forms at the site of injury to an artery.

k. Death of brain tissue that results from insufficient blood supply due to blockage or damage of a cerebral vessel.

l. Diseases of the systemic arteries and veins, especially those to the extremities, that impede adequate blood flow.

m. Early lipid deposits within blood vessels.

n. Diseases involving one or more of the heart valves.

o. A temporary deficiency of blood to a specific area of the body.

p. A cerebral vascular accident, a condition in which blood supply to some part of the brain is impaired, so that the tissue is damaged; typically due to infarction or hemorrhage.

q. Abnormally high blood pressure.

Coronary Artery Disease

After reading pages 638 to 639 of *Physiology of Sport and Exercise*, draw a flowchart (on a separate piece of paper) depicting the sequence of events that lead to myocardial infarction via coronary artery disease. Begin with fatty streaks in childhood, and progress through atherosclerosis to myocardial infarction.

Hypertension

After reading page 639 of *Physiology of Sport and Exercise*, draw a flowchart depicting the sequence of events that lead to heart attack, heart failure, stroke, and kidney failure via hypertension.

Stroke

There are two main causes of strokes—cerebral infarction and hemorrhage. List and explain the three ways that cerebral infarction occurs:

List and explain the two types of hemorrhage that can cause a stroke:

Congestive Heart Failure

After reading page 641 of *Physiology of Sport and Exercise*, draw a flowchart depicting the sequence of events that lead to the need for a heart transplant via congestive heart failure. Begin with the events that can damage the heart, and progress through resulting symptoms to the point of irreversible heart damage.

| Activity 20.3 | # Pathophysiology of Cardiovascular Disease |

Do this activity after reading pages 642-644 of *Physiology of Sport and Exercise.*

Understanding the pathophysiology of a disease—that is, the physiology of a specific disease process—gives us insight into how physical activity might alter the disease process. Complete this activity to learn more about the pathophysiology of coronary artery disease and hypertension.

Coronary Artery Disease

1. Without looking in *Physiology of Sport and Exercise*, write in the correct labels for the figure located on the next page.

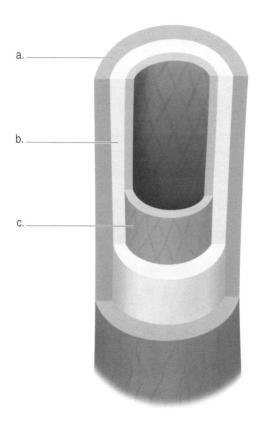

2. Two hypotheses exist for how atherosclerosis develops in the coronary arteries: the arterial injury hypothesis and the lipid-infiltration hypothesis. The lipid-infiltration hypothesis is quite complex and beyond the scope of this course. Jot notes here showing the sequence of events underlying the arterial injury hypothesis:

Hypertension

3. The pathophysiology of hypertension is not well understood. In fact, more than 90% of people with hypertension have idiopathic hypertension, meaning its cause is unknown. List the six possible causes of hypertension mentioned in *Physiology of Sport and Exercise*:

a. _____   d. _____

b. _____   e. _____

c. _____   f. _____

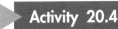

Determining Individual Risk for Cardiovascular Disease

Do this activity after reading pages 645-649 of *Physiology of Sport and Exercise.*

Determining our risk for cardiovascular disease is of great interest to many people, because if we can lessen our risk, we can prevent death due to this disease. In this activity, we will look closely at the risk factors for coronary artery disease and hypertension.

Coronary Artery Disease

Match each term with its correct definition by writing the letter of the corresponding definition in the blank.

Terms

_____ 1. Primary risk factors

_____ 2. Blood lipids

_____ 3. Triglycerides

_____ 4. Lipoproteins

_____ 5. Low-density-lipoprotein cholesterol (LDL-C)

_____ 6. High-density-lipoprotein cholesterol (HDL-C)

_____ 7. Very-low-density-lipoprotein cholesterol (VLDL-C)

Definitions

a. The body's most concentrated energy source and the form in which most fats are stored in the body.

b. The cholesterol carried by the cholesterol carrier that is regarded as a scavenger and is theorized to remove cholesterol from the arterial wall and transport it to the liver to be metabolized.

c. The cholesterol carried by very-low-density lipoproteins in the blood from the small intestines or liver to adipose tissue or muscle for storage.

d. The cholesterol carried by the cholesterol carrier that is theorized to be responsible for depositing cholesterol in the arterial wall.

e. Risk factors that have been conclusively shown to have a strong association with a certain disease.

f. The proteins that carry the blood lipids.

g. Blood-borne fats, such as triglycerides and cholesterol.

After reading page 645 of *Physiology of Sport and Exercise,* see how many risk factors of coronary artery disease you can remember. Write them in the spaces provided below.

Alterable primary risk factors	Alterable secondary risk factors	Unalterable secondary risk factors
8. _____	12. _____	14. _____
9. _____	13. _____	15. _____
10. _____		16. _____
11. _____		

17. The ratio of Total-C to HDL-C may be the best index of risk for coronary artery disease. If Subject A has a Total-C of 180 mg/dl and an HDL-C of 30 mg/dl, what is Subject A's Total-C to HDL-C ratio?

18. If Subject B has a Total-C of 220 mg/dl and an HDL-C of 80 mg/dl, what is Subject B's Total-C to HDL-C ratio?

19. Based only on this ratio, which subject is at lower risk for coronary artery disease?

Hypertension

After reading page 648 of *Physiology of Sport and Exercise,* see how many risk factors of hypertension you can remember. Write them in the spaces provided below.

Alterable risk factors:

20. _____

21. _____

22. _____

23. _____

24. _____

Unalterable risk factors:

25. _____

26. _____

27. _____

The Role of Physical Activity in Preventing Cardiovascular Disease

Activity 20.5

Do this activity after reading pages 650-656 of *Physiology of Sport and Exercise.*

How much does physical activity reduce the risk of coronary artery disease? Furthermore, how much physical activity does it take to reduce the risk of cardiovascular disease? And what physiological adaptations from physical activity cause these risk reductions? Researchers have been studying these issues for several decades. Complete this activity to discover their findings.

Coronary Artery Disease

1. How much more likely are those who are occupationally sedentary (not physically active at work) to die from coronary artery disease than those who are occupationally active?

2. How much more likely are those who are inactive in leisure-time pursuits to die from coronary artery disease than those who are active in their leisure?

3. What level of physical activity or fitness is necessary to reduce one's risk of coronary artery disease?

4. Skim through pages 651 to 653 of *Physiology of Sport and Exercise,* and list all of the ways in which physical activity might help to prevent coronary artery disease. Include training adaptations that might reduce the risk, as well as changes in risk factors that result from exercise training.

Hypertension

5. How do the blood pressures of more active people compare to those of less active people?

6. In the follow-up study from Cooper Clinic, how much more likely were people with low fitness levels to develop hypertension than those who were highly fit?

7. Skim page 655 of *Physiology of Sport and Exercise*, and list all of the ways in which physical activity might help to prevent hypertension. Include training adaptations that might reduce the risk, as well as changes in risk factors that result from exercise training.

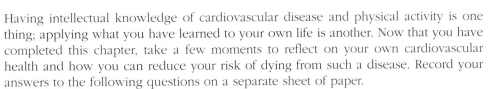

Putting It All Together: Cardiovascular Disease and Physical Activity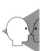

Activity 20.6

Do this activity after reading chapter 20 of *Physiology of Sport and Exercise.*

Having intellectual knowledge of cardiovascular disease and physical activity is one thing; applying what you have learned to your own life is another. Now that you have completed this chapter, take a few moments to reflect on your own cardiovascular health and how you can reduce your risk of dying from such a disease. Record your answers to the following questions on a separate sheet of paper.

1. Look back at activity 20.4. What risk factors do you have for coronary artery disease?

2. In the above list, circle the coronary risk factors that you can alter.

3. What are the possible consequences of not altering these risk factors?

4. Look back at activity 20.4. What risk factors do you have for hypertension?

5. In the above list, circle the hypertension risk factors that you can alter.

6. What are the possible consequences of not altering these risk factors?

7. Create a brief plan of action for altering your coronary artery disease and hypertension risk factors.

Sample Test Questions for Chapter 20

Test yourself on your knowledge of this chapter by taking this self-test. Write the correct answers on a separate sheet of paper.

Multiple Choice

1. Which of the following problems is *not* a consequence of congestive heart failure?

   a. edema
   b. shortness of breath
   c. need for a heart transplant
   d. high blood pressure

2. Based only on race and gender, who of the following is most likely to develop coronary artery disease?

   a. African American female
   b. Hispanic female
   c. African American male
   d. White male

3. Based only on information provided here, who of the following is most likely to develop coronary artery disease?

   a. A female executive who has mild hypertension and no family history of coronary artery disease.
   b. A male farmer who drinks occasionally and plays golf two times a week.
   c. A female computer programmer who smokes and whose mother died of cancer at age 55.
   d. A male computer programmer who smokes and whose father died of a heart attack at age 49.

4. Which of the following is *not* a training adaptation that might reduce the risk of coronary artery disease?

   a. decreased stroke volume
   b. hypertrophy of the heart
   c. increased coronary circulation capacity
   d. improved collateral circulation of the heart

True-False

5. Physical inactivity has not been established as a primary risk factor for coronary artery disease.

6. Atherosclerosis begins in childhood.

7. Varicose veins result from high blood pressure.

8. The process of atherosclerosis appears to begin with injury to or disruption of the endothelial cells lining the intima.

9. It has been conclusively proven that stress is the major cause of hypertension.

10. There is no increased risk of heart attack during the actual period of exercise.

11. The use of oral contraceptives poses no increased risk of cardiovascular diseases.

12. Most patients with heart disease can safely benefit from exercise.

Fill in the Blank

13. The clinical condition in which the heart muscle becomes too weak to maintain an adequate cardiac output to meet the body's oxygen needs is called

_____.

14. _____ is a process in which arteries become progressively narrower due to changes in the lining of the arteries and plaque accumulation.

Short Answer

15. Explain how insulin resistance might contribute to and interrelate with hypertension, coronary artery disease, upper-body obesity, and type II diabetes.

16. Explain how a person can have moderately high levels of total cholesterol yet be at a relatively low risk of coronary artery disease.

Essay

17. Describe motor and behavioral deficits that can result from a stroke.

18. If plasma volume increases with endurance training, why does this not increase blood pressure?

Answers to Selected Chapter 20 Activities

20.2   Forms of Cardiovascular Disease

1. d;   2. j;   3. g;   4. o;   5. a;   6. m;   7. q;   8. e;   9. h;   10. p;   11. k;   12. c;   13. l;   14. b;   15. n;   16. f;   17. i

18. Cerebral thrombosis—a thrombus (blood clot) forms in a cerebral vessel, often at the site of atherosclerotic damage to the vessel.

19. Cerebral embolism—an embolus (an undissolved mass of material) breaks loose from another site in the body and lodges in a cerebral artery.

20. Atherosclerosis that leads to narrowing of and damage to a cerebral artery.

21. Cerebral hemorrhage—one of the cerebral arteries ruptures in the brain.

22. Subarachnoid hemorrhage—one of the brain's surface vessels ruptures, dumping blood into the space between the brain and the skull.

20.3   Pathophysiology of Cardiovascular Diseases

1. a. Tunica adventitia; b. Tunica media; c. Tunica intima (endothelium)

2. *Arterial injury hypothesis:* scratching of inner lining of a coronary artery causes endothelial cells to slough off, exposing underlying connective tissue; blood platelets are attracted to the injury site and adhere to the exposed connective tissue; the platelets release PDGF, which promotes migration of smooth muscle cells from the media into the intima; a plaque, formed of these smooth muscle cells, connective tissue, and debris, forms at the site of injury; as the plaque grows, it narrows the arterial opening, impeding blood flow; lipids, especially LDL-C are deposited in the plaque.

3. genetic factors, high sodium intake, obesity, insulin resistance, physical inactivity, psychological stress

20.4 Determining Individual Risk for Cardiovascular Disease

1. e; **2.** g; **3.** a; **4.** f; **5.** d **6.** b; **7.** c; **8-11:** smoking, hypertension, unfavorable blood lipids, physical inactivity; **12-13:** obesity, diabetes/hyperinsulinemia; **14-16:** heredity, male gender, advanced age; **17.** 6.0; **18.** 2.75; **19.** Subject B; **20-24:** insulin resistance, obesity, diet/sodium intake, use of oral contraceptives, physical inactivity; **25-26:** heredity, advanced age, race

20.5 The Role of Physical Activity in Preventing Cardiovascular Disease

1. Two times as likely.

2. Two to three times as likely.

3. Low-intensity activity is sufficient to reduce the risk of CAD.

5. More active people have lower systolic and diastolic blood pressures.

6. Less fit people were 1.5 times more likely to develop hypertension than highly fit people.

Answers to Selected Chapter 20 Test Questions

Multiple Choice

1. d;   2. c;   3. d;   4. a

True-False

5. False   6. True;   7. False;   8. True;   9. False;   10. False;   11. False;   12. True

Fill in the Blank

13. congestive heart failure

14. Atherosclerosis

Short Answer and Essay

For questions 15 to 18, check your answers against the explanations given in the textbook.

Obesity, Diabetes, and Physical Activity

concepts

- A sedentary lifestyle has been associated with an increased risk of obesity and type II diabetes.

- Obesity and diabetes are strongly associated with other diseases that have high mortality rates.

- Obesity can be caused by a combination of many factors, including heredity.

- Diabetes is a disorder of carbohydrate metabolism that develops when there is inadequate insulin secretion or utilization.

- Physical activity is important in both weight maintenance and weight loss. It also has many desirable effects for people with diabetes, particularly those with type II diabetes.

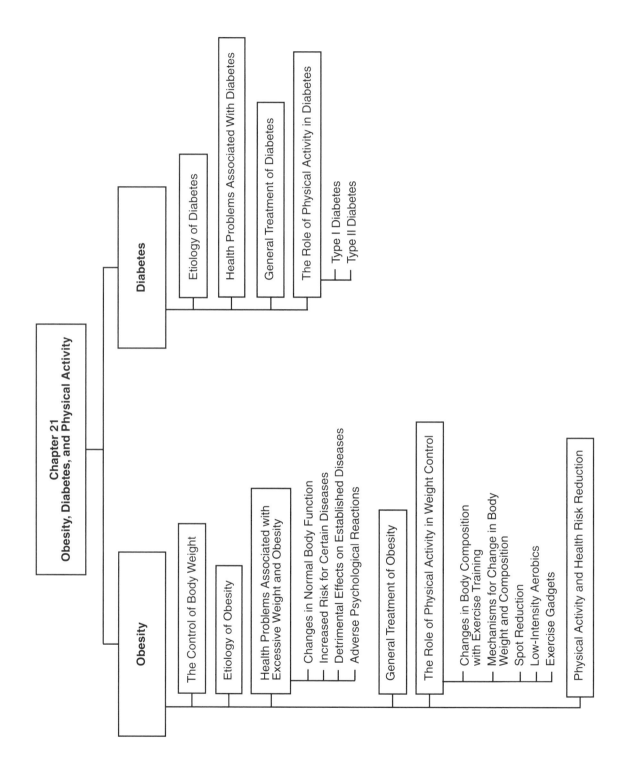

Chapter 21
Obesity, Diabetes, and Physical Activity

Obesity

The Control of Body Weight

Etiology of Obesity

Health Problems Associated with Excessive Weight and Obesity

- Changes in Normal Body Function
- Increased Risk for Certain Diseases
- Detrimental Effects on Established Diseases
- Adverse Psychological Reactions

General Treatment of Obesity

The Role of Physical Activity in Weight Control

- Changes in Body Composition with Exercise Training
- Mechanisms for Change in Body Weight and Composition
- Spot Reduction
- Low-Intensity Aerobics
- Exercise Gadgets

Physical Activity and Health Risk Reduction

Diabetes

Etiology of Diabetes

Health Problems Associated With Diabetes

General Treatment of Diabetes

The Role of Physical Activity in Diabetes

- Type I Diabetes
- Type II Diabetes

Activity 21.1

Defining Obesity-Related Terms

Do this activity after reading pages 664-682 of *Physiology of Sport and Exercise*.

Many terms related to obesity are incorrectly used or used interchangeably. To get off to a good start with this chapter, test yourself by matching the terms with their definitions. In the blank by each term, write the letter of the corresponding definition.

Term

_____ 1. Overweight

_____ 2. Obesity

_____ 3. Relative weight

_____ 4. Body mass index

_____ 5. Resting metabolic rate (RMR)

_____ 6. Thermic effect of a meal (TEM)

_____ 7. Thermic effect of activity (TEA)

_____ 8. Upper-body (android) obesity

_____ 9. Lower-body (gynoid) obesity

_____ 10. Excess postexercise oxygen consumption (EPOC)

Definition

a. The body's rate of energy expenditure early in the morning following an overnight fast and 8 h of sleep and prior to any activity.

b. The percentage by which an individual is either overweight or underweight, generally determined by dividing the person's weight by the mean weight for the medium frame category for his or her height (from standard weight tables).

c. Elevated oxygen consumption above resting levels after exercise; at one time referred to as oxygen debt.

d. Obesity that follows the typically male pattern of fat storage, in which fat is stored primarily in the upper body, particularly in the abdomen.

e. Body weight that exceeds the normal or standard weight for a particular individual based on sex, height, and frame size.

f. A measurement of body overweight or obesity determined by dividing weight (in kilograms) by height (in meters) squared. Highly correlated with body composition.

g. The energy expended in excess of the resting metabolic rate to accomplish a given task or activity.

h. Obesity that follows the typically female pattern of fat storage, in which fat is stored primarily in the lower body, particularly in the hips, buttocks, and thighs.

i. An excessive amount of body fat, generally defined as more than 25% in men and more than 35% in women.

j. The increase in the rate of energy expenditure associated with digestion, absorption, transport, metabolism, and storage of ingested food.

Activity 21.2

Controlling Body Weight

Do this activity after reading pages 666-668 of *Physiology of Sport and Exercise*.

Physiology of Sport and Exercise states that the body has the ability to balance energy intake and expenditure to within 10 to 15 kcal per day, about the equivalent of one potato chip! If this is true, why do so many people have trouble controlling their weight? The concepts of daily energy expenditure and the set-point theory may help explain this.

On the next page is a bar graph that shows the possible sum of resting metabolic rate (RMR), the thermic effect of a meal (TEM), and the thermic effect of activity (TEA) for an average-fed, relatively active person. In general, the energy expenditure components adapt to match changes in caloric intake.

1. In the space to the right of the first bar, draw a second bar to illustrate how this person's body might adapt to fasting or a very-low-calorie diet. Assume a 1,000 kcal/day diet with the same percentages of energy expenditure.

2. Draw a third bar to illustrate how the body adapts to overeating. Assume a 3,500 kcal/day diet.

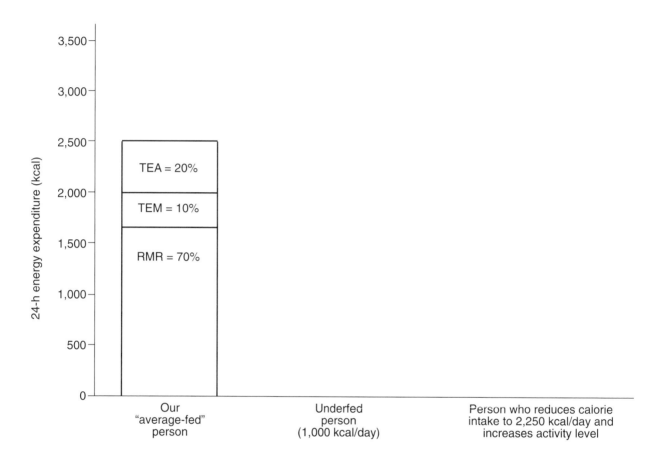

3. If a person consumes more calories than needed (as in your "overfed" bar) for a long period of time, what is the theorized effect on that person's set-point weight?

4. Suppose the person illustrated in the first left-hand bar (the one already drawn for you) restricts her diet to 2,250 kcal/day and increases her daily activity level. Draw a fourth bar on the graph to illustrate the possible ratios of the three components of energy expenditure.

Causes and Health Risks of Obesity

Do this activity after reading pages 668-674 of *Physiology of Sport and Exercise.*

The causes of obesity are quite complex, and the resulting health problems are quite detrimental. Answer the questions below to develop a more complete understanding of the causes and health risks of obesity.

1. It is easy to incorrectly ascribe obesity to laziness or gluttony; on the other hand, it is also easy to incorrectly ascribe obesity to only genetics over which we have no control. The truth for most people is much more complex. Skim through pages 668 and 669 of *Physiology of Sport and Exercise* and list (on a separate sheet of paper) eight possible causes of obesity mentioned in this text.

2. Overweight and obesity are associated with an increased overall rate of death (mortality). Even though overweight and obesity in and of themselves do not cause death, what five diseases associated with overweight and obesity can lead to early death? (See page 672 of *Physiology of Sport and Exercise.*)

3. Draw a brief flowchart depicting the cycle of weight gain that can lead to respiratory problems and severe cardiovascular illnesses. (See pages 672-673 of *Physiology of Sport and Exercise.*)

4. So far we have looked at diseases that obesity can *cause*. But what about its effects on existing diseases? See page 674 of *Physiology of Sport and Exercise*, and list the health problems that generally benefit from weight reduction.

Methods of Estimating Obesity

Do this activity after reading pages 664-674 of *Physiology of Sport and Exercise.*

Because obesity refers to the condition of having an excessive amount of body fat, body composition measures are some of the best ways to assess obesity. Because we studied body composition measures in an earlier chapter, we will concentrate here on measuring obesity using relative weight, body mass index, and waist-to-hip ratio. To complete the following exercises, you will need this data:

Subject A = female, 168 cm (5 ft 6 in.) tall, 66 kg (145 lb), 107 cm (42 in.) waist, 96.5 cm (38 in.) hips

Relative Weight

1. Calculate the relative weight for Subject A.

2. Calculate your own relative weight.

Body Mass Index

3. Calculate the BMI for Subject A.

4. Calculate your own BMI.

Waist-to-Hip Ratio

5. Calculate the waist-to-hip ratio for Subject A.

6. Calculate your waist-to-hip ratio.

Conclusions

7. In summary, what do these measurements tell you about Subject A's level of obesity?

8. In summary, what do these measurements tell you about your own level of obesity?

Physical Activity and Weight Control

Do this activity after reading pages 676-682 of *Physiology of Sport and Exercise*.

Exercise is an essential component in any program of weight reduction or weight control. Skim pages 676 to 682 of *Physiology of Sport and Exercise* and draw an "up arrow" if exercise increases the parameter listed below and a "down arrow" if exercise decreases it.

Parameter	Increase or decrease with exercise? (Use ↑ or ↓)
1. Metabolism rate during exercise	
2. Metabolism rate after exercise ends	
3. Total body weight	
4. Amount of body fat	
5. Amount of fat-free (lean) body mass	
6. Appetite, when exercise is intense enough to increase body temperature	
7. Resting metabolic rate	
8. Thermic effect of a meal preceded or followed by a bout of exercise	
9. Fatty acid mobilization	

Diabetes Mellitus

Do this activity after reading pages 683-687 of *Physiology of Sport and Exercise*.

Diabetes mellitus, often simply called diabetes, affects a sizable portion of the population—15 million people in the United States alone and 25% of the population age 85 and older. People with diabetes have a relatively high mortality rate. Read pages 683 to 687 of *Physiology of Sport and Exercise* and take notes in the table on the next page. Use these notes as a study tool for your class's exam on this topic.

	Insulin-dependent (type I)	Non-insulin-dependent (type II)
Etiology When occurs in life		
Why occurs (causes of)		
Associated health problems		
Treatment		
Role of exercise in treatment		

Putting It All Together: Obesity, Diabetes, and Physical Activity

Activity 21.7

Do this activity after reading chapter 21 of *Physiology of Sport and Exercise.*

Now that you have gained an understanding of obesity and diabetes, it is important to apply what you have learned to your own life. Take a few moments to reflect on your own health and how you can reduce health problems related to these disorders. Write your responses to the following questions on a separate sheet of paper.

1. Look back at Activity 21.4. What do your answers tell you about your own level of overweight or obesity?

2. Look back at Activity 21.3. Which of your answers to 21.3, question 1, might be affecting your own weight?

3. In the above listing, circle the possible causes of obesity that you can alter.

4. What are the possible consequences of not altering these causes?

5. Look back at Activity 21.6. What risk factors do you have for getting type II diabetes? Write them here. (If you have type I diabetes, questions 5, 6, and 7 will not apply to you.)

6. In the above listing, circle the diabetes risk factors that you can alter.

7. What are the possible consequences of not altering these risk factors?

8. Create a brief plan of action for altering your risk of obesity and type II diabetes. Be sure to include physical activity in your plan.

Sample Test Questions for Chapter 21

Test yourself on your knowledge of this chapter by taking this self-test. Write the correct answers on a separate sheet of paper.

Multiple Choice

1. A person desiring to lose 11 kg (24 lb) should attempt to reach this goal no faster than in

   a. 4 to 6 weeks (1 to 1-1/2 months)
   b. 6 to 8 weeks (1-1/2 to 2 months)
   c. 8 to 12 weeks (2 to 3 months)
   d. 12 to 24 weeks (3 to 6 months)

2. Which best expresses the body mass index of a female who weighs 70 kg and is 175 cm tall?

   a. 32.5 kg/m^2
   b. 24.5 kg/m^2
   c. 22.9 kg/m^2
   d. 43.3 kg/m^2

3. Which of the following items does *not* characterize type II diabetes?

   a. Delayed or impaired insulin secretion.
   b. Impaired insulin action in the insulin-responsive tissues of the body, including muscle.
   c. Overactive insulin action in the insulin-responsive tissues of the body, including muscle.
   d. Excessive glucose output from the liver.

True-False

4. A person can be overweight according to standard height/weight tables and yet have a lower-than-normal body-fat content.

5. A person can be within the normal range of body weight for his or her height and frame size by standard height/weight tables and yet be obese.

6. When a specific area of the body is exercised, only the fat in that area will be utilized, reducing only the locally stored fat.

7. An active lifestyle can reduce the risk of dying from coronary artery disease even if a person remains overweight or obese.

8. Heredity has little or no impact on one's tendency to become obese.

9. Glycemic control is generally not improved by exercise in most people with type I diabetes.

Fill in the Blank

10. _____ is the condition of having an excessive amount of body fat.

11. _____ refers to having a body weight that exceeds the normal or standard weight for a particular person based on height and frame size.

12. _____ is a term used to express the percentage by which an individual is either overweight or underweight.

Short Answer

13. List three possible causes of fatty acid mobilization during exercise.

14. Contrast the etiology and characteristics of type I and type II diabetes.

Essay

15. Explain how undereating, overeating, and physical activity can affect the three components of energy expenditure.

16. Describe the risks and benefits of physical activity for people with type I and type II diabetes.

17. Describe how physical activity affects various physiological parameters that, in turn, contribute to weight maintenance and weight loss. Include a discussion of metabolic rates, body fat, body mass, body weight, appetite, thermic effect of a meal, and fatty acid mobilization.

Answers to Selected Chapter 21 Activities

21.1 Defining Obesity-Related Terms

1. e; 2. i; 3. b; 4. f; 5. a; 6. j; 7. g; 8. d; 9. h; 10. c

21.2 Controlling Body Weight

1. The graph you drew should show a TEA of 200, a TEM of 100, and an RMR of 700.

2. The graph you drew should show a TEA of 700, a TEM of 350, and an RMR of 2,450.

3. It is theorized that this person's set point would stabilize at a much higher weight than the previous set point.

4. The person's TEA would increase, perhaps to 30% or more (675), and the RMR would likely decrease as a percentage of the overall total, perhaps to 60% (1,350).

21.3 Causes and Health Risks of Obesity

1. heredity/genetics, hormonal imbalances that lower metabolic rate, emotional trauma, alterations in basic homeostatic mechanisms, cultural habits, inadequate physical activity, improper diets

2. heart disease, hypertension, certain types of cancer, gallbladder disease, diabetes

3. obesity $\rightarrow$ respiratory problems $\rightarrow$ lower exercise tolerance $\rightarrow$ additional weight gains $\rightarrow$ lower exercise tolerance $\rightarrow$ lethargy due to increased plasma CO_2 and polycythemia in response to lower blood oxygenation $\rightarrow$ thrombosis, enlargement of the heart, or congestive heart failure

4. angina pectoris, hypertension, congestive heart disease, recurrent myocardial infarction, varicose veins, diabetes, orthopedic problems

21.4 Methods of Estimating Obesity

1. 66 kg/57.88 kg = 1.140 = 114% or 145 lb/127.5 lb = 1.137 = 114%

2. Answers will vary.

3. 66 kg/(1.68 m)^2 = 66 kg/2.82 m^2 = 23.4 kg/m^2

4. Answers will vary.

5. 107 cm/96.5 cm = 1.1 or 42 in./38 in. = 1.1

6. Answers will vary.

7. All measures indicate that Subject A has more body fat than is optimal, although she is not obese; that is, she does not have more than 35% body fat. In addition, Subject A's extra fat is in her upper body, so she is at increased risk for diabetes and cardiovascular diseases.

8. Answers will vary.

21.5 Physical Activity and Weight Control

1. ↑, 2. ↑, 3. ↓, 4. ↓, 5. ↑, 6. ↓, 7. ↑, though studies are not conclusive, 8. ↑, 9. ↑

Answers to Selected Chapter 21 Test Questions

Multiple Choice

1. d; 2. c; 3. c

True-False

4. True   5. True;   6. False;   7. True;   8. False;   9. True

Fill in the Blank

10. Obesity;

11 Overweight

12. Relative weight

Short Answer and Essay

For questions 13 to 17, check your answers against the explanations given in the textbook.

CONCLUDING ACTIVITY

A Good Workout Revisited

Do this activity after reading *Physiology of Sport and Exercise*.

Now that you have completed your study of *Physiology of Sport and Exercise,* you have a much more complete view of how your body responds, adjusts, and adapts to physical activity. Prior to taking this course, you probably recognized some of these changes—your heart beating faster, your respiration increasing, your muscles aching—without understanding what caused these adjustments.

Look back at your answers to the Introductory Activity, "A Good Workout," on page xi of this book. Do you see how much more you understand these adaptations now that you have completed this course? Let us revisit that Introductory Activity and reflect on all that you have learned.

Choose your favorite physical activity, whether it be running, cycling, doing aerobics, playing basketball, or whatever you find most enjoyable. Spend a few minutes warming up, and then do this activity at a relatively high intensity for 15 minutes or so. End your workout by cooling down for a couple of minutes. Pay close attention to how different parts of your body react and adapt to the physical activity.

Once you finish your workout, take some time to reflect on these different parts of your body and how they respond, adjust, and adapt to exercise. Recall from early chapters the underlying body structures, physiology, and other factors that causes these adaptations:

Muscles: Structure and function, slow-twitch and fast-twitch muscle fibers, muscle fiber recruitment

Nervous system: Neurons, nerve impulses, synapses and neurotransmitters, central nervous system, peripheral nervous system, sensory-motor integration, motor response, muscle size, hypertrophy, atrophy, muscle soreness, resistance-training programs

Metabolism: Energy sources, energy expenditure, ATP production, fatigue, adaptations to aerobic training, adaptations to anaerobic training

Hormonal responses

Cardiovascular system: Structure and function, cardiovascular responses and adaptations to exercise

Respiratory system: Ventilation, diffusion, gas exchange at muscles, respiratory responses and adaptations to exercise

Environment: Exercise in the heat, in the cold, at altitude, under water, in microgravity (in space)

Training: Volume, intensity, overtraining, tapering for peak performance, detraining

Ergogenic aids: Pharmacological, hormonal, physiological, nutritional

Nutrition: Six nutrient classes, water and electrolyte balance, the athlete's diet, gastrointestinal function during exercise, sports drinks

Body build, body size, body composition

Age: Growth and development in the young athlete, performance abilities and changes in older athletes

Gender differences and similarities

Designing an exercise prescription for health and fitness

Cardiovascular disease, obesity, diabetes

It is amazing how much you have learned, isn't it? Throughout this course, *Physiology of Sport and Exercise* has taken you on a fascinating journey of how your body adapts to exercise and what factors affect those adaptations. Perhaps this course has changed your view of the importance of physical activity in your life. Or perhaps you have developed such an interest in this topic that you want to pursue a physiology-related career. In either case, this course has provided you with a solid foundation in attaining your goals.